Mobilisation of the Spine

Mobilisation of the Spine
Notes on examination, assessment and clinical method

Gregory P. Grieve

FCSP DipTP
Former Postgraduate Tutor,
Department of Rheumatology and
Rehabilitation,
Norfolk and Norwich Hospital, Norwich.
Former Supervisor and Clinical Tutor, Spinal
Treatment Unit,
Royal National Orthopaedic Hospital, London

FOREWORD BY

Hugh Phillips

BSc(Hons) MB FRCS
Consultant Orthopaedic Surgeon,
Norfolk and Norwich Hospital, Norwich.

FOURTH EDITION

CHURCHILL LIVINGSTONE
EDINBURGH LONDON MELBOURNE AND NEW YORK 1984

CHURCHILL LIVINGSTONE
Medical Division of Longman Group Limited

Distributed in the United States of America by Churchill
Livingstone Inc., 1560 Broadway, New York, N.Y. 10036, and
by associated companies, branches and representatives
throughout the world.

First Edition 1975
Second Edition 1977
Third Edition 1979
Fourth Edition 1984
  Reprinted 1986

ISBN 0-443-02795-1

British Library Cataloguing in Publication Data
Grieve, Gregory P.
  Mobilisation of the spine. — 4th ed.
  1. Spinal adjustment
  I. Title
  615.8'22   RZ341

Library of Congress Cataloging in Publication Data
Grieve, Gregory P.
  Mobilisation of the spine.
  1. Spine. 2. Manipulation (Therapeutics) I. Title.
[DNLM: 1. Manipulation, Orthopedic WB 535 G848m]
RD768.G74 1984   617'.560622   83-21063

Produced by Longman Singapore Publishers Pte Ltd
Printed in Singapore

Foreword

This excellent book, originally a synthesis of the author's unique teaching courses, has now matured into a classic practical text, a triumph of orderly thought and presentation. Whilst written for both student and post-registration chartered physiotherapists, any professional with an interest in spinal disorders will learn from it.

Mr Grieve's rightful emphasis on clinical history and thorough examination before and during treatment is clear and recognises that the therapist's assessment is no less important than that of the referring colleague.

The new generation of physiotherapists will welcome this further edition as an essential guide to their practice in manipulative and mobilising techniques. It is the best substitute for a personal experience of observing Mr Grieve at work, a privilege I have so often enjoyed.

H. P.

Acknowledgements

Mr. Hugh Phillips, in whose agreeable company I have learnt much, and have also enjoyed the best of teamwork between surgeon and physiotherapist, has kindly honoured me by writing the Foreword to this edition.

The Editor of Physiotherapy, and Messrs Churchill Livingstone, have kindly agreed to the reproduction of selected passages and illustrations from my CSP Journal articles and my book *Common Vertebral Joint Problems* (1981).

I am most grateful to those who patiently modelled during long and tedious photographic sessions, viz: the late Moira Pakenham-Walsh, Sarah Key, Jenifer Horsfall, Gillian Brown, Denise Poultney, Fiona Percival, Sue Williams and Diana Start, and acknowledge with pleasure my fruitful working relationship, for more than twenty years, with Geoffrey Maitland, who in 1961 visited St. Thomas' Hospital in London, where I was then working.

Margaret Moore and Bridget Cole, Librarian and Assistant Librarian of the Medical Teaching Centre, Norfolk and Norwich Hospital, have unstintingly helped my searches through the literature. I cannot thank them enough.

Many of the illustrations are the work of John Tydeman, Medical photographer, and I pay tribute to his interest, patience and technical skill; also to Uta Boundy, of the Royal National Orthopaedic Hospital, London and the late Dr John Graves of the Graves Audiovisual Medical Library. For the other half of the team, Barbara Grieve, I need only mention our deep pleasure and real companionship in working together.

Halesworth, Suffolk, 1984   G.P.G.

Preface to Fourth Edition

Continuing demand for this little text, rearranged and expanded, indicates appreciation of manual mobilisation and manipulation as an integral part of physiotherapy,[69] in fact for some thirty per cent of our patients[70] who are numbered in millions.

Like its predecessors, it is not intended to 'teach students how to manipulate' since that is the job of their teachers, incorporating such parts of currently available texts as suit their particular purpose and mode of teaching.

While it is desirable that students begin with one or other integrated system of manual treatment, the big and rumbustious world outside must sooner or later be confronted, and I seek to encourage *self-education* in those important basic skills — examination, assessment and clinical method — also to provide a body of succinct information, with some digression on salient aspects, for those seeking to gain a first foothold in the clinical practice of this speciality.

As knowledge increases, imparting it to students in small compass becomes more difficult. One can provide stark but handy lists of mindless procedural drills for examination and treatment, as desirable *aides-memoires* for use in conjunction with practical classes, or strike a fuller balance between mass and portability. Preferring the latter, this edition, like Topsy, just growed. Signposts to more knowledge are in the References and Further Reading section.

Recent developments are (i) the use of post-isometric relaxation techniques[140] (ii) a long-overdue lessening of the importance of the localised manipulative thrust[13,42,92] (iii) increasing recognition of the value of correcting chronic imbalance between phasic and postural muscle groups[90] and (iv) the effectiveness of a properly co-ordinated lumbar extension regime, when indicated, for low back pain.[125] Yet it remains wise to be wise, for there is nothing new under the sun. 'One is never so avant-garde as when young, when what is said to be new really seems new, and one lacks the experience to recognise old hat refreshed with new trimmings.'[21]

Thus proprioceptive neuromuscular facilitation techniques, evolved by physiotherapists some thirty or more years ago,[101] are now employed in a modified way together with combined-movement positioning for individual vertebral segments, and given a new and not very sensible label of 'muscle-energy' or functional techniques. 'Post-isometric relaxation' techniques is a more suitable term.

Essentially, they are still passive movement in the real sense that movement to get 'release', or gain range, is gently imposed by the therapist during the short relaxation (inhibition) phase following isometric contraction, which merely prepares the ground for the movement, as it were.

Knowledge slowly increases, yet the remarks of that gifted naturalist, Gilbert White, who over 200 years ago wrote *The Natural History of Selborne*, remain relevant today to some aspects of the management of musculo-skeletal conditions. 'Ingenious men will readily advance plausible arguments to support whatever theory they shall choose to maintain; but then the misfortune is, every one's hypothesis is each as good as another's since they are all founded on conjecture.'

Two hundred years later, this discomforting state of affairs still applies, as Prowse's observations in our own Journal[160] on *respiratory* disease, for example, will show. 'The literature on the effects of intermittent positive pressure breathing is vast and inconclusive. The striking feature is the absence of clear proof of its effects on the one hand, and the almost religious belief of its adherents, be they patients, doctors or physiotherapists, on the other ... Even with conditions as common as asthma and chronic bronchitis, definition is difficult, assessment and diagnosis are hard, many aspects of aetiology and treatment are ill-understood and all in all our knowledge is woefully inadequate.'

The same could be, and has been, said about spinal joint problems and in his foreword to a recent comprehensive book[121] Professor Ian Macnab, a very experienced orthopaedic surgeon, has suggested that if we honestly question ourselves, we can only be disturbed at our remarkable ignorance.

After the basic biological sciences have been mastered by students of any clinical discipline, medical or paramedical, the way in which general practitioners, physicians, surgeons, physiotherapists and other manipulators conceive the nature of musculo-skeletal problems may sharply differ, and this often unrecognised dichotomy underlies a great deal of the difficulty in understanding what each protagonist is talking about, since what people know is less important than how they think.

Dialogue is patchy and misunderstood, and the various rationales of treatment are not always explained to others in easily understood terms which have a sound scientific basis.

Some of the more vocal, however authoritative, may actually have had little real experience of *handling* these joint problems on the clinical shop-floor.

Also, 'logic' and 'science' are sometimes strenuously invoked for treatment procedures which are more truly described as 'This is my preferred way of treating the patient and it really does work sometimes.' Our difficulty is that *everything* works, for some of the patients, for some of the time, if the wind is in the right direction. In our enthusiasm for this or that therapeutic revelation we sometimes overlook the infinite range of biological plasticity of response, and of individual uniqueness, which makes fools of us all at one time or another.

In 1732, Tom Fuller MD observed that one good head is better than a hundred strong hands; and life does not change. 'Manipulation' is not manhandling a joint into submission by vigorous and sometimes rough treatment, and in any case manipulation, with the whole range of treatment methods embraced by that emotive word, is not *per se* all that important. *What is of lasting, fundamental value is the way the would-be 'manipulators' are trained, in the sense of learning how to look, how to perceive, how to handle, to test, to palpate and to assess,* and later how to discriminate.

Like teachers, the primary objective of therapists is to make themselves superfluous, not to keep patients coming back every week or month, for years in some cases.

The occasional patient may require attention on a regular basis, but the numbers ensnared in this 'must-keep-going-regularly-to-my-manipulator' syndrome is scandalously high. Even if there *is* one born every minute, it is poor clinical practice to suggest to patients that regular attendance is a necessity in the interests of their musculo-skeletal health. This deception is too common. Thorough initial analysis and well-planned work reduce the need for more work, and the majority of patients can be taught in a very few sessions how to look after themselves.

Halesworth, Suffolk, 1984   G.P.G.

Contents

Surface anatomy

Palpation of the vertebral column and limb girdle structures is a vital part of examination for spinal joint problems; thus there should be familiarity with what underlies the surface terrain on both the dorsal and ventral aspects, and this is best gained by having a skeleton to hand while palpating the structures of the living model.

CERVICAL SPINE

The posterior tubercle of the *atlas* (C1) may be felt in the mid-line (Fig. 1.1), under the 'eaves' of the overhanging occiput, in a small proportion of people, but for the most part it is an impalpable bony point, unless considerable and uncomfortable pressure is unwisely applied. Its surface mark is thus the soft-tissue sulcus between the occiput and the prominent spinous process of the axis (C2).

Unless the patient's cervical tissues are very thickened, the posterior arches of atlas (C1) can be palpated posterolaterally immediately under the occiput. It is necessary to direct the fingertip anteromedially and slightly upward, and to ensure that there is muscle relaxation. The *lateral tip of the transverse process of the atlas* is palpable, in most people, between the angle of the jaw and the mastoid process (See Fig. 11.16, p. 138). In a few, it is not easy to find, and less so when upper cervical tenderness is such as to make even the most gentle probing difficult.

The little sulcus, which is formed by the adjacent bony points of mastoid process and atlas, allows a comparison of the position of C1 in relation to the skull, and also of movement in the craniovertebral joints; 'abnormalities' are not necessarily significant.

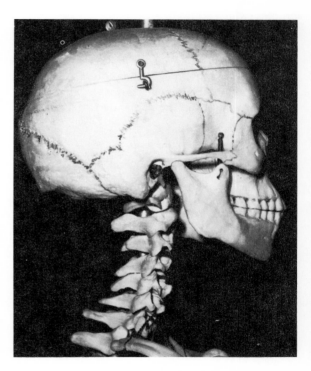

Fig. 1.1 Lateral aspect of cervical spine. Note the large and prominent spinous process of C2, the distance between the posterior tubercle of the arch of atlas and the C2 spinous process, and the somewhat depressed spinous processes of C3, C4 and C5. Tip of lateral mass of atlas is palpable between mastoid process and mandibular angle (see Fig. 11.16).

The axis

The axis (C2) is marked by a large beaked spinous process; this terminates in an inverted-V which can sometimes be verified by careful palpation. While on inspection it is not as evident as that of C7, it often *feels* as large. The C2 transverse process can be identified through the soft tissues.

C3 spinous process

This is a shy little bony point (Figs. 1.2, 1.3) almost concealed by the overhanging beak of C2, and may therefore be missed when palpating the neck of the prone patient from cranial to caudal. It is most easily felt by directing the thumbtip pressure anteriorly and slightly cranially.

The remaining cervical spinous processes may be asymmetrically bifid, and may give the impression of rotation if unusually prominent on one side. Doubt about whether one is palpating C6 or C7 spinous process (which seems to arise more frequently when treating degenerative joint disease than when palpating fellow-students!) can be resolved by placing a fingertip so that it lies between the two spinous processes. On extending the subject's neck, C7 spinous process remains palpable while that of C6 glides away from the palpating finger.

C2 to C6 spinous processes

The tips of C2 to C6 spinous processes lie on the same level as the lower margin of the inferior articular facet, which is thus the lower margin of the facet-joint. Thus the tip of C4 spinous process, for example, overlies the lower margin of the C4–C5 facet-joint. Since the inter-articular bony mass is marked dorsally by a little bony hump, it is quite easy to run the thumbtips down the para-vertebral sulcus on either side, some 2–3 cm from the midline, and locate these humps which overlie the facet-joints.

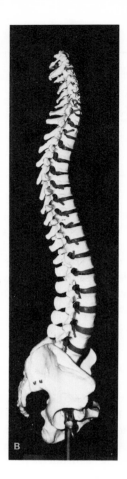

Fig. 1.2 Lateral aspect of the vertebral column. Note the varying configurations and size of spinous processes.

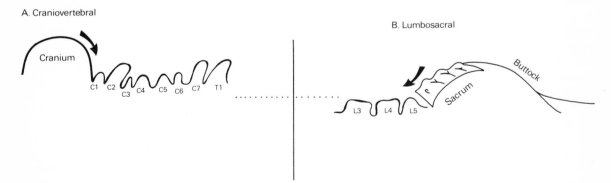

A. Craniovertebral

Cranium

C1 C2 C3 C4 C5 C6 C7 T1

B. Lumbosacral

Buttock

Sacrum

L3 L4 L5

Fig. 1.3 Similarities between cranio-vertebral and lumbo-sacral configuration on sagittal palpation. (A) As the palpating finger moves caudally off the occiput, C1 posterior tubercle is 'the little blunt church tower at the bottom of the valley' and C2 is large and unmistakeable. (B) Similarly, as one moves cranially down the fused dorsal spines of the sacrum, L5 is 'the little blunt church tower at the bottom of the valley' and L4 is large and unmistakeable.

They are easiest to feel at C4 and above, and are most easily palpated with the patient in prone-lying or in side-lying.

Facetal osteophytes are usually shelf-like projections and when marked they, with their covering of thickened soft tissues, may simulate these normal bony prominences.

The lateral extremities of the transverse processes are easily located through the soft tissues on either side, although this becomes less easy below C6.

With the patient supine, the anterior aspect of the cervical transverse processes can be palpated, and unilateral or bilateral anteroposterior contact mobilising techniques employed. Locating the most comfortable point for pressure should be carefully done, with the musculature pushed to one side. Some patients may experience proximal arm pain, and some a feeling of impending syncope, if the pressure is not considerate.

C7 spinous process

The spinous process of C7 is prominent, but so is that of T1, and perhaps the term 'vertebra prominens' should be written 'vertebrae' and applied to both of them, instead of customarily to C7 (Fig. 1.1). Those of C6 and C7 are usually not bifid; further, the transverse processes of C7 extend laterally as far as those of C2, so that a paramedian perpendicular would join their tips. Those of C3 to C6 would not extend laterally to reach this perpendicular line.

C7 transverse process can be identified in front of trapezius muscle but palpation is uncomfortable, and it is often simpler to locate it through the broad, triangular median aponeurosis of the middle fibres of trapezius.

In the prone patient, palpation of a cervical rib at C7 may require strong probing since it will lie anteriorly, i.e. deep, to the transverse process. It is much easier to compare sides when the patient is supine.

Cord segments

In the typical cervical region, the tip of the spinous process corresponds to the level of the *succeeding* spinal cord segment, i.e. C6 spinous process is level with the C7 cord segment (Fig. 1.4).

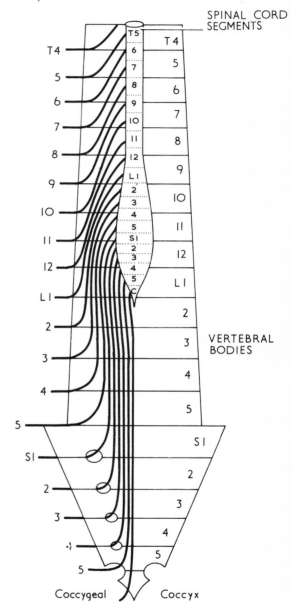

SPINAL NERVES
(shown on this
side only)

SPINAL CORD
SEGMENTS

VERTEBRAL
BODIES

Fig. 1.4 Vertebral column and nerve roots. The spinal cord terminates at L1/2.

THORACIC SPINE AND RIBS

The anterior concavity of the thoracic spine varies quite considerably between individuals. While it is obvious that the region's general configuration must conform to the patient's body type so far as sagittal curvature is concerned, there will be found a surprising variety of mid/upper thoracic curvature. Quite commonly, the interscapular region is flat and in some it will be markedly so, and this with radiographic appearance reported as 'normal'. In many, this apparent postural deviant is associated with upper thoracic and cervical joint problems but by no means invariably.

Thoracic spinous processes

These characteristically 'lie down the back like the scales of a fish' so that the tip of a spinous process lies level with the subjacent vertebral body, but this does not apply to the upper two or three, and lower two or three segments, i.e. the lower margin of these spinous processes lies roughly on the same level as the lower margin of the same body. (Fig. 1.2).

It is seldom appreciated how variable these levels of horizontal relationship can be, and why descriptions can only be generalised; comparison of three newly articulated skeletons will make the point. In the middle seven or eight thoracic levels, the tip of the spinous process lies more or less level with the laminae of the subjacent vertebra. The tips of the spines are not bifid but slightly bulbous, and progressively become more ridge-like towards the thoracolumbar junction.

Anomalies are common, and deviation of a spine to one side or other is frequently palpable; these should not be taken as positional evidence of rotation since comparison of the relationship of the laminae will demonstrate there is no fixed rotation.

The facts that the acromioclavicular joint lies level with the C7–T1 interspace, the spine of scapula lies approximately level with T3 spinous process and its inferior angle approximately level with T7 spinous process, provide a rough guide only. For accuracy it is necessary to count downwards from T1 or upwards from L5.

A practical method of counting is to place the tips of two adjacent fingers on the interspinous depression above and below one spinous process, and to shift the two fingertips as one when transferring to the next spinous process. There can still be difficulty if the spines are very close and virtually fixed thus by chronic segmental stiffening. Caudally, the spines become progressively more short, and project more dorsally; this shorter level will influence the type of movement induced by transverse pressures on the side of the spinous process.

The lower parts of the thoracic laminae

These are easily felt in the paravertebral sulci as a series of flattened ridges, and it is important to remember that the ridge palpated is the dorsal aspect of the interarticular part; it overlies the lower facet-joint of that vertebra.

The first rib

The first rib articulates only with the first thoracic vertebra; the spinous and transverse processes of T1, and angles of the first rib, are on the same horizontal level. Palpation of the first rib *angle* through the trapezius muscle, which may be in some spasm, can be painful for the patient; the flat upper surface of the rib is easily felt in the prone patient by lifting the upper fibres of trapezius and palpating immediately beneath. By careful probing, the transverse process of T1 can also be identified.

Anteriorly, the first palpable rib below the clavicle is the first rib. Frequently, the anterior shafts of the *2nd ribs* are unduly prominent, and simple observation from the front as well as palpation will confirm the fact.

Unilateral prominence, associated with marked local tenderness anteriorly, may occur in lesions of a second rib.

For all ribs, the intercostal spaces are somewhat wider in front than behind.

On a posterior view of the trunk, the line of the *rib angles* is not vertical; that of the *8th rib* is usually furthest from the mid-line, and both above and below this level a line joining them deviates slightly inwards, more so above the 8th rib.

Grant[66] states, 'Since the deep muscles of the back diminish in bulk as they ascend, it follows that the angles become progressively nearer the tubercles from below upwards, till the first rib is reached.' The important point is that generally they are nearer the tubercle more cranially, and further away more caudally.

Down to the 8th or 9th thoracic vertebra, the transverse process is level with the *upper* border of its vertebral body, and since the head of a typical rib articulates with (i) its numerically corresponding vertebral body and the one above, and (ii) the tubercle articulates with the numerically corresponding transverse process, it follows that the *rib angles* will be palpated just below, or at the same level of, the *transverse processes*.

One should be careful not to mistake a small soft-tissue nodule or fasciculus, which may be acutely tender, for 'a rib angle'; it is necessary to push the overlying soft tissues to one side to be sure one is indeed feeling an immovable bony point.

Doubts as to *which* rib angle must always be clarified by counting upwards or downwards. The single costal facet on T11 and T12 vertebral bodies is virtually level with the transverse process, but the associated rib does not articulate with it. The slight angle of the 11th rib is easily palpated at about the horizontal level of T12 spinous process, but the 12th rib, which may be 2–20 cm long, is virtually featureless and not so easy to find, especially in women.

Cord segments

In the upper thoracic region, the tip of the spinous process corresponds to the *second* succeeding segment, e.g. the spinous process of T4 overlies the T6 spinal segment. In the lower thoracic spine, there is a three-segment discrepancy, i.e. T10 spinous process overlies the first lumbar cord segment. At the last two segments, T11 spinous process overlies L3 cord segment and T12 overlies the first sacral cord segment.

As with all biological measurements, there is a normal range of variation as to the precise level of caudal termination of the human spinal cord, relative to the vertebral canal. The adult cord may terminate anywhere between the last thoracic and the third lumbar vertebra. Spinal cords in the female, and those of negro races, tend to be slightly longer than those of white males (Fig. 1.4).

In the newborn child, the spinal cord extends to the upper border of L3.

THE LUMBAR SPINE

The iliac crests do not invariably lie level with the L4 vertrebral body, and more frequently (about 60 per cent of cases) they lie in the same plane as the L4–L5 interspace. In some 20 per cent they are level with the L5 vertebral body, and this is sometimes referred to as 'a high-riding L5'. Only in the remaining 20 per cent of cases do the iliac crests lie in the same plane as the L4 vertebral body.

For this reason, it is more accurate to localise the L4 spinous process by first finding that of L5, which in most cases can be identified by sliding the tip of finger or thumb cranially along the fused spines of the sacrum (Fig. 1.3). The blunted and often small bony point, lying at the centre of the lumbosacral depression is the fifth lumbar spinous process.

Because anomalies (in the form of transitional vertebrae and spina bifida) are common in this region, there may be difficulty in deciding which is the fifth lumbar spinous process. The first segment with palable movement will decide the issue, and the vertebra immediately above the first movable joint will be the lowest lumbar vertebra, whether it is L4, L5 or 'L6'.

Palpation of the prone patient's lumbosacral region can sometimes be difficult because of anomalies, and when there is the real likelihood of confusion in identifying bony points, the patient's position should be changed to that shown in Figure 14.7 (p. 202).

The important points about the lumbar spinous processes are:

1. That of L5 is surprisingly often a deep, small and blunted bony point, while that of L4 is a comparatively large and sagitally ridged eminence.
2. The ridged eminences from L4 upwards (including the lower thoracic spines) are often a little depressed at about their middles, and it is embarrassingly easy to assume that one is palpating an interspinous gap when, in fact, one's finger is in the depression which marks the middle of a quadrangular lumbar spinous process.
3. The palpable ridge of one middle or upper lumbar spinous process may be considerably broadened, giving the impression of 'osteophytosis' of the bony point; this is a normal structural variation and should not be given any special significance.

The lumbar transverse processes

These generally lie level with the interspace between the spinous processes, and they are larger in the middle of the region than at the upper and lower ends. The palpable eminences which can be detected through the soft tissues on either side are not the laminae, but are the prominent dorsal aspects of the inferior articular processes. They mark the level of the facet-joints, and lie on either side of the lower third of the spinous processes.

The facet-joints

The facet-joints lie at a depth of some 5 cm below the skin surface, although this dimension is considerably reduced by firm digital pressure when palpating through the soft tissues.

THE PELVIS

Directly beneath a skin dimple on each side, the most eminent part of the *posterior superior iliac spines* lies opposite the second sacral segment, the 'spinous process' of which is not always palpable as a discrete bony point.

The posterior superior iliac spines do not invariably present with a detectable and localised eminence, but may remain simply as flatly curved bony ridges; medial to them the palpable depression is the sulcus overlying the sacro-iliac joint. At this point, the synovial cavity of the joint itself lies some 3 cm or more beneath the palpating finger, this space being occupied by the massive interosseous sacroiliac ligament; yet during testing movements the rhythmically changing relationship between the sacrum and the iliac spine is readily detectable in young, and many older, adults.

Some 5 or 6 cm below, and slightly laterally, the *posterior inferior iliac spines* are palpable through the upper mass of the buttock, and immediately medial to this point the lowest part of the sacroiliac joint can easily be felt.

The *sacrococcygeal joint* lies slightly higher than a horizontal line joining the upper tips of the greater trochanters; the *sacral hiatus,* lying between the cornua, is easily identified as a median depression over the apex of the sacrum.

Near the highest point of the buttock in young people, the *sacrotuberous ligaments* can be detected through the gluteal mass, and with a little practice it is not difficult to note differences in tension between them. In maturer patients, the palpation point will lie a little above the highest point of the buttock mass.

Difficulties of orientation can be resolved by identifying the *ischial tuberosities* and marking out the known attachments of the ligaments between these two eminences and the lateral borders of the sacrum.

Anteriorly, *Baer's point* (q.v.) lies a little below McBurney's point, the latter being situated at the junction of the outer and middle thirds of a line joining the anterior superior iliac spine and the umbilicus. Medial to and slightly below the anterior superior iliac spine, the iliacus and psoas major muscles form a palpable longitudinal bundle, and in the medial plane the uppermost part of the sulcus formed by the symphysis pubis is easily felt.

In passing, the notion that the vermiform appendix lies more or less directly under McBurney's point is fallacious. The structure can variously be situated some 10 cm or more from this surface mark, this circumstance helping in assessment of referred pains of spinal origin, so frequently simulating visceral disease.

2

Vertebral movement

Observations on the movement of special segments and vertebral regions are usually included with anatomical descriptions of the joints concerned, but by reason of the prime importance of the *functional interdependence of the vertebral column,* these matters may usefully be gathered together as a single section.

Campbell and Parsons[24] provide an illustration of functional interdependence, drawing attention to balance and stabilisation of the skull on the atlas by the deep group of small suboccipital muscles (Fig. 2.1) comprising the anterior, lateral and posterior recti and the superior and inferior obliques, together with the ligaments and fascia of this region, but also by an external group of long hypaxial muscles, e.g. semispinalis capitis, spinalis capitis (Fig. 2.2), trapezius and sternomastoid. Radiation of pain from

the middle and lower cervical and upper thoracic segments to the occipital and other cranial regions is explicable when the morphology and actions of these muscles are considered.

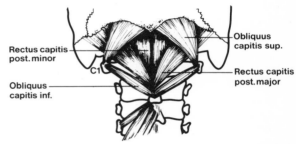

Fig. 2.1 Posterior aspect of the cranio-vertebral region and the small sub-occipital muscles. Note the lateral tip of atlas extending well beyond the transverse process of C2.

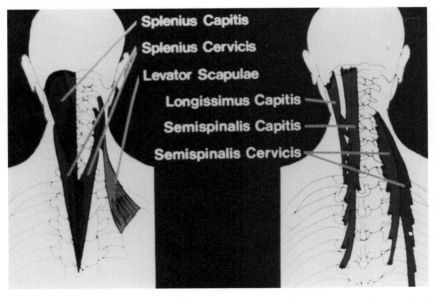

Fig. 2.2 Posterior aspect of the cervico-thoracic region. These deep, long, strap-like muscles may have a tethering effect upon neck movement, as well as initiating 'rib-joint lesions', by reason of chronic hypertonicity.

'Irritation at any spinal segment, but the cervical ones in particular, may result in hypertonus of these long muscles and traction on their collagenous attachments to the occipital cranium. In this way thoracic and even lumbosacral lesions such as postural malalignments and arthrosis, or myofasciitis from local or remote (visceral) causes, have been shown to produce cephalalgia and its concomitants.'

In passing, the neurophysiological interdependence of vertebral movement is of equal importance. *In three-dimensional space, the spine has six degrees of freedom (Fig. 2.3) —a vertebral body can move in six different ways:*

1. In the longitudinal axis of the spine, e.g. under compression or distraction effects.
2. Forwards or backwards in the sagittal plane — e.g. a degree of gliding or translation motion.
3. Laterally, in the frontal plane, by similar slight gliding motions.
4. Forwards and backwards tilt around a frontal axis, i.e. flexion and extension.
5. Lateral tilting, or rotation around a sagittal axis, i.e. movement in the frontal plane.
6. Rotation in the horizontal plane, around a vertical axis.

A vertebra may thus rotate about, or translate (glide) along, any of these three axes, or move in various combinations of these motions 'since the division of a movement into these planes at right angles to each other is a descriptive device which nature does not recognise.'[13]

A consideration of cervical flexion and extension (Fig. 2.4 (a) and (b)) shows a characteristic of movement in that each typical vertebra not only tilts forward and backward (rotation about a frontal axis) but also translates forward and backwards in the median plane, making a series of steps in the anterior curved line during flexion when seen on lateral films.

Pure movement in any of the three principal planes very seldom occurs, since orientation of facet-joint surfaces does not exactly coincide with the plane of motion and therefore modifies it, to a greater or lesser extent. Tilt or rotation cannot occur at an interbody joint without some disc deflection. The axis about which the rotation and/or tilt occurs is the *'centre of rotation'*. This point changes with the movement, being differently placed from one instant to another; we can therefore only speak of 'the instantaneous centre of rotation'; vertebral movement becomes more capable of analysis, and understandable, as the instantaneous centre or

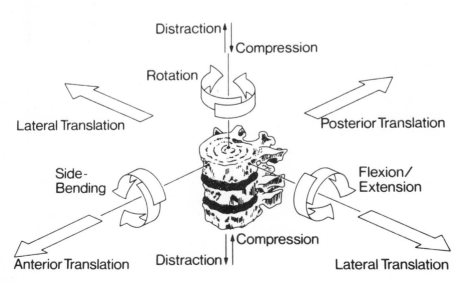

Fig. 2.3 Scheme to illustrate the six degrees of freedom of vertebral segments. (After White A A, Panjabi M M 1978 Clinical biomechanics of the spine. Lippincott, Philadelphia).

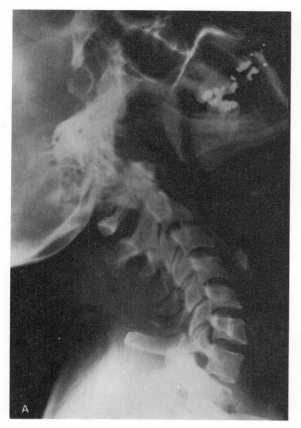

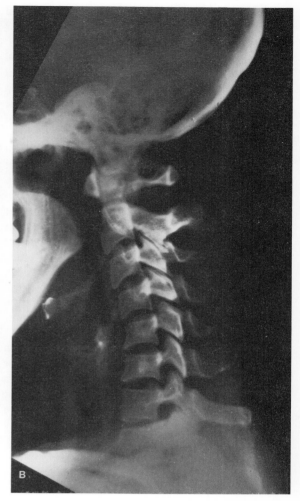

Fig. 2.4 (A) and (B) Ranges of extension (A) and flexion (B) of cervical spine in a 42-year-old female. Note that the smooth curve of an imaginary line, joining the fronts of the vertebral bodies in extension, becomes broken during flexion, and forms a series of steps, particularly evident at the C4–5 segment but also above and below it. The discs are thus horizontally distorted by these shearing effects which occur during sagittal movement of the neck. The mechanics are disturbed by C2–3 stiffness, evident on the flexion film.

rotation becomes more completely understood. Spinal movement is complex, and the intricacies of changing relationship observed on cineradiographic and other studies are sometimes difficult to explain.

Further to the observations of Campbell and Parsons, this difficulty may partly be because of the unwitting tendency to visualise factors governing joint movement* in terms of localised articular and ligamentous morphology *only,* and to overlook the

numerous muscular and connective tissue structures which attach at one end to either of the two moving bones but which may span several segments before attaching elsewhere. Simple examples of this guy-rope effect are (a) the tendency for elevation of the arms to impose extension on the thoracic and lumbar regions, by tension applied to latissimus dorsi and pectoralis major, and (b) the tendency for the knee to bend during straight-leg-raising because of tight hamstrings. It seems insufficiently appreciated that these factors, familiar enough in the examples given, may well act in more subtle but equally important ways during movement of a vertebral segment.

Thus far, the vertebra has been considered as a

*Further observations are given in 'Perceiving the nature of factors limiting movement' (p. 12).

rigid body, but this is not so. The phrase vertebral movement must be taken to include *deformation of the bone itself,* as well as the cartilage covering it.

Radin *et al.*[161] subjected plugs of subchondral bone and articular cartilage to compressive tests, and demonstrated that bone is capable of deforming under pressure and thus attenuating peak dynamic forces applied; the cancellous bone is capable of making a contribution equal to that of articular cartilage. In a single vertebra the deformation must be a small proportion of 'movement' of the whole vertebral body, yet this depends on the movement. Distortion of the neural arch during rotation strains of the lumbar spine is plainly detectable[49] and the accumulation of the increments of distortion effects are obviously a factor contributing to amounts of movement of whole spinal regions. Dynamic experiments on the vertebral bodies of sheep *in vivo*, and on bovine articular cartilage and subchondral bone, clearly demonstrate that bone is a structural component with plasticity, deforming under comparatively light loads.

Rolander[164] showed that with solid neural arch fusion, there is enough elasticity in the bone anterior to the pedicles to allow movement between vertebra and disc on vertical loading. While a 'solid' posterior fusion corrects gross instability, it should not be expected to completely immobilise a mobility segment.

GENERAL CONSIDERATIONS

The presence of arthrotic changes in facet-planes do not, of themselves, *necessarily* have any effect upon ranges of movement, neither does the presence of osteophytosis.

In general terms, the *relative amplitude of movement* available at the three regions (Figs. 2.5 and 2.6) is dictated by the proportion of disc height to the vertebral body height, broadly as follows:

	Cervical	*Thoracic*	*Lumbar*
Disc height	1/4	1/7	1/3
Body height	3/4	6/7	2/3

Consideration of the greatest regional range being apparent at the cervical spine must include the factors of (a) the translation occurring in sagittal movements and (b) the upper two atypical cervical

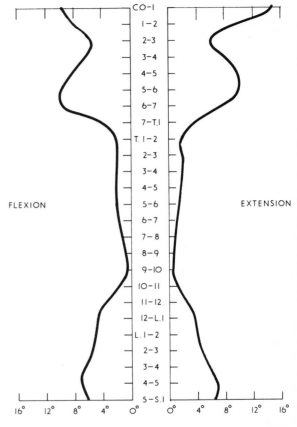

Fig. 2.5 Average ranges of segmental movement. (A general impression of *relative* segmental mobility averaged out from a variety of sources. Individuals may vary widely from the values given and the factors of age and body type should be borne in mind.)

N.B. Apart from the upper cervical spine, ranges of flexion and extension depicted are average total excursions and not the excess of flexion over extension, or vice versa, at individual segments.

segments having no disc, yet a greater range of some movements, including translation at C1–C2.

An important factor governing the *direction* and the *nature,* and sometimes the *amplitude,* of movement between adjacent vertebrae is the orientation of facet-joint planes, e.g. the almost vertical 'set' of the thoracic facets would preclude any great degree of flexion, even without the factor of ribs crowding together anteriorly.

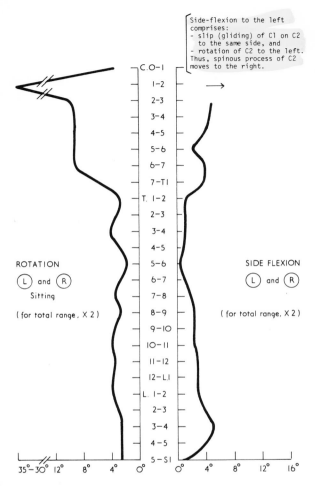

Side-flexion to the left
comprises:
- slip (gliding) of C1 on C2
  to the same side, and
- rotation of C2 to the left.
Thus, spinous process of C2
moves to the right.

ROTATION
(L) and (R)
Sitting
(for total range, X 2)

SIDE FLEXION
(L) and (R)
(for total range, X 2)

35°–30° 12°   8°   4°   0°   0°   4°   8°   12°   16°

Fig. 2.6 Average ranges of segmental movement. (A general impression of *relative* segmental mobility averaged out from a variety of sources. Individuals may vary widely from the values given and the factors of age and body type should be borne in mind.)

Side-flexion to the left comprises:
—slip (gliding) of C1 on C2 to the same side, and
—rotation of C2 to the left.
Thus, spinous process of C2 moves to the right.

It is clinically useful to have a working knowledge of *relative* ranges of individual segmental movements (Figs 2.5 and 2.6) also of the differing factors limiting movement at the three regions and the especially important junctional areas, but after the simple relative values are known, they should not be given too much importance. Patients will differ very widely from the values given, and concepts of normal or average are of minor importance. Tables or schemes of ranges of movement of this kind, abstracted mean values of movement from a variety of sources, are of much less clinical usefulness than the informed and practised ability to assess the movement of a spinal segment in dynamic relationship to its immediate neighbours, and in general terms of the patient's body-type. Only in this context does the degree of movement have meaning, as when assessing hip mobility in different individuals, for example.

Regional movement characteristics are dependent upon factors which differ between regions, e.g. (a) the annulus fibrosus and longitudinal ligaments govern the amplitude of sagittal lumbar movement, (b) contact of facet-joint planes limits lumbar rotation, like the flanges on train-wheels, more so in extension, and (c) approximation of spinous and articular processes limits thoracic extension.

There is a wide variation of normal mobility between individuals, according to body type and to age and sex, hence assessment is important during clinical examination. An initial increase in thoracic and lumbar mobility occurs, for example, during the decade 15 to 24 years, followed by a progressive decrease with advancing years, often by as much as 50 per cent.[141]

Van Adrichem and van der Korst[178] measured lumbar flexibility in 248 healthy youngsters between 6–18 years, and reported a more marked increase of lumbar flexion range with age in boys than in girls.

After studies of a population of normal males (142) and normal females (142) between the second and ninth decade, Sturrock *et al.*[170] reported that up to age 65, the total sagittal mobility of thoracic and lumbar spines was about 10 per cent greater in males; after 65 the position is reversed. Up to 65, men can flex about 15° more than women; after, women bend 5° more than men. Through-out the age range, women were able to extend more than men. This background should be borne in mind when assessing the more detailed aspects of regional movement.

Generally, male mobility exceeds female mobility in sagittal movements, and female mobility in side-flexion movements exceeds that of males. While it is well appreciated that the length of the hamstrings, and/or the degree of their tension normally existing at the time of the test, should be taken into account during assessment of lumbar flexion mobility, it is surprising how often these factors appear to be overlooked, or insufficiently noted, during examination. The occasional patient can bend to touch the floor without any appreciable change of segmental relationship in the low lumbar spine.

Characteristic movement combinations

Coupling, i.e. two types of motion occurring at the same time, is very common in spinal function, and frequently three motions will simultaneously take place during normal physiological movement. Pure movement in one plane perhaps does not exist.

Only *sagittal spinal movements* roughly approximate to motion in one plane, assuming that no abnormal curvature exists.

In rotation and side-bending movements, after the first degree or two of motion, one induces a portion of the other, and they are inseparable. It *is* possible to bend the neck sideways and keep one's nose pointing straight to the front, but vertebral rotation to the same side will occur to a degree anyway, and this voluntary resistance of the natural tendencies of cervical movement will be accompanied by a feeling of strain.

It is these natural, or physiological, combined-movement tendencies which require further examination.

1. *Flexion* reduces side-bending and rotation ranges; it eradicates the cervical curve, usually most noticeably at segments C4–5–6, and sometimes slightly reverses the lumbar curve from the L3 segment upwards.
2. *Extension* also reduces the range of side-bending and rotation.
3. *Side-bending* restricts flexion and extension, and while the vertebral region concerned is held in the position of side-bending, the following tendencies will be noted:
   a. in the cervical spine, side-bending makes rotation easier to the concavity (i.e. to the same side) than to the convexity, whether the neck be in neutral, flexion or extension
   b. in the thoracic spine below T3 and in the lumbar spine, side-bending makes rotation easier to the convexity (i.e. to the opposite side) than the concavity, when side-bending occurs in neutral or extended position. If the thoracic and lumbar spine be flexed, and then bent to one side, rotation will be easier to the concavity, as in the cervical spine.
4. *Rotation* restricts flexion and extension, and is invariably accompanied by a degree of side-bending.

The physiological tendencies are thus: *Typical cervical region* (C2–C6) side-bending is invariably accompanied by rotation to the same side, and vice versa, from all positions of sagittal movement, i.e. whether the neck be flexed, neutral or extended.

Cervicothoracic region (C6–T3). Although movement rapidly diminishes from above downwards, side-flexion is accompanied by rotation to the same side, and vice versa.

Thoracic and lumbar regions. Side-bending is accompanied by rotation to the same side (and vice versa) only in flexion. In the neutral or extended position, side-bending is naturally accompanied by rotation to the opposite side, and vice versa.

Summarised, in all sagittal starting positions of the cervical spine, and in the flexed thoracic (below T3) and lumbar spines, side-bending is perforce accompanied by rotation to the same side, and vice versa; in the neutral or extended thoracic (below T3) and lumbar spines, side-bending is perforce accompanied by rotation to the opposite side.

These regional combinations of movement are the normal physiological tendencies when the vertebral column is side-flexed or rotated from the flexed, extended or neutral position.

For those who may be unfamiliar with these movement combinations, it is important not to accept the statements at their face value, but to meticulously work their own spines through the various positions and verify for themselves the tendencies described. A useful exercise is for the experimenter to sit or stand, put the spine into the positions described and note the resistance encountered when a movement *opposite* to the physiological tendency is tried.

The distinctive nature of upper cervical movement, and sacro-iliac movement, has been discussed in more detail elsewhere.[70]

The only other point to mention is that *flexion* of the cervical region produces a degree of movement restriction, by ligamentous tension at the typical segments, and thus the range of head-rotation on a flexed neck is likely to represent, for the most part, atlantoaxial range.

Perceiving the nature of factors limiting movement

Distinguishing between *types* of movement limitation is easy when handling normal mobile peripheral joints, e.g. the abrupt stop when testing full extension of elbow or knee is quite different to the squashy feel of soft-tissue approximation when the same joints are flexed to their limit.

As MacConaill[119] has shown, flexed joints are loose-packed and movement is limited by soft-tissue contact, whereas extension movements are limited by close-packing, when the female surface is in most complete congruence with the male surface, the capsule and ligaments are in maximal tension and it is difficult, although not impossible, to separate the bones by traction.[179] A moment's examination of the close-packed humeroulnar joint in fullest extension reveals that a measure of accessory abduction and adduction range can still be passively produced, without releasing the degree of extension — the limit of extreme movement is always something of a movable feast and this ability to accurately assess, by observation and by feeling, what is normal and abnormal in peripheral joint movement is served basically by applied anatomical knowledge, the assessment becoming more accurate with clinical experience; this too applies to the vertebral joints.

On giving overpressure at the extremes of voluntary movement of spinal regions. The 'end-feel' in normal young subjects is mostly that of soft-tissue tension, i.e. the combined resistance in varying degrees of muscle with its attachment-tissues, fascial planes, ligaments, joint capsules and the annulus fibrosus of discs. We know, for example, that the main limiting factor in sagittal lumbar movement is the annulus, although other soft tissues are put on tension; rotation and side-flexion of the three regions, with flexion of the lumbar and thoracic regions, have an elastic resistance to manual attempts to increase range, and the precise end-of-range is difficult to pinpoint; however, comparison between sides allows assessment, and range abnormalities can readily be perceived on overpressure, if not by simple observation beforehand, or both.

That cervical and thoracic extension are limited by bone-to-contact (or cartilage-covered bone contact, in the normal) and not especially by soft-tissue tension, cannot fully be perceived manually because all one can feel is a somewhat harder and less elastic stop to the movement, although a degree of elastic resilience remaining is easily detected.

Gently forcing cervical extension produces unpleasant discomfort before a solid limitation, if a normal subject allows this degree of questing. Cervical flexion is limited by approximation of mandible and sternum compressing the soft tissue between, yet movement can be continued for a few degrees as the posterior vertebral tissues are stretched by the 'beer-handle' effect of pressing downwards on the occiput.

Craniovertebral extension is limited by the posterior edge of the atlantal facets engaging the condylar fossae of the occiput; the same movement is limited at the cervicothoracic junction by the inferior articular processes of C7 engaging horizontal grooves below and behind the superior facets of T1. Thoracic extension is limited by contact of inferior articular processes with the laminae below, and by contact of the spinous process.

At the thoracolumbar junctional region, a 'mortise' effect is produced in full extension by engagement of the articular facets of T11 and T12 (sometimes T12 and L1) and this is one of the few articular mechanisms in the body where a practically solid bony-contact lock occurs at the extreme of movement.[34]

Practically all other so-called bone-to-bone locks, with the exception of dental occlusion and lumbar rotation in neutral or extension, occur to a degree only.

When testing vertebral accessory-movement ranges by rhythmic pressures against the bony prominences available to palpation, with the patient lying prone in a neutral position, the anatomical and functional criteria governing *voluntary-movement* assessments do not apply on a one-to-one basis at each segment. (See Figs. 2.5, 2.6).

For example, (i) the 35°–45° range of rotation at C1–C2 is not reflected in the degree of movement palpable on postero-anterior pressure on the C2 spinous process — the odontoid prevents this — and to appreciate the limit of available range of rotation it is necessary to turn the patient's head through 90°, and feel how far short of this amplitude the spine of C2 has moved. Nevertheless, should voluntary cervical rotation to one side be limited to 30° or less, by pain arising from changes at the C1–C2 segment of that side, this will be very accurately reflected in the ease with which involuntary spasm and voluntary muscle guarding are provoked on applying unilateral pressures to C1 on the painful side, and transverse pressures to the spine of C2 towards the painful side, with the patient lying in the neutral position.

Again, (ii) in the presence of pain referred forward to the pectoral region and breast which is arising from thoracic joint changes at interscapular levels, cursory examination of voluntary thoracic movement does not invariably reveal positive signs, neither does overpressure at the limit of the customary regional movements always reveal abnormality.

Limitation at individual segments is sometimes concealed from detection during observation of regional movements, only to be revealed on searching tests of combined movements or more surely on careful and systematic palpation at segments T345.

Further, (iii) stiffness spanning three mobility-segments between L1 and L4 is often detectable by careful observation of the patient's back during active tests, but not invariably so; yet after active tests which may be somewhat inconclusive, a flat-handed downward pressure on the lumbar region declares the probability at once, and segmental palpation confirms it.

3

Segmental innervation

Nerve root irritation or compression will disturb neurological function giving rise to signs and symptoms in the tissues supplied by that root.

Root involvement affecting *muscle strength,* if present, is invariable revealed without testing every muscle and every joint action.

Concerning muscle weakness, the absence or presence of neurological deficit can be confirmed by testing only one muscle, or joint action, as representative of a given cord segment supply.

The distal reference of so-called 'root' pain, arising from involvement of a single root, is likely to lie in the distributions presented in Figures 3.1–3.6 but not invariably so, because the size and boundaries of dermatomes appear to have a tendency to fluctuate according to the changing levels of facilitation existing at the spinal cord segments and there is also some variation between individuals in patterns of pain reference or projection.

The *paraesthesiae* of root involvement are likely to be most evident in the distal part of the dermatome.

In the broadest terms, the table will help to indicate the probable level of involvement. The precise nature of the lesion affecting the nerve root often remains in doubt in non-surgical cases, and occasionally in surgical cases.

The following factors should be borne in mind:

(i) overlap of cutaneous supply
(ii) pre- and post-fixation of plexuses
(iii) numerical discrepancy between vertebrae and roots in the cervical region
(iv) the great obliquity of the lumbo-sacral roots (Fig. 1.4), because of which two adjacent roots may be disturbed by tissue trespass at a single intervertebral segment.

Referred pain of musculo-skeletal origin from a vertebral segment, *without root involvement* by mechanical irritation or compression, is by no means always confined to the dermatome areas outlined in the table which follows and depicted in Figures 3.1–3.6.

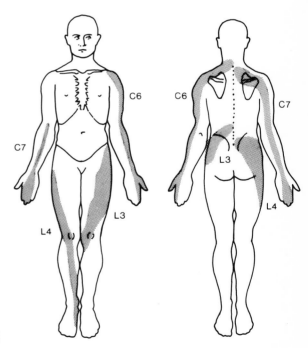

Fig. 3.1 Limb Dermatomes. Because dermatomes are not fixed territorial or anatomical entities, but *neurophysiological* entities, whose boundaries fluctuate according to the prevailing levels of cord segment facilitation, the areas delineated above are those corresponding to body regions in which pain and other symptoms may often be partly or wholly distributed from joint problems in the general neighbourhood of associated vertebral segments.[99]

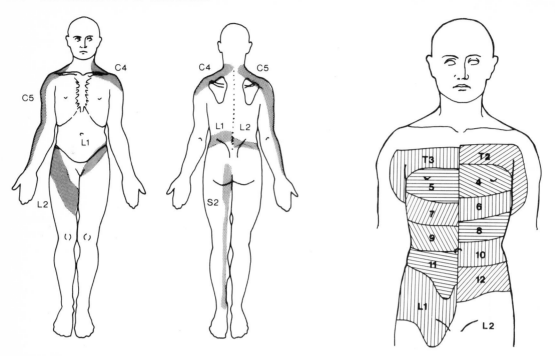

Fig. 3.2 Limb Dermatomes.

Fig. 3.4 Trunk Dermatomes

Fig. 3.3 Dermatomes generally overlie myotomes, e.g. the skin innervated by segments L2-3-4 (via the lateral, intermediate and medial femoral cutaneous nerves) broadly overlies the muscle supplied by L234, and both correspond roughly to the L2, 3 and 4 sclerotomes; but there are several body regions where innervation of skin differs from that of deeper structures, and among them are: the face, pectoral region, heart and diaphragm, scapular region, thenar eminence and buttock. They are evident on comparison of a classical dermatome chart with myotomes, the segmental innervation of muscles (p. 18). For example, the skin of the face is innervated by the 5th cranial nerve, and the muscles of expression by the 7th cranial; the intrinsic scapular muscles are supplied by C5-6, and the skin covering the region is innervated by T234, the heart is derived from the T123 somites, the diaphragm from C345, and the trunk dermatomes covering the region are derived from somites T5678. The important point is that superficial tissue and the underlying structures have broadly the same innervation in some places; in other places they do not, *and it happens that the latter body regions are those frequently involved in vertebral pain syndromes.*

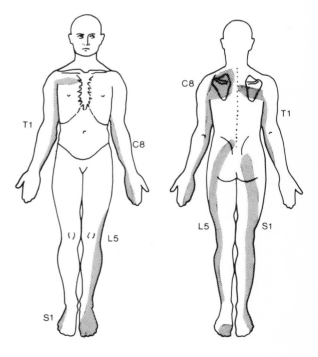

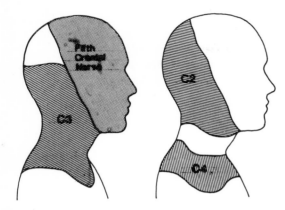

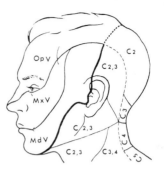

Fig. 3.5 To show extent of overlap of dermatomes.

Fig. 3.6 Areas of cutaneous supply by the V cranial nerve (ophthalmic, maxillary and mandibular divisions) and the 2nd, 3rd and 4th cervical nerves. (Reproduced by kind permission of Wyke B D 1968 The neurology of facial pain, and the Editor, British Journal of Hospital Medicine.)

Further, this type of pain may be referred into a sclerotome distribution (Figs. 3.7 and 3.8) and it is wise to keep an open mind when assessing the probable level of vertebral involvement on the basis of patterns of distal reference of pain and other symptoms.

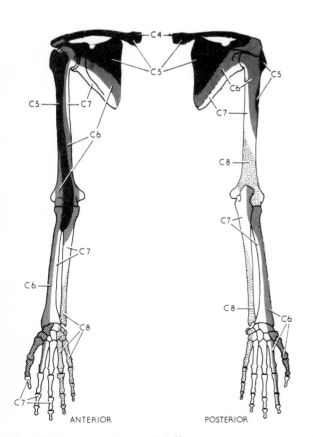

Fig. 3.7 Sclerotomes of upper limb.[89]

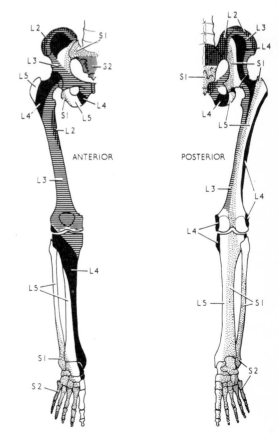

Fig. 3.8 Sclerotomes of lower limb.[89]

PATTERNS OF SOMATIC NERVE ROOT SUPPLY

N.B. Above the C4 segment it is wise to test muscles supplied by both a.p.r. and p.p.r. Below this, it suffices to test those supplied by a.p.r. only. Pain referred from a single vertebral segment is not always confined to the related dermatome areas outlined below but they are a help in localising vertebral joint problems (see Figs. 3.1–3.6)

Spinal cord segment	Dermatome	Representative muscle(s)	Joint action	Reflex
C1	—	*a.p.r. C1–2* rect. cap. ant. longus capitis	tuck chin in	—
C2 + V. cranial	vertex occiput forehead temple	*p.p.r. C1–2* rect. cap. post. maj. & minor obliquus sup.	push chin up	—
		V. cranial mastication	jaw movement	V. cranial[65] jaw jerk[153] corneal reflex
C3 + V. cranial	neck jaw throat inner clav.	*a.p.r. C3–4* scaleni *p.p.r. C3–4* Upper extensions of erector spinae	press head and neck laterally	v. cranial[65] jaw jerk[153]
C4	clavicle supraspinous fossa proximal deltoid	*a.p.r. C4* levator scap. trapezius	elevate shdr. girdle	—
C5	upper trapezius deltoid and lateral arm to wrist	deltoid	abduction of arm	biceps jerk
C6	upper trapezius lateral arm & forearm to two lateral digits	biceps	elbow flexion	biceps and brachio- radialis jerks
C7	mid-scapula post. arm to middle three digits	triceps	elbow extension	triceps jerk

Spinal cord segment	Dermatome	Representative muscle(s)	Joint action	Reflex

C8	scapula
	inner arm to
	   medial two
	     digits
		thumb
		  extensor
		finger
		  flexor
			thumb
			  extension
			finger
			  flexion
				—

T1	lower
	  scapula
	inner arm to
	  medial wrist
		intrinsic
		  hand
		  muscles
			finger
			  adduction
			  and
			  abduction
				—

T2	inverted 'T'
	  with limbs to
	  inner arm,
	  pectoral and
	  scapular areas
		—	—	—

T4	sloping band at nipple level	—	—	—
T7	sloping band at xiphoid level	much overlapping of		upper abdominal (T7–T10)
T10	sloping band at umbilical level	adjacent dermatomes		lower abdominal (T10–T12)
L1	Sloping band at inguinal level	—		—

Spinal Cord Segment	Dermatome	Representative Muscle or Group	Joint Action	Root Traction	Reflex
L2	sloping band around upper buttock to front upper thigh	psoas-iliacus	hip flexion	? femoral nerve stretch test	—
L3	upper buttock front thigh to inner knee and below	quadriceps	knee extension	femoral nerve stretch	knee jerk

L4	middle
	buttock
	Outer lower
	thigh
	Shin and
	dorsum to
	great toe
		tibialis
		  anterior
			foot
			  dorsiflexion
				? femoral
				nerve stretch
				also
				straight-leg-
				raising
					knee
					jerk

Spinal Cord Segment	Dermatome	Representative Muscle or Group	Joint Action	Root Traction	Reflex
L5	Mid-buttock Post. thigh Outer leg All toes (dorsum) and medial plantar	toe extensors tibialis posterior	extension of big toe Inversion with plantar-flexion of foot	Straight-leg-raising	Great toe jerk[173]
S1	lower mid-buttock Posterior thigh, behind lateral malleolus to fifth toe and lateral plantar	(a) peronei (b) glut. max. (c) hamstrings (d) calf	(a) eversion (b) contract buttock (c) knee-flexion	straight-leg-raising	Ankle jerk
S2	postero-medial strip from buttock to heel	hamstrings calf	knee-flexion (d) toe standing	? straight-leg-raising	—
S3–4 (somatic)	'saddle' area upper inner thigh	muscles of pelvic floor bladder and genital function			
S2–3–4 (parasymp.)	genitals perineum				

4

Autonomic nerves in vertebral pain syndromes

The principle of metameric segmentation, linking vertebral segment to the spinal cord segment, spinal roots and sympathetic trunk, includes the innervation of internal organs.[104]

Thus, general visceral afferent fibres occur in the vagus, glossopharyngeal and possibly other cranial nerves, and in the second, third and fourth sacral nerves, i.e. the *parasympathetic pathways*. In general, the afferent fibres occupying the pre- and post-ganglionic pathways of the *sympathetic system* from soma and viscera have a segmental arrangement as follows:[179]

Head and neck	T1–5
Upper limb	T2–5
Lower limb	T10–L2
Heart	T1–5
Bronchi and lung	T2–4
Oesophagus (caudal part)	T5–6
Stomach	T6–10
Small intestine	T9–10
Large intestine as far as splenic flexure	T11–L1
Splenic flexure to sigmoid colon and rectum	L1–2
Liver and gall bladder	T7–9
Spleen	T6–10
Pancreas	T6–10
Kidney	T10–L1
Ureter	T11–L2
Suprarenal	T8–L1
Testis and ovary	T10–11
Epididymis, ductus deferens and seminal vessels	T11–12
Urinary bladder	T11–L2
Prostate and prostatic urethra	T11–L1
Uterus	T12–L1
Uterine tube	T10–L1

Lamina V. cells of the substantia gelatinosa thus receive multiple inputs, from both soma and viscera.[147] The relation between input at the posterior horns from soma and viscera was reported by Kostyuk[102] who demonstrated that afferents from the viscera can cause presynaptic inhibition upon somatic afferent impulse traffic, and also exert post-synaptic inhibition which is under supraspinal modulatory control from the bulbar reticular formation.

It was also shown that visceral afferents inhibit the effect of converging afferent impulse traffic from the skin, and conversely, stimuli to the skin can cause inhibition of Lamina V. neurones on which visceral afferents terminate.[159]

There was the same mutual inhibition exhibited by Group 111 afferents from skeletal muscles and skin.

MacKenzie[123] postulated that both visceral and somatic afferents are capable of acting on common spinal cord pools of neurones, which are subject to summation, facilitation and inhibition effects, and this view is supported by more recent experimental findings.[41]

Thus in disease of a viscus, the patient will very frequently experience cutaneous pain; this painful skin area will often be acutely tender and cutaneous vasoconstriction may also be evident. Further, the underlying muscle will show a greater or lesser degree of hypertonus, i.e. spasm.

The skin areas of the body wall which have the same segmental innervation as a particular viscus, one somatic, the other autonomic, and which show the changes mentioned in visceral disease, are termed 'zones of secondary hyperalgesia'.[96]

As Head[81, 82] discovered in his studies of herpes zoster these zones or segments are garland-shaped zones of skin. The zones of secondary hyperalgesia of Head, Kappis-Lawen and Lemaire are tabulated below, and if these are compared with each other and also with the table it will be evident that (a) the zones roughly accord with the trunk dermatomes, and (b) there is considerable variation within a broadly generalised pattern.[104]

external environment, the three main categories of events (with their consequences) likely to occur in the deeper musculo-skeletal tissues are (a) mechanical trauma, distraction or trespass by related tissues, (b) infectious invasion, and (c) non-infectious but noxious changes in their biochemical environment. If this notion is correct, the degree of

Table 4.1

	Head	Kappis-Lawen	Lemaire
Heart	C3–C4 T1–T8	—	C3–C4 T1–T5
Descending aorta and aortic arch	C3–C4 T1–T3	—	C3–C4 T1–T3
Thoracic aorta	—	—	T4–T7
Pleura	—	—	T2–T12
Oesophagus	(T5)–T8	T5–T6	T1–T5–T8
Stomach	C3–C4 (T6) T7–T8	T6–T8 (T9)	(T5) T6–T9
Liver and Biliary tract	C3–C4 T7–T10	T9–T10	(T5) T6–T9 (T10)
Pancreas	—	T8	T6–T9
Intestine	T9–T12	—	—
Small intestine	—	T9–T10	T9–T11
Large intestine	—	T11–T12	—
Transverse colon	—	—	T9–T10
Descending colon	—	—	T11–T12
Rectum	S2–S4	—	—
Kidneys and ureters	T10–L1 (L2)	T11	T1–L1
Adnexa	T11–L1	T12–L1	—
Peritoneum	—	—	T5–T12

Kunert[104] observed that hyperalgesic zones are more commonly found in acute and sub-acute visceral disease than in the more chronic disorders. *There is evidence that the same visceral afferent fibres subserve both normal visceral sensation and also pain.* Nathan[147] observed 'one can suggest that the signalling of events from the viscera is simple, because there are only simple events to report; but the events occurring to the outside of the body are of many kinds and they may require a more complicated system to report them.'

The 'simple events' affecting viscera and amounting to noxious stimuli are mainly distension and traction; cutting or burning the bowel, for example, does not cause pain, although ischaemia of cardiac muscle is intensely painful.

In animals the same visceral fibres are slightly activated by passive disturbances of a viscus, and more intensely activated by active contraction. Intense contractions of these viscera, e.g. the stomach, in man causes pain. One may hypothesise that, in comparison to the cutaneous ability to register the wealth and variety of changes in man's

organisation and sophistication of the musculo-skeletal tissue nociceptors together with their peripheral connections is possibly somewhere between those of skin and viscera, although both appear to share an enormous wealth of spinal and supraspinal synaptic pathways.

Knowledge of the intimate link between soma and viscera does not mean that manual treatment of the vertebral column necessarily implies acceptance of the notion that one of its purposes is to influence visceral disease. Since treatment without indication is a speculation, and since ordinary, workaday clinical competence to recognise and assess comprehensive indications in the whole field of thoracic and visceral disease would require the combined skills of physicians, and abdominal and thoracic surgeon, it is probably unwise to profess, or imply, this as part of the basis of physical treatment of the spinal column.

All those experienced in manipulation can report numerous examples of migrainous headaches, dysequilibrium (vertigo), subjective visual disturbances, feelings of retro-orbital pressure, dysphagia, dysphonia, heaviness of a limb, extra-segmental paraesthesiae, restriction of respiratory excursion, abdominal nausea and the cold sciatic leg being relieved by manual or mechanical treatment of the vertebral column; but while these effects are noted, and the underlying mechanisms investigated with the purpose of understanding better what we do, they are insufficient reason to put the cart before the horse.

In other words, the prime impulse for physical treatment of the vertebral column is properly vertebral column disorder, and not visceral disorder.

Yet we must recognise the importance of autonomic neurone involvement[103] in spinal changes of neural trespass, which often initiates chronic changes in the soft tissues of the limbs, and very frequently simulates visceral disease, in that respiratory, cardiac, hepatic, renal and pelvic conditions may be suspected, so 'real' are the counterfeit symptoms produced and referred by benign spinal joint conditions. Peripheral associated changes, for example in the shoulder and elbow regions, can very frequently be eradicated by mobilisation and manipulation of the vertebral joints, the restoration of pain-free movement in the peripheral joint occurring together with improvement of the spinal joint abnormality. This is not always the case; a common clinical experience is that the more chronic are the associated changes in the vertebral and peripheral joints, the more frequently is it necessary to attend to both spinal and peripheral joint changes.

Common examples are 'capsulitis' of the glenohumeral joint, bicipital tendinitis, supraspinatus tendinitis, lateral epicondylitis (tennis elbow), etc., associated with C5–C6, and often T2–T3–T4 joint problems; likewise, medial epicondylitis (golfer's elbow) associated with C5–C6–C7–T1 vertebral joints, and painful restrictions of hip-joint mobility associated with L3–L4 segment abnormalities. Further, the association of painful temporomandibular joint conditions (in the absence of defects of dental occlusion) and upper cervical joint changes, may be more than coincidence, although the mechanism of production may not be quite the same. Clinical observations indicate that reflex sympathetic effects without frank dystrophy, the shoulder-hand syndrome, the ubiquitous low-grade collagenosis in peripheral tissues, the 'frozen' shoulder and chronic 'capsulitis' of the shoulder, carpal-tunnel syndrome, etc., may on many occasions be manifestations, *to a greater or lesser degree,* of the same malign, self-inflicted wound of chronic facilitatory states of lower cervical and upper thoracic cord segments, as a consequence of trauma to limb girdle and/or silent, degenerative spondylotic change, inducing connective-tissue changes in the limb.

5

Referred pain

The phenomenon of referred or projected pain, i.e. that felt at a greater or lesser distance from the lesion producing it, is well recognised but not fully understood. It is a frequent source of difficulty in identification of the vertebral segments involved and therefore in the correct location of treatment.

> One of the difficulties arises from the fact that the symptoms produced by a spinal joint derangement can be surprisingly diverse and are often manifest at a distance from the spine rather than in the spine itself.[13]

Serious visceral disease can produce spinal pain which mimics that of relatively innocent vertebral joint problems and conversely, pain referred around the chest wall from vertebral and rib joint involvement can very easily simulate the pains of visceral disease such as pleurisy and cardiac ischaemia.

Pain from somatic structures can faithfully reproduce the character and distribution of visceral pain, of angina and breathlessness, abdominal pains with nausea and vomiting, the flatulence of cholecystitis and the frequency of renal disease; additionally, visceral signs such as abdominal tenderness and abdominal rigidity are often produced.

In many of these cases active spinal movements, even with overpressure, are painless and it is not until the spine is examined segment by segment that the pain is provoked, either locally and/or peripherally.

Lewis and Kellgren[109] observed that all the essential features of renal colic, pain diffused from loin to scrotum, iliac and testicular tenderness and cremasteric retraction, can be provoked by a stimulus confined to the somatic structures of the spine. The stimulus was injection of spinal ligaments with hypertonic saline.

Kirkaldy-Willis and Hill[100] mention that lower abdominal and scrotal pain, from upper lumbar disc herniations, is not infrequently confused with renal or ureteric disorders.

Feinstein et al.[51] describe patients with frontal headache referred from the cranio-vertebral junction.

Familiar examples of pain perceived at a distance from the site of tissue damage are:

1. Upper limb pain in neck and also shoulder lesion.
2. Headache from cervical and temporo mandibular joint problems.
3. Pectoral and costochondral pain from thoracic joint conditions.
4. Pain in the epigastrium, and/or posterior body wall, in gallbladder disease.
5. Groin pain from joint problems at the thoracolumbar junction.
6. Low backache in osteoporosis of the lower thoracic spine.
7. Pain in posterior thigh and upper calf from sacroiilitis.
8. Pain referred to the foot from lumbar intervertebral disc disease.
9. Thigh and knee pain in arthrosis or tuberculosis of the hip.

It is unwise to expect that referred pain from a single vertebral segment will occupy the classical dermatome associated with that segment. The receptive field of a single dermatome, surgically isolated by cutting spinal roots above and below the intact root, can be much widened by experimentally enhancing cord segment facilitation.[99]

This is a clear reminder that the concept of

dermatomes, as segmentally numbered and finite territories, is like describing an iceberg while looking only at its tip. Cord segment facilitation is an integral part of the pain process itself, of course.

Inman and Saunders[89] made 160 observations on referred pain and showed that the radiation of pain in the experimental and clinical cases *never* (my italics):

— followed the distribution of a major nerve trunk
— corresponded with the overlying dermatome, or
— followed the exact pattern of the vascular tree.

There are several observations about wide variability in the territorial spread of referred pain from vertebral lesions:

1. Pain is not always distributed to the expected dermatomes, but may spread over a wider area.[19]
2. Pain of cervical spondylosis may be felt in myotome areas and not necessarily in dermatomes.[165]
3. Pain referred from deep somatic tissues differs in location from the conventional dermatome.[51]
4. Pain caused by irritation of one spinal nerve root may extend in some cases more widely than the recognised distribution.[15]
5. Referred pains are not invariably of segmental root distribution. They may miss out a segment and then spread into two adjacent segments.[85]

It appears clear that actual damage to the segmental nerve root is not necessary in order to produce referred pain. This pain need not be confined to the dermatome or the sclerotome of that level.[13]

Pain happens *within* the central nervous system, not residing 'in' the damaged locality, though it may be perceived so by the patient. 'Pains do not really happen in hands or feet or heads; they happen in the *images* of heads and feet and hands.'[139]

The injection of hypertonic saline into the lumbosacral supraspinous ligament may give pain radiating down the leg as far as the calf. It may also be associated with tender points commonly situated over the sacroiliac joint and the upper outer quadrant of the buttock.[120]

Sympathetic pathways and central connections, as well as somatic nerves, may be involved in mechanisms of pain reference (see p. 21).

Regarding the upper thorax, *Brain and Wilkinson*[16] observe that:

> The upper thoracic nerves also contribute sensory fibres and the distribution of pain down the medial border of the arm, forearm and hand and radiation up in the neck towards the lobe of the left ear suggests that there are communications between the sympathetic nerves and somatic afferent fibres at the levels of the superior, middle and inferior cervical sympathetic ganglia.

Clinical experience, of shoulder and arm symptoms being relieved by mobilisation of thoracic segments as low as T8, is not rare.

> The evidence of the experimental work is said to suggest that there is not only a distal but also a central mechanism involved in the production of referred pain, and the suggestion is made that the central mechanism is both in the higher centres and in the (spinal) cord itself.[13]

Pain is *not* referred or projectd along nerve trunks to the site of reference:

1. Cases are reported of anginal pain being referred to a phantom upper limb.[27]
2. Anginal pain referred to the left arm is not abolished by a complete brachial plexus block with local anaesthesia.[79]
3. Harman[78] succeeded in provoking *pain* and *paraesthesiae* in phantom limbs by saline injection.
4. Referred pain to the tip of the shoulder, initiated by phrenic nerve irritation, occurs just the same when all the cutaneous nerves to the shoulder-tip have been excised.[40]
5. Referred pain was experimentally evoked in areas previously anaesthetised by regional nerve block.[51]

While an injection of local anaesthetic into a peripheral attachment-tissue, e.g. a tendon, or other musculo-skeletal soft tissue, may relieve pain in that vicinity, the true source of that pain has not necessarily been demonstrated.

That pain of proximal origin may be reduced by injection at its peripheral site of reference is a decided advantage, and has many clinical applications, but it is basically important to increase our understanding of the mechanisms underlying these phenomena, because their nature is not yet fully elucidated.[70]

The complaint of pain and the demonstration of local tenderness may obscure the fact that the offending pathologic lesion is centrally placed, and may lead to the clinician to believe, erroneously, that the disease process underlies the site of the patient's complaint. This erroneous belief may be apparently confirmed by the temporary relief of pain by the injection of local anaesthetic. Such pain relief may be maintained for a surprisingly long period of time. These points must be borne in mind when considering soft tissue lesions.[120]

Referred pain may or may not be accompanied by secondary hyperalgesia . . . injection of procaine into the superficial or deep hyperalgesic structures will reduce the amount of pain. When cutaneous hyperalgesia is marked, pain originating from deep structures may be greatly relieved by spraying ethyl chloride coolant on the affected area. Spread of excitation in the central nervous system may produce widespread painful contractions of skeletal muscle remote from the noxious stimulus. Procaine injected into the affected muscles abolishes this type of pain.[96]

Reliance on the infallibility of dermatomes, or sclerotomes, as distal territories immutably related to a single vertebral segment, can cause difficulty. Hockaday and Whitty[85] describe how the location of referred pain can be influenced by pre-existing pain in another segment.

Deciding, by a process of Sherlock Holmes detection, that the lesion lies here or there because that is where it *ought* to be, without careful and systematic vertebral palpation, is not enough.

It is a profound mistake to arbitrarily apply conventional anatomical description to all individuals, whilst holding 'all is based on simple anatomy'. Anatomy is not simple, it is very complicated and so are the neurophysiological mechanisms underlying it. Our understanding of them is far from complete. There are so many considerations and variables:

1. The wandering of the sinuvertebral nerve, up and down the neural canal before terminating in receptors.
2. The variability of dermatomes.
3. The 'untidiness' of sclerotomes.
4. Pre- and postfixation of plexuses.
5. Differing myotomes — deltoid, for example, may be supplied by C3, C4 or C7, and not necessarily by C5–6.[18]
6. Differing pain tolerances.
7. The nature of the lesion, about which we can often only make an intelligent guess.
8. The fact that individual responses vary quite widely.
9. The somewhat fulsome descriptions given by patients.

Three-quarters of the emphasis, in assessing where to work in mobilising or manipulating the vertebral column, should perhaps rest on what is found by palpation, following regional active, and passive segmental, tests of movement.

During examination therefore, a standard clinical method might include these basic principles:
1. The suspension of disbelief while listening to the patient.
2. Examination by a process of exclusion from proximal to distal.
3. The inclusion of all tissues and structures from which pain *could* be arising.
4. Allowances for the odd fact which does not fit in.
5. A careful search over several segments to either side of the suspected level, by detailed palpation.

6

Introduction to examination

Either at the time of the initial clinical examination, which is essentially a sorting procedure, or at a subsequent examination conducted by the clinical worker who is going to treat the patient, it is necessary to give fullest attention to an 'indications' examination, which is concerned solely with the *manner* in which the diagnosed joint problem is manifesting itself, and with localising the vertebral segment(s) involved.

Arranged in logical sequence, comprehensive examination by the therapist is the foundation of effective treatment, and it is necessary to acquire an orderly and systematic approach.

Examination should always follow a basic pattern, in strict sequence; this enables the therapist to build up a firmly grasped technique of investigating joint problems and will give increasing confidence in assessment as skill is progressively acquired:

1. *'Listen'* History
2. *'Look'* Observation
3. *'Test'* Test
4. *'Feel'* Palpation
5. *Record* Write an account of examination
6. *Assess* Sort out priorities of information derived, and therefore of treatment.

Attention should be concentrated on only one aspect at a time.

N.B. Sections 1, 2, 3 and 4 are elaborated as needed to elicit full information.

Aims of this fundamentally important procedure are:

a. *Subjective examination* — to gather all relevant information about the site, nature, behaviour and onset of the *current* symptoms, with their behaviour in the past and details of previous treatment, if any, and to formulate the next step of physical tests accordingly. A 'symptom' requires the patient's testimony and usually cannot be perceived by the examiner, although its effects may be perceptible.

b. *Objective examination* — to seek abnormalities of function, using active, passive, neurological and special tests of all tissues likely to be involved, guided by the history. A 'sign' is an objective thing and can be perceived by the examiner.

c. To apply this information in planning treatment.

Disturbances of function in the musculo-skeletal and nervous system, and their effects, are noted, and the more precise and full is examination the more likely is correct localisation of the joint problem, with a clear appreciation of how movements of the vertebral segment(s) are abnormal.

EXAMINATION

Having established the salient features for which the patient is attending, i.e. pain, movement-restriction, painless loss of function, lateral spinal deviation, dysequilibrium, listing or instability, loss of confidence, anxiety about locomotor function, walking difficulties, attendance following inpatient invasive or outpatient procedures (removal of POP cast, for example), the particular form of examination will differ according to the nature of the dominant features.

In every physical examination there is a theoretical ideal. The examiner tests all anatomic and dynamic aspects of the joint in question (bones, soft tissues, range of motion, muscle strength, vascular and neurological integrity). In a practical examination, however, the key to an accurate diagnosis is often based not on a step by step analysis of all possible factors, but on a specific investigation of the patient's subjective complaint. A thorough, complete examination is always performed, but emphasis is naturally placed on that portion of the examination that has the greatest clinical relevance.[88]

Planning the most efficient and productive form of examination, from patient to patient, becomes easier with clinical experience, but first there *must* be a foundation, i.e. practical realisation of Hoppenfeld's 'theoretical ideal', and a good beginning is to thoroughly drill oneself in the systematic approach of examining *all* the separate tissues from which pain and other symptoms *might* be arising. Thus basic procedures are described below.

Knowledgeable trimming and speeding up of procedure follows naturally in time, as the worker gains clinical experience, but the informed and responsible use of short cuts rests on competence, and the beginner's obligation is to steadily acquire this by orderly self-discipline and dedicated practice.

Principle governing procedure

Confronted by recommended basic examination drills for each vertebral district and associated peripheral joints, there is the question of efficiently combining them, when both a spinal and a particular peripheral joint require detailed investigation over and above a routine check.

Since pain is very frequently referred from proximal to distal, and since joints which are situated in areas to which pain of spinal origin is commonly referred often develop secondary dysfunction which contributes to the total picture of signs and symptoms, all examinations should invariably proceed from the spine to the distal body parts.

Therefore, *examination* of patients for mobilisation treatment includes a comprehensive examination of suspected joints and a routine examination of associated joints and tissues, though the latter is frequently varied and added to by the content of the history — hence the need to *plan* examination of peripheral joints.

Even though the temporo-mandibular joint, for example, requires comprehensive and detailed examination in its own right, it is a good plan to regard the *temporo-mandibular* joints, and *sacro-iliac* joints, as 'peripheral' joints in the sense that the former naturally belongs in the general forequarter examination and the latter is part of the general hindquarter examination.

The upper limbs also then become peripheral joints associated with the upper half of the thoracic spine as well as the forequarter, while the lower limbs (apart from their place in the basic hindquarter examination) should always be checked neurologically if there is the suspicion or probability of cord interference by cervical and/or thoracic joint problems.

The worker with much clinical experience may sometimes, on the basis of reasonable likelihoods evident during the history and on observation, start examination at the 'peripheral' joints named (e.g. sterno-clavicular, acromio-clavicular, temporo-mandibular and sacro-iliac) and then check the associated vertebral district and other appropriate peripheral joints, but this is no field for the beginner; it is full of pitfalls, even for the experienced.

It is good sense to begin by sticking to the methodical, unvarying basic routine of completing the whole forequarter or hindquarter examination and *then* going back to complete such comprehensive examination of individual joints as may have been indicated during methodical completion of the basic drills suggested.

Only in this way will the student steadily accumulate knowledge of the infinite variety of clinical presentations, the infinite permutations of signs and symptoms, and the yawning discrepancy between what is understood from pre-packaged teaching programmes and what actually transpires on the clinical shop-floor.

It is enlightened self-interest *to teach oneself* by plodding method — the facile short-cut teaches nothing.

My preference is not to teach short cuts to beginners, or to anybody else, however experienced. It is much better for these eventually to be developed by the individual as expertise is gained; in this way they retain a sound clinical basis for what they do, rather than willy-nilly adopting more experienced clinicians' methods, which may tend unjustifiably to be used when in a hurry or feeling tired. *What is learned during the handling of patients is paramount — these are the best lessons, and remain with us long after the tutorials, the book, and the practical classes are assimilated and forgotten.* This philosophy is reflected in arrangement of the examination drills suggested. (p. 53) which at times may necessitate going over a roughly similar drill already completed, this time with a different emphasis.

SUBJECTIVE EXAMINATION — HISTORY

Because the therapist's examination is not always an initial sorting procedure, emphasis on particular aspects, and thus the sequence of examination, are different; it is important to appreciate the reason for this.

This little text is concerned less with the whole range of vertebral column disease than with introducing beginners to the treatment, by physical means, of common patterns of vertebral pain and movement-restriction; these with other signs and symptoms are, for the most part, the sequelae of degenerative change, in its many forms.

The particular *sequence* of examination suggested reflects this emphasis, because degeneration of musculo-skeletal tissue has existence in time as well as space.

Most patients genuinely — a few obsessively — believe they can 'begin at the beginning' and provide a clear, chronological and meaningful sequence of development of their clinical features, together with the precise cause of their difficulties. Some can, many cannot.

Needless emphasis, often derived from patent medicine advertisements, is given to events and symptoms which are of no great import, including what the doctor said about their 'arthritis' or what the osteopath said about 'three slipped discs', while salient traumatic episodes, for example, are quite overlooked during the rambling tale of 'how it all began'.

By *first* fully comprehending how the patient is presently troubled and restricted, and *then* tracking back over time by specific questioning, therapists are much more likely to get a workmanlike grasp of what they are dealing with, together with its context of the patient's life-style, past history and temperament.

Assessment and continuing re-assessment are the basis from which constructive treatment evolves, and because *pain* and *its behaviour* are the dominant factors

a. compelling the majority of patients to seek treatment

b. guiding the selection and modification of treatment

a clear grasp of both the distribution and the behaviour of pain are of first significance.

Since patients depressed by pain tend to describe the onset in a rambling and sometimes emotionally-charged fashion, which may thoroughly confuse the therapist with a host of 'red herrings' and prejudice the orderly grasp of essentials, the sequence of history-taking suggested is:

(i) patient's daily activity, at work and play

(ii) the pain, and other symptoms, *currently* troubling the patient

(iii) the onset of the attack, and previous attacks, if any

(iv) previous treatment, if any, and its effects (see Table 6.1).

The patient should be kept to the point, kindly but firmly, and irrelevant elaboration discouraged. The therapist should *listen*, make no assumptions, try to clarify the information being gathered, (Fig. 6.1) and help the patient to be as precise as is reasonably possible, by:

— keeping the questions simple

— asking one at a time

— getting an answer before proceeding to the next one

— avoiding putting words into the patient's mouth

— giving equal value to awkward points in the history, though they may be unwelcome in that they negate favourite theories and bias on the therapist's part.

APOTHEGM

I KNOW THAT YOU BELIEVE
YOU UNDERSTAND
WHAT YOU THINK I SAID
BUT I AM NOT SURE YOU REALISE
THAT WHAT YOU THINK YOU HEARD
IS NOT WHAT I MEANT

Fig. 6.1 Since it is vital for the patient to understand what the question is about, the therapist must put it clearly and simply.

Table 6.1 The skeletal framework of orderly history-taking

---

1. Patient's occupation

2. Pain   Where? (and where *not*)   Trunk?   Trunk and limb(s)?   Limb(s) only?
                     Where worst?
                     Nature?
                     Behaviour – related to   **Time**   **Posture**   **Activity**

Constant pain?

Yes   No

Does it vary? — Yes

NO*

What aggravates?
How much?
Trunk > Limb(s)?
Trunk/Limb(s) equally?
Limb(s) > Trunk?
Immediately?
Later?
For how long?
What eases?
Promptly?
Later?

3. Paraesthesiae and concomitant symptoms
          (e.g tingling, 'pins and needles', formication,
          dizziness, numbness, 'uselessness', 'heaviness',
          'coldness', localised 'burning' etc.)

          Nature?
          Where?
          Behaviour?

4. Mandatory questions (see p. 32)

5. Onset   This episode?
                      Previous episodes?

6. General health, previous history and treatment results

---

*Raises suspicion of neoplastic disease,
 inflammatory arthritis or psychogenic pain.

1. Patient's occupation

The nature and degree of the patient's work and recreation activity should be known. The varied physical work of a housewife who shops, cooks, cleans and helps to garden for a large growing family; the packer or assembler who sits handling materials all day; the chair-bound administrator; the plough-man who is sitting and continually turning one way to watch the furrow; the fruit-picker; the over-keen Yoga exerciser, the commercial representative who spends most of every workday in a car —each will be prone to different forms of musculo-skeletal stress, the nature of which influences both plans of treatment and emphasis in prophylaxis.

2. Pain

Always *listen* to a complaint of pain, and remember that the pain point has the same wide individual variation as pain itself . . . modify treatment according to necessity . . . failure to listen to a complaint of pain may, incidentally, lead to serious errors in treatment.[155]

The important information is that concerning the *current* distribution of pain and where it is worst; outlined by the patient pointing with one finger if possible (where it is *not* is also important), its nature and characteristics, i.e. its behaviour related to time, posture and activity (p. 30) and the degree of joint and/or root irritability (p. 130). Distinctions must be made between:
— constant pain, with areas of radiation at times
— periodic or episodic pain
— elicited pain, i.e. that which is produced only by certain postures, movements or by later testing examination and/or palpation.

Distribution should be interpreted in relation to dermatomes, myotomes and sclerotomes as a likely, but not infallible, help to localisation of cause.

The distribution of pain may be important, yet its segmental significance is not always easy to clarify because:
a. dermatomes are neurophysiological entities, whose boundaries can fluctuate with the levels of facilitation at cord segments
b. patients vary considerably in their patterns of pain reference or projection from apparently similar, common joint abnormalities
c. pain may be referred to sclerotome areas, which differ from dermatomes.

For example, the symptom-area outlined by the patient often indicates the need to investigate two or more possible sources, e.g. back pain over the lumbo-sacral segment, with an ache spreading across anterior thigh from postero-lateral buttock to medial knee, should lead to comprehensive examination of hip as well as lumbar spine. *Thus the content of History dictates the scope and planning of subsequent testing.*

Nature

The pain may be:
— a dull, persistent ache, lying deep and hard to outline
— transient, severe pain superimposed on this at times
— a mild catch or twinge, or a severe jab or 'shoot' on movement
— sickening, severe and disabling 'root' pain
— inseparably associated as painful paraesthesiae, i.e. prickling, 'burning' or disagreeable hyperaesthesia, and more severely as hyperpathia.

Irritability

An initial assessment of the degree of joint and/or root irritability (q.v.) should be made.

Characteristics

In seeking the behaviour of pain related to time, posture and activity, a logical sequence of enquiry can assist the patient as well as the therapist, e.g.:

How has the pain behaved during the last fortnight
— increasing — static — decreasing?

Night pain
— how do they lie? Most/least comfortable position?
— sleep disturbed?
— how? because *pain* wakes the patient without changing position or has patient disturbed joint by changing position?
— painful paraesthesiae wakes patient in early hours?
— type of bed base, mattress and pillows?

Rising a.m.
— painfree, but weight-bearing provokes?
— painfully stiff?
— how long to loosen up?

Day pain
— does pain increase steadily as day goes on, or depend upon activity (i.e. time dependent/stress dependent)? Trunk > limb(s) or vice versa?
— which posture or activity aggravates/eases? Sitting (and standing from) — standing — bending and lifting — arms above head — reaching — housework — coughing and sneezing — deep breath — sustained flexion and returning from — driving — reversing car — sewing — reading — theatre — walking?

Evening pain

— does pain build up regularly in evening? Trunk >
 limb(s) or vice versa?
— eases now because can rest?

Understanding the characteristics of pain and the
pattern of its aggravation and relief does not
necessarily make accurate identification of the tissue
responsible any easier, but provides the therapist
with the vital criteria which are of fundamental
importance in assessment of efficacy of treatment.
Painstaking exercise of discernment and a grasp of
small detail are infinitely worthwhile, because in
time they provide an understanding of joint problem
behaviour which no other exercise or education can
give.

3. Abnormalities of feeling

The *distribution* in head, neck, throat, trunk and
limbs of dysaesthesia, paraesthesiae, hyperpathia
and areas of loss of sensation must be noted, together
with their characteristics related to time, posture and
activity. Swallowing difficulties (dysphagia)?
Speech difficulties (dysphonia)? Lump in the
throat? Feeling of weight on the head? Difficulties of
concentration and remembering? Blurred vision?
Head feels 'heavy'? Arm feels 'useless'?

4. Mandatory questions

There are some questions which are mandatory, and
it is unwise to begin treatment without the required
information (see Contraindications).

Cervical region

— any dizziness (vertigo), blackouts or 'drop'
 attacks?
— history of upper respiratory tract infection? (In
 juniors)
— any history of rheumatoid arthritis or other
 inflammatory arthritis? Treated by systemic
 steroids?
— anticoagulant drugs?
*— any neurological symptoms in legs?

Thoracic region

— has the patient been treated recently by systemic

steroid drugs? Anticoagulants?
*— any neurological symptoms in legs?

Lumbar region

— any perineal or 'saddle area' anaesthesia or
 paraesthesiae?
— any change in micturition habits associated with
 the back trouble, or sphincter disturbance?
— steroids or anticoagulants?

N.B.

a. It is desirable that the therapist sees the X-ray,
 but the more important information is that the
 patient *has* been recently X-rayed, and the films
 have been seen by a radiologist.
b. General health and possible co-existent disease
 should be enquired about.
c. The significance of inexorable night pain should
 be borne in mind.

A frivolous mnemonic may help the forgetful (i.e. all
of us) to bear these in mind.

*'XXX Ale dizzily steers 'urting rheumatoid legs to
night watering place'*

XXX Ale	— X-ray and anticoagulant drugs
Dizzily	— Dizziness
Steers	— Steroids
'Urting	— Upper respiratory tract infection
Rheumatoid	— Rheumatoid arthritis
Legs to	— Leg symptoms
Night	— Night pain
Watering place	— Micturition disturbance, 'saddle' anaesthesia.

5. Onset

(i) This may be *insidious*, a mild and sporadic ache
demanding attention as it becomes painfully more
continuous; the patient may have no recollection of
injury or stress, but frequently, long forgotten

---

*These questions are additional to the routine neurological
examination of arms with cervical and thoracic regions, and legs
with thoracic, lumbar and sacral regions (q.v.).

trauma may be recalled which can reasonably be associated with a current joint condition. This pattern often indicates a problem easier to help than not.

(ii) Onset may be *slow or delayed*, in that symptoms begin some hours or days following stress (see p. 232); this fact can assist in selecting treatment, e.g. lumbar traction.

(iii) *Sudden onset*, in the form of recent severe trauma sufficient to fracture bones, after which the symptoms arising from joints were of secondary importance, can indicate that treatment of the joint condition will progress only slowly.

(iv) *Sudden onsets of joint locking* are commonly easier to help than slow onsets over hours or days, but a history of recurrent locking shows the need for treatment-emphasis on preventing recurrence rather than reduction of the derangement. Concerning recent stress and injury, it is surprising how often patients will initially disclaim this, to recall by the next treatment session a severe fall three days previously.

6. Previous history

Degenerative joint conditions, like chronic bronchitis, exist in time as well as space. Knowledge of the past behaviour of joint troubles can help in assessing the nature of the problem and therefore in planning treatment more appropriately. When asked about similar troubles in the past, the answer may include information about 'only odd attacks of fibrositis and rheumatism' or 'stiffness only'. It is probable that the patient is unwittingly relating information about spondylotic episodes and the significance of this history should be clear to the therapist.

Questions should therefore include:

— similar trouble before?
— if 'no' —episodes of stiff neck? Stiff back?
— onset of previous attacks, if any?
— trauma? Site of pain? Radiation?
— how long to recover?
— recovered completely?
— treatment given, if any? How effective was treatment?
— general health? Weight loss recently?

The answers to these questions indicate the likely pathology and stage of progression, the likely percentage and the rate of improvement, and the possibility of recurrence. The information helps in assessment.

OBJECTIVE EXAMINATION — OBSERVATION

Much information can be gathered by observation, which begins on first sight of the patient and continues throughout the physical tests of the examination.

Initially:

— way of moving
— gait
— general posture
— manner
— willingness to co-operate

are noted, and following the 'subjective' examination the patient undresses sufficiently for the body region to be adequately observed. The patient should be examined in a warm room with a good light; the therapist should be placed to see well, and basic procedures should follow the same sequence every time.

When looking for small alterations of position of this nature it is important that the master eye should be over the midline of the patient. To determine your master eye, make a circle with the index finger and thumb of one hand and hold it out in front at arm's length. With both eyes open observe what is seen clearly through the circle. Then close each eye in turn. When the object originally seen remains in view, you are looking with your master eye. When the object changes the master eye is closed.[13]

Changes in:

— attitude (deformity)
— contour (swelling, wasting, muscle spasm)
— colour (circulation, inflammation)
— skin appearance generally
  are noted, taking into account general build and age.

Clinical examination of pelvic posture in standing and sitting, and comparison of leg lengths can be completed quite quickly and should form part of the examination for *all* vertebral regions (see 'Other postures, (a) Standing and sitting', p. 35). The reasons for stressing the importance of this measure are, of course, the mechanical and neurophysiological *interdependence* of the vertebral column, which declares itself in a variety of ways, some of them subtle; unless borne in mind during examination, the small signs and portents may be missed, and the therapist's grasp of the genesis of clinical features would be incomplete.

The important point is that it is not possible to know in advance just how big a factor, in production of symptoms and signs remote from the pelvic levels, the consequences of pelvic asymmetry may be from patient to patient. Stoddard[169] describes three patients with obscure anterior thoracic pains, whose symptoms were relieved by no other treatment than an appropriate heel lift.

While location of the *source* of backache, or a cervical, thoracic or lumbar pain is necessary, there is also the question of the *genesis* of these pains, and the functional inter-dependence of the spine should always be considered.

In no way does this detract from the importance of accurately localised treatment, but it does clarify the context of that treatment, and might considerably improve an understanding of why vertebral joint problems behave as they do.

Adequate appreciation of this basic premise seems fairly thin on the ground, even among those with some experience of handling vertebral joint problems.

Neck and thoracic region

Patient sits sideways on treatment couch or on stool, with hands on thighs so that all aspects of head and trunk may be seen.

From the front:

Relate head, neck and trunk to an imaginary perpendicular or a purpose-designed 'grid' background. Note horizontal level of eyes, position of chin and neck, contour and symmetry of clavicular joints, shoulder joints, sub-clavicular hollows and the mass of neck, pectoral and arm muscles. Note symmetry of waist contours related to arms. Observe and handle the patient's hands for intrinsic muscle wasting and temperature.

From the side:

Relate head and neck posture to trunk posture, and note increased or decreased curvature, e.g. note any flattening of interscapular region, undue prominence of one or both medial borders of scapula or localised increase of upper thoracic kyphosis.

From behind:

Check contour of posterior cervical muscle, Trapezius, Latissimus Dorsi and Sacrospinalis muscles. Note bulk and symmetry, especially of medial 'yoke' region. Check levels and attitude of scapulae, horizontal body curves (ribs) and back muscle contours.

Palpation:

Feel sides and back of neck and 'yoke' area for palpable asymmetry, and Trapezius with pectoral muscle for postural spasm.

Lumbar and pelvic region

Patient stands with feet a little apart and parallel and the minimum of covering.

From behind:

Relate spine and gluteal cleft to imaginary perpendicular, and horizontal level of shoulders and scapulae with pelvic levels. Observe waist contours, symmetry of rib cage and Sacrospinalis muscle masses. Check attitude of whole pelvis, level of iliac crests, dimples over posterior superior iliac spines; observe buttock contours, level of gluteal folds, and posterior limb muscles for wasting.

Palpation:

Iliac crests and posterior iliac spine levels, muscle mass of Sacrospinalis for postural spasm.

From the side:

Check if patient stands with pelvis rotated, and with increased/decreased spinal curvature.

From the front:

Check symmetry of anterior superior iliac spines, contours of abdomen and muscle mass of thigh, leg and foot.

Palpation:

Anterior iliac spines and tubercles of iliac crest.

Other postures

It is necessary to observe the contours and attitudes of body parts in postures other than sitting or standing, and to compare changes in these two factors when different postures are assumed. These further positions involving movement are described under 'observation' because it is this aspect of the clinical examination which should be given the most attention during the tests described. The particular arrangement of physical tests will vary from patient to patient; it is essential that examination procedures are *planned* on the basis of initial observations and history, and different aspects of the examination may need to be combined if the patient is in much pain. Patients in moderate or more severe pain should not be subjected to prolonged inspection while they endeavour to hold difficult and painful postures, and during the early stages of treatment it is often necessary to make these postural observations *during* the normal tests of movement.

a. *Standing and sitting.* A simple method of determining whether a compensated lateral tilt of the pelvis in young people is probably due to a leg length inequality is to assess the degree of tilt in standing, and then to assess it again with the patient sitting on a hard horizontal surface such as a gymnastic stool. When sitting, the patient is supported on ischial tuberosities, and should the tilt be eradicated and the pelvis then assessed as level, a reasonable assumption is that the cause of the tilt lies in unequal leg lengths. The test is less reliable for the more mature patient in whom adaptive shortening may have occurred, and in any event can never be more than a quick and

simple test which is less satisfactory than antero-posterior films of the hip joints, whole pelvis and lumbar spine in the standing position. Ideally, whole-spine erect films allow the superimposition of vertical and horizontal plane lines, and the most accurate assessment.

b. *Flexion during standing and sitting.* Besides comparison of vertebral and pelvic posture in the coronal, sagittal and horizontal planes in *standing* and *sitting*, comparisons may need to be made when the patient bends forward when standing, and bends forward when sitting (Figs. 6.2, 6.3).

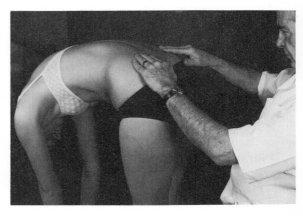

Fig. 6.2 Observing possible asymmetry of movement, contour and attitude on flexion when standing.

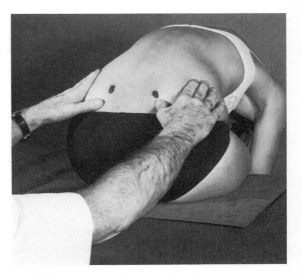

Fig. 6.3 Observing possible asymmetry of movement, contour and attitude on flexion when sitting.

A tangential view, from behind or in front as is most suitable, will not infrequently demonstrate one or more of pelvic rotation, alteration in the horizontal relationship of posterior superior iliac spines (Piedallu's sign[158]) flattening of one paravertebral muscle mass, vertebral rotation, visibly disparate amounts of movement occurring in different regions, maintenance of a rigid low lumbar lordosis and lateral deviation to one or the other side. Sometimes a postural lateral deviation in standing will be eradicated in the flexed position, and in other patients a straight spine in standing or sitting will deviate on flexion, either momentarily or progressively throughout the movement (see p. 147).

c. *Contour and attitude in supine lying.* These should be compared to posture when standing and sitting, and the alterations noted. Body contours should be viewed tangentially. The supporting surface should be uniformly even, and care taken that the patient is lying in a neutral position, so far as this is possible. Many elderly patients will require three or more pillows.

The contours of the neck, the position of the clavicles and the pectoral region together with shoulders, should be observed, and the sides of the thorax compared. Pelvic posture and the horizontal relationship of anterior superior iliac spines should be noted.

With a 'horse-shoe' grasp over the neck of each talus of the supine patient, the examiner places his thumbs immediately beneath each medial malleolus and bends the patient's knees so that the soles of the feet are rested side-by-side on the plinth, with the operator's thumbs in neutral side-by-side contact. The patient is then instructed to gently raise the pelvis off the couch, move it from side to side, and then settle it down again in the most neutral position. The patient's legs are then extended and the relative position of the operator's thumbs, still grasping as above, are compared. Equality or inequality of leg lengths in the supine position should be noted.

Standardised tests should not lead to standardised conclusions, and 'leg length discrepancy' observed by this test has no significance unless incorporated into the overall assessment of posture in the standing and sitting positions; the two ubiquitous factors of (i) lumbo-sacral/pelvic anomaly and (ii) asymmetrical adaptive shortening of strong connective-tissue and muscle, should temporise a ready tendency to

ascribe the cause to changes in sacro-iliac joints.[68]

Pelvic rotation observed in supine lying which was not present on standing may be due to wasting of the gluteal muscle mass on one side. This is not always easily detectable in standing, and an apparently normal but 'soft' gluteal mass, due to gluteus maximus weakness, is more easily squashed by pelvic weight when lying than its opposite fellow with normal tone.

d. *Prone lying.* With the patient in a neutral prone-lying position, body contours should again be noted by a tangential view.

With a 'horse-shoe' grasp now over the tendo-calcaneus, and the examiner's thumb and index finger lying immediately under the medial and lateral malleolus respectively, leg lengths should be compared (a) with the legs in neutral position, and (b) after the grasp has been changed so that the thumbs rest on the middle sole of foot and fingers rest on dorsum of foot, with the knees flexed to 90°. Before assessing a leg-length discrepancy in the position (b), both legs should be moved as one, forward and backward and to the left and right, before being stabilised at 90°. The movements should not be large enough to grossly disturb the resting position of the pelvis. Minor apparent discrepancies in leg length may occur if this preparatory 'settling down' is not completed.

A lateral view of the alignment of tibial tubercles in this position completes the observation of posture in prone lying.

N.B. Asymmetry of contour and attitude need not be of any significance in the context of symptoms reported by the patient. The sometimes unwitting tendency to assume that 'symmetry is all', and that asymmetry must always be 'normalised' for symptoms to be relieved, is an insufficient basis for planning treatment.[68]

OBJECTIVE EXAMINATION — PHYSICAL TESTS

Tests of the tissues mentioned below are related to their function.

a. Joint function is *movement*, and both active and passive tests of voluntary range, and passive tests of accessory range, are necessary.

b. Muscle function, with its tissue of attachment,

is first to *develop* and then to *sustain* tension. By resisted isometric contractions, weakness and/or pain on applied tension are noted.

c. Ligaments and capsule *sustain tension, limit and also guide movement and maintain the integrity of joint structures.*

Tension is applied by passive movement, noting whether pain is caused, movement is limited or the peri-articular structures allow undue movement. It should be noted that *localised* tension is much easier to apply to the structures of single peripheral joints than to those of the multi-jointed vertebral segments.

d. Neurones *conduct impulses*, and the conduction is tested by methods which disclose loss or abnormalities of conduction, i.e., questioning the patient regarding sensation and equilibration changes, difficulties of walking, observing possible vasomotor disturbance and muscle wasting, observing and palpating for muscle spasm, testing for neurological deficit as muscle weakness and diminution or loss of tendon jerks, and testing skin for sensory diminution or loss.

e. Some *special tests,* e.g. straight-leg-raising, prone-knee bending and others are applied to test the freedom of movements of spinal nerve roots and neural canal structures, but are not conduction tests. Special tests may include, for example, (i) trunk rotation with the head stabilised, and (ii) successively tapping the spinous processes with a patella hammer. It should be noted that a single testing procedure, i.e. *resisted isometric contraction of muscle,* may be employed both in (b) to seek abnormalities in the muscle and its attachment-tissues, and in (d) to determine whether motor nerve conduction is normal.

Tests of movement

When symptoms and their behaviour are understood and postural abnormalities noted, the next step is to clarify which vertebral movements, or carefully applied stresses:

(i) reproduce or aggravate the patient's symptoms
(ii) are in themselves abnormal.

Since arthrosis and spondylosis are largely benign diseases of the joints, consideration of the movement abnormalities resulting is fundamental to devising treatment. They can be manifested in many ways,

sometimes obvious during an active test and sometimes remaining undetected until passive tests (q.v.) of both voluntary and accessory movements are completed.

Mobility in multi-joint articulations

The physiological range of movement at each vertebral joint, however small in comparison to the larger peripheral joints, is just as important to healthy joint function; when diminished by various causes, limitation at an individual segment is rather more difficult to detect than in peripheral joints in that it cannot readily be seen, although with practice it can easily be palpated. A typical cervical vertebra takes part in the formation of ten separate joints. One thoracic vertebra takes part in twelve joints (counting each demi-facet) and each lumbar vertebra, six joints. During degeneration changes and after trauma the natural apportioning of movement to each small component of this kind of complex articulation may be upset, and what appears on cursory examination to be normal movement in gross terms is actually movement achieved by extra strains on those joints adjacent to the stiff segments of the articulation. This abnormality tends to be self-perpetuating, and cannot always be remedied by the patient who has little influence, by way of voluntary effort, upon this defect. Movement may be limited, of full or limited range but distorted, and sometimes excessive in hypermobile joints.

Limitation may be due to:
— pain
— spasm of antagonistic muscle-groups
— other tissue-tension, e.g. as stretch on adhesion formation or other soft-tissue contracture
— tissue-compression, e.g. as squeeze on marginal chrondro-osteophytes, peri-articular thickening or intra-articular tissue changes.

Testing movement of vertebral regions

During examination of a joint, one *can* only do:
(i) Functional test (active movement)
(ii) Passive test
— of functional range (especially the 'end-feel' of the movement) i.e. passive physiological-movement tests (PP-MT)
— of accessory movement and joint char-

acteristics i.e. passive accessory-movement tests (PA-MT)

— of surrounding fibrous and other soft tissues

(iii) Muscle power test

Each part contributes information about the state of the joint and its immediate neighbourhood, though the importance of each part varies according to the position and nature of the joint.

While it is not possible to suggest a rigid testing sequence applicable to all joints, a basic *spinal* testing procedure must include the following tests:

Joint movement
— active, functional test
— passive test of active and accessory movement

Joint structures
— by local stress—tension, compression, torsion, unilateral approximation

Muscle testing
— for muscle and attachments ⎱ by localised
— for neurological deficit ⎰ isometric tension

Other neurological tests
— tendon jerks, plantar response, sensation

Special tests, e.g.
— straight-leg-raising (*N.B.* This is not an exclusively neurological test)
— rotation test for giddiness
— spinal tapping test, etc.

and these are modified according to the nature and characteristics of the joint under examination.

Since pain is very frequently referred from proximal to distal, and since joints which are situated in areas to which pain of spinal origin is commonly referred often develop secondary dysfunction which contributes to the total picture of signs and symptoms, all examinations should invariably proceed from the spine to the distal body parts.

Therefore, **examination** of patients for mobilisation treatment includes a comprehensive examination of suspected joints and a *routine* examination of associated joints and tissues, though the latter is frequently varied and added to by the content of the history—*hence the need to* **plan** *examination of peripheral joints.*

Factors to be noted are:
— willingness to move
— quality of the movement (deviation, asymmetry, adventitious movement)
— limitations of normal range, if any
— amount of limitation

— nature of the limitation
— reluctance
— increasing pain
— spasm
— pain and spasm simultaneously
— inert tissue-tension
— tissue compression
— muscle weakness
— if painful
  — *when?* (e.g. 'arc' of pain, or towards the end of range?)
  — how quickly does pain increase during movement, if at all?
  — how much pain is caused, or how easily exacerbated? (Initial assessment of irritability)
  — does it limit the movement? (It need not)
  — *where* is the pain?
  — is it exacerbation of presenting pain only, or spreading further, or a pain not previously reported?
  — extent of spread into a limb?
— paraesthesiae and concomitant symptoms
  — elicited or aggravated by movement? Or posture?
  — which movement? Which posture?

It is important to establish the *factor primarily responsible* for the abnormal movement, because appropriate treatment procedures should be based on this knowledge; frequently only one of these factors is primarily responsible, although at times this is not so. When a particular test elicits poorly localised pain, try modifying the testing movement to clarify the source of pain.

Normal movement

To prove that movement is normal, it is necessary to:
— repeat quickly
— add pressure at extreme range, which should be tolerable
— give sustained pressure at end of range
— sustain pressure on movement towards the side of pain, and it may also be necessary to:
— give compression on movement towards the side of pain
— test 'corner' or combined movements

Cursory examination of movement is insufficient, and therefore ranges which appear full and painless should be tested by passive overpressure at the extremes of active range before being accepted as normal (Figs. 6.4 and 6.5). Overpressure may cause

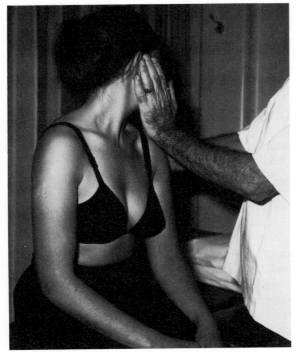

Fig. 6.4 Overpressure at the limit of active range of left cervical rotation.

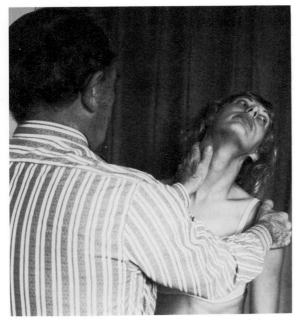

Fig. 6.5 Overpressure to the combined movement of extension and left-side flexion of the cervico-thoracic junction.

discomfort in normal joints, but this test should not hurt; if it does, the joint is suspect and its degree of involvement requires clarification by further examination.

Again, the orthodox single testing movements, e.g. flexion, extension, rotation etc. may frequently be insufficient to reproduce or aggravate the patient's symptoms, or to reveal latent joint abnormalities which are underlying the patient's complaint; because of inadequate examination of movement, therefore, joint problems amenable to treatment may remain undetected.

More searching tests of movement include:

(i) combined movements, e.g. extension with side-flexion, or flexion with side-flexion (conveniently termed 'quadrant' testing movements) (Fig. 7.30).

(ii) applying compression or overpressure at the extremes of single or combined movements

(iii) gently holding a vertebral region at the extremes of range of an active movement, single or combined, so that possible delayed or latent effects may be elicited. This test is of value when the presence or absence of 'root' pain (see p. 40) remains undetermined by less searching tests.

Descriptions of combined (or 'quadrant') movements, are as follows:

Upper cervical spine

Sit or stand at side of sitting patient
— extend at cranio-vertebral junction
— then rotate towards one side
— then side-flex towards that side
— add moderate compression if test is to be more searching

Lower cervical spine

Stand facing sitting patient—one hand on (R) frontal area and other on (L) scapula. (Can do from behind, if facing mirror and can see patient's face)
— approximate occiput to (L) scapula, then add rotation to the same side

Cervico-thoracic

Stand facing sitting patient, place (L) hand on (R)

shoulder and (R) hand on (L) low neck, so that palmar aspect of metacarpal heads bears against low cervical transverse processes

— press into extension and (R) side flexion, then rotate (R)

Thoracic, spine

Stand behind sitting patient (use mirror if possible)
— extend, side-flex to (L) then rotate (L)

Lumbar spine

Stand behind standing patient with hands on shoulders
— extend, side flex to (L), then rotate to (L).
All tests should be repeated to the opposite side.

N.B. Do not lose tension or approximation as additional movements successively are imposed.

Limit of range

This is virtually indefinable in an absolute sense, since the limit of *active* movement varies with the state of the tissues, the time of day, the willingness of the patient, and the speed of the movement performed, and the limit of *passive* movement varies with the tolerance of the patient, the courage or indiscretion of the operator, and the metabolic or vascular state and temperature of the patient's tissues at the material time. Probably a useful working definition is: 'Limit of range is reached when the therapist, the patient, and the joint decide that the movement has proceeded far enough'!

The intensity and duration of increased pain on movement depends upon the degree of joint and/or root irritability

Accurate assessment of this is important, because pain which is easily exacerbated indicates the need for careful handling, both in examination and treatment. The three factors to be considered are:

— the amount of movement required to exacerbate pain
— the intensity of the added pain
— how long it takes to recede to normal levels.

A small unguarded movement stirring up intense pain for some hours indicates a highly irritable joint.

Irritability is also manifest when a quick testing movement elicits spasm earlier in the range than does a more sedate testing movement, and also when both *pain and spasm,* either of which is of sufficient magnitude to limit range, are elicited simultaneously. Pain which is not easily provoked and which settles down very quickly after provocation by a gross movement indicates a much less irritable joint.

Spasm of antagonistic muscle-groups can be elicited, as the primary movement-limiting factor, notwithstanding a degree of pain beginning either before the limitation or being elicited as the point of limitation is reached. The accompanying pain is frequently not sufficient of itself to stop the movement. The variety of ways in which joint irritabiity can be evidenced is due not only to the state of the joint but also to the variations in central nervous system excitability from patient to patient. In less irritable joints, pain may be limiting the movement at any point on the range. Pain may also begin during a movement and rise only moderately until the movement is fully completed. A painful 'arc' of movement, of greater or lesser amplitude, may be traversed during an otherwise uneventful movement, as may sudden 'jabs' or 'catches'. If the two factors of inert tissue-tension and tissue-compression are taken together as *'resistance'*, it is commonly found that arthrotic and spondylotic vertebral segments, giving rise to the complaint of a dull persistent ache, can be limited by this resistance as the primary factor, without eliciting further pain of any consequence. The resistance may be due to changes of long standing or be of more recent origin.

Distortion also occurs during movements, and when asymmetry or deviation from normal paths is noted during active tests, it is important to clarify its significance. If it is the patient's natural way of moving, manual prevention of the deviation during testing will produce discomfort but no pain; when the deviation is an involuntary guarding response against pain during movement, its manual prevention during movement will hurt, and this information helps in selection and accurate assessment of treatment procedures.

Crepitus on movement is more likely to be arising from the synovial joints.

Hypermobility of vertebral segments can either be *acquired,* when pathological instability is underlying it, or be inherited as in those patients who are naturally loose-jointed.

Testing muscle function

Static isometric contractions, of vertebral and paravertebral muscle, are more frequently employed as neurological tests, i.e. of motor nerve conduction than as tests of intrinsic changes in muscle and/or its attachment-tissues, but where weakness of paravertebral muscle, e.g. the abdominal wall, is believed part of a postural defect, an assessment of muscle-power is necessary, and similarly where it is suspected that forces sustained by joints may have produced tissue-damage to muscles.

Resisted 'static' (isometric) contractions

It is probably wise to accept that while this may be the aim, it is an extremely difficult thing to arrange in practice. (See Figs. 6.6–6.11.)

Joint·movement always occurs, joint surface compression occurs, and surrounding non-contractile joint structures are almost always disturbed in some way. It is practically impossible to *keep joints quite still* while muscles around them are put into strong 'static' contractions. Thus, when examining the peri-articular contractile tissues (of peripheral

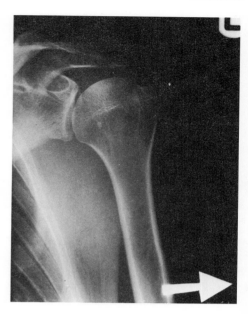

Fig. 6.7 Effects on joint relationship of isometric contractions: strong 'static' *abduction*. Shoulder girdle has moved proximally in relation to rib cage. Humeral head has approximated to glenoid and has descended a little, besides rotating a little.

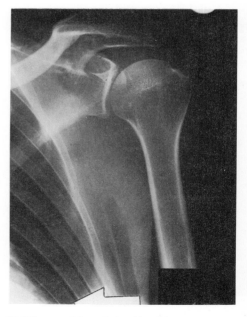

Fig. 6.8 Effects on joint relationship of isometric contractions: strong 'static' *adduction*. Shoulder girdle has moved proximally. Humerous has rotated (see white spot) and is approximated to glenoid.

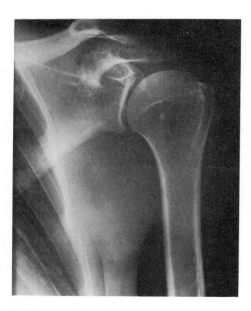

Fig. 6.6 Effects on joint relationship of isometric contractions: resting gleno-humeral joint.

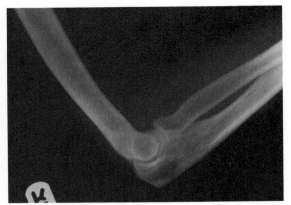

Fig. 6.9 Effects on joint relationship of isometric contractions: resting elbow joint.

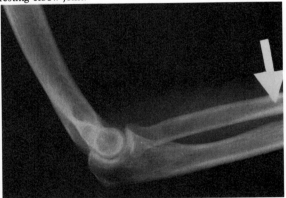

Fig. 6.10 Effects on joint relationship of isometric contractions: strong 'static' elbow extension. Head of radius depressed, in relation to ulna. Change in contour of neck of radius demonstrates rotation of radius.

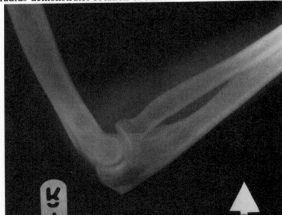

Fig. 6.11 Effects on joint relationship of isometric contractions: strong 'static' elbow flexion. Radial head is strongly approximated to capitulum and has been elevated. Humero-ulnar joint space is narrowed. Compare to Fig. 6.9. (Figs. 6.6–6.11 are reproduced by courtesy of N. Philbrook who kindly arranged the radiography.)

joints) such as muscle, tendon and teno-periosteal junction, by applying local tension, the fact that joint compression and joint shearing invariably occurs should be borne in mind. Aggravation of pain by these tests need not necessarily indicate that the lesion lies in these contractile tissues. Meticulous examination will reveal that it is not often a muscle attachment near a joint is abnormal without the joint also being abnormal, and the precise nature of the changes occurring is not as clear-cut as is sometimes asserted, especially so in upper limb areas commonly involved in referred pain (and other symptoms) from more proximal vertebral lesions.

The equivocality of positive signs

The notion that joints remain 'still', while surrounding muscle groups are statically (isometrically) contracted against resistance, is a fallacy, as Figures 6.6–6.11 will show.

This principle of musculo-skeletal diagnosis, or rule-of-thumb method of attempting to 'localise' the tissue at fault—more particularly in peripheral joints—is not as reliable as many believe, and does not infallibly indicate (i) the precise site of the lesion, nor (ii) invariably differentiate it from lesions in closely-related tissues.

It is, in fact, a further example of the *equivocality of positive signs*, of which there are many.

For example:

— alteration of reflex behaviour can occur with and also without disc trespass involving the associated lumbar nerve root[47] (p. 46)
— individual muscle weakness and a depressed tendon jerk can be normalised by injection of local anaesthetic into lumbar facet-joint capsules (p. 46)[142]
— each of the straight-leg-raising, prone-knee-bending and femoral nerve stretch tests may be positive for differing reasons, with or without nerve root involvement (p. 48)
— a painful arc on abduction of the arm may inculpate the sub-deltoid bursa, the tendons of supraspinatus and/or subscapularis, the acromio-clavicular joint or any combination of these
— 'dizziness' on combined cervical extension and rotation may be due to:
  (i) vertebro-basilar ischaemia (p. 48)

(ii) cranio-vertebral joint conditions not involving trespass (p. 49)

(iii) both

In the whole field of musculo-skeletal testing,
there are very few positive signs which relieve us of
the obligation to *assess*.

Testing connective-tissue structures

Local tension (by passive movement or resisted
contraction). The term 'selective tension' is not used,
since it is extremely difficult to arrange that a single
tissue has tension selectively applied to it only. It is
usually only possible to dispose the patient in such a
way that tension is applied to a whole group of
tissues, *including* the tissues one is presently
interested in. Active movements apply normal stress
and tensions to all soft tissues. When muscles are
relaxed the range of passive movement exceeds that
which is possible actively, and for this reason the
inert capsular, ligamentous and aponeurotic tissues
are additionally tested by passively applying further
tension; this is regionally localised, so far as possible,
by careful hand-placing and grasps.

When assessing the responses to these tests, i.e. in
terms of which tissue be giving rise to the pain or
spasm thereby elicited, two factors should be borne
in mind:

(i) Movement of a rigid structure, i.e. a vertebral
body, must also move *all* structures attached to
it

(ii) Pain may be elicited on passive stretching of one
aspect of a spinal region, and be re-elicited on
following resisted isometric contraction of
muscles on the same aspect. This does not
necessarily indicate that the lesion must
therefore lie in vertebral muscle.

The tests are:

(i) The passive overpressure to *apparently normal*
gross active movements (described above)

(ii) Passive questing movements of vertebral
regions, to try and ascertain more clearly the
nature of factors *limiting* gross active movements,
or of other responses, e.g. a test of cervical
rotation or flat-handed pressure on the spine of a
prone patient (see p. 107). More localised
passive tests are described under 'palpation'.

*Because any applied movement, by way of
examination (or treatment) technique, may indeed be
moving the tissue in which we are presently interested,
we cannot exclude from our factors for assessment the
other structures also being moved. This especially
applies to unilateral and combined lumbo-sacral —
sacro-iliac — hip conditions.*[70] *In hot pursuit of 'proof'
of this or that theory of the effects of manual treatment,
this somewhat inconvenient consideration tends to fall
by the wayside.*

Neurological tests

Information that the signs and symptoms of root
involvement are appearing, have become established,
or are regressing, is an important factor in
assessment, as is the *distribution* of neurological
signs. Evidence that more than one root is
unilaterally involved, or that there is bilateral
evidence of root changes, generally contraindicate
many treatments.

Root involvement affecting *muscle strength*, if
present, is invariably revealed without testing every
muscle and every joint action. Concerning muscle
weakness, the absence or presence of neurological
deficit is confirmed by testing only one muscle, or
joint action, as representative of a given cord
segment. In broad terms, the pattern of nerve root
supply will *help* to indicate the *probable* level of
involvement. During the therapist's 'indications'
examination, the neurological tests employed are
restricted to those providing guides for treatment,
and normally the only *tendon reflexes* tested are the
biceps, supinator, triceps, knee, ankle and great toe
jerks (Figs. 6.12(a)(b)(c)(g)(h)(i)). Plantar responses
are also tested and the absence of ankle clonus must
be determined (Figs. 6.12(j)(k)). Incipient root
involvement may be missed if reflexes are tested
once only, and routine 'indications' examinations
should include tapping the tendon *six successive
times*, to uncover the fading reflex response which
indicates developing root signs.

The jaw jerk (p. 18) can be of importance to the
neurologist in distinguishing cervical myelopathy —
normal jaw jerk with exaggerated limb reflexes —
from the possibility of an intracranial lesion, when
the jaw jerk also is exaggerated in the same
circumstances.

While the medial (L5, S1) and the lateral (S1)
hamstring reflexes (Figs. 6.12(e)(f)) may at times
assist in decisions about involvement of these roots,

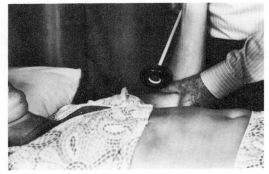

Fig. 6.12
(a) The biceps jerk

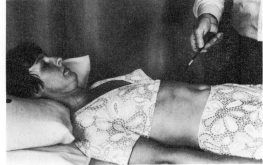

(d) Testing abdominal cutaneous reflexes

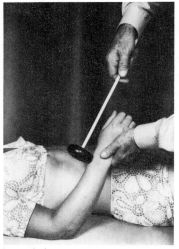

(b) The supinator jerk

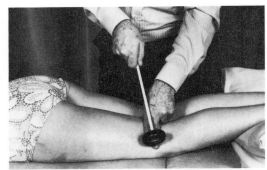

(e) The lateral hamstrings jerk

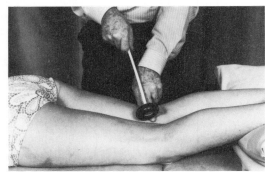

(f) The medial hamstrings jerk

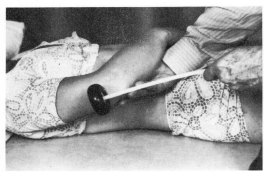

(c) The triceps jerk

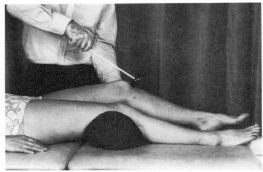

(g) The knee jerk

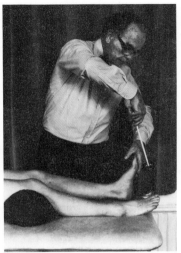

(h) The ankle jerk

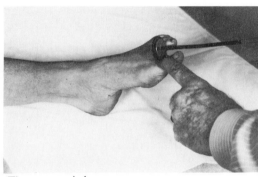

(i) The great toe jerk

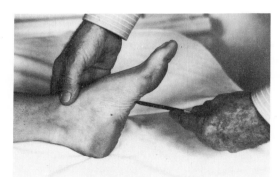

(j) Testing for the plantar response

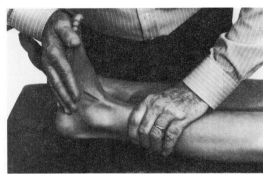

(k) Testing for ankle clonus

they are not routinely tested.

When testing for *sensory changes* leading questions should be avoided. Patients should be asked to report, with eyes closed, when tactile sensation is stimulated by simple stroking tests. When areas of complete anaesthesia are reported, or suspected, the testing of skin sensitivity to pin-prick is necessary.

N.B. When attempting to localise the segmental level of root involvement by distribution of root signs, the overlap of cutaneous supply, and pre- and post-fixation of plexuses should be borne in mind, also the discrepancy between vertebrae and roots in the cervical region and the great obliquity of the lumbo-sacral roots. The precise nature of the lesion affecting the nerve root often remains in doubt in non-surgical cases, and sometimes in surgical cases, also.

Specifying the precise level of vertebral abnormalities, and/or nerve root involvement, solely on the basis of distribution of neurological signs in a limb, is an inexact science. Clinical localisation of a lesion producing radicular pain is not always certain, e.g. the neurological findings may be identical irrespective of whether discogenic trespass is at L3-4 or L4-5. For example: Phillips[157] observes: ' . . . neurological features in the upper limbs are not very helpful in localising the level of significant invertebral disc pathology . . . we early came to the conclusion, reinforced by long experience, that contrary to the statements of many physicians on this topic — but in agreement with Brain et al.[14] — 'neurological findings are of extremely limited use in assessment of the precise level of cord and root involvement, and may be misleading.'

Sunderland[171] mentions that a single spot on the thoracic body wall may be innervated by fibres from five adjacent spinal nerve roots.

In a series of 560 patients, surgically treated for lumbar disc disease, correct preoperative *clinical* localisation was achieved in only 39.2 per cent.[105]

Hanraets[77] also stressed this aspect, i.e. the diagnostic unreliability of peripheral distribution of neurological symptoms and signs, in clinical determination of the precise level of root involvement.

While confusion and mistakes may sometimes be due to the presence of thoraco-lumbar and lumbo-sacral transitional vertebrae[183] bony anomalies alone are insufficient to explain the unreliability of depending upon neurological deficit to inculpate a particular vertebral segment. That a depressed or absent ankle jerk, or a weak muscle, may be the sequel of facet-joint changes[142] is a further pointer to the probability that neurological signs are not so much 'mechanical' sequelae of root trespass as evidence of *central nervous system inhibition*, which can be caused by more than one type of spinal musculo-skeletal change.

Expressed otherwise, we need to think like telecommunication, as well as mechanical engineers.

While reflex alterations accompanying sciatic pain, for example, are diagnostically significant, they are neither constant nor entirely reliable; their presence is not incontrovertible proof of nerve-root compression. The possibility that diminished reflex responses may be due to segmental central nervous system disturbance, and not entirely to physical trespass upon nerve roots, is strongly suggested by a report of four patients with bilaterally diminished ankle jerks, in whom surgically verified unilateral disc lesions did not approach the nerve root.[47]

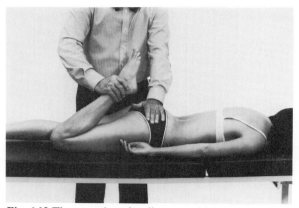

Fig. 6.13 The prone-knee-bending test, which goes by a variety of names. Some clinicians bend both knees together, this being more a provocation test for spinal stenosis than much else. Besides 'stretching the femoral nerve' it imposes tension upon a whole lot of other structures, too, and reduces the vertical dimensions of *all* lumbar intervertebral foramina.

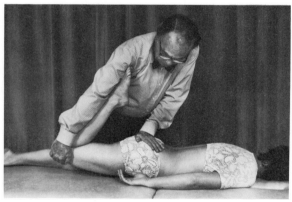

Fig. 6.14 Prone-knee-bending with hip-extension, the so-called 'femoral nerve stretch test'. Provocation of pain by this test is not, of itself, pathognomonic of any single segmental lesion, of joint or spinal root, because it often provokes the pain from lesions anywhere between L1 and S1.

Special tests

Passive testing movements such as:
— straight-leg-raising in supine lying
— knee extension in sitting
— neck flexion in supine lying and in sitting
— knee bending with hip extension in prone lying (Figures 6.13, 6.14)
either alone or in combination, can exert tension on the spinal nerve roots with their dural sleeves. Thus they provide information on the freedom of movement of those structures, and on the extent of entrapment or restriction imposed by trespass of related structures and/or by intrinsic changes in the tissues themselves. The degree of root irritability is likewise indicated by limitation occurring simultaneously with aggravation of 'root' pain, co-existing with loss-of-conduction signs in that root.

(i) *The straight-leg-raising-test* places a varying degree of tension on each of the lumbo-sacral roots, from L4 to S2 inclusive, the most traction being exerted on the first sacral root. Further, a degree of lumbo-sacral plexus and root traction must occur when the foot is dorsiflexed in addition (Bragard's sign), but it is a mistake to ascribe the increased calf pain, willy-nilly, to the pain of increased root tension. Exacerbation of 'sciatic' pain, by forcible foot dorsiflexion near the end of a painfully-limited straight-leg-raising range[68] is not always a reliable indication that the extra pain is due to further sciatic nerve stretch; foot dorsiflexion will often produce calf pain at 60°–70° on a normal leg, and simple calf-tenderness often accompanies purely sacro-iliac conditions, being exacerbated by the dorsiflexion text. Allowing the knee to flex relieves the pain elicited when the knee is kept straight—while this knee-flexion relieves tension on the sciatic nerve, it also relieves tension on the hamstrings, of course; thus the manoeuvre does not provide any more specific information about the *cause* of painfully-limited straight-leg-raising.

Similarly, while it is known that internal rotation of the lower limb exerts tension on the root components of the sciatic nerve, the test is of negligible additional clinical value provided the straight-leg-raising test has been meticulously performed in the first place, i.e. with the knee extended, the foot at 90°, the leg slightly adducted and with neutral rotation. The point at which painful root tension limits further movement (if this *is* the limiting factor) can be adequately determined one way or another, and need not require alternative tests which essentially give the same information. Many people have 5°–10° normal discrepancy between limits of left and right straight-leg-raising, and the normal full range can be anything between an angle of 75°–120°, measured between longitudinal axis of leg and horizontal surface of couch. The one important factor to note is *the character of the response* and to use this as a criterion for assessing the efficacy of treatment techniques.

(ii) *If knee-extension in sitting* is passively tested, the mechanics of the cord, meninges and root traction are broadly similar to (i), with exceptions that gravitational compression, adding to intra-discal pressure, now tends to increase the effect of any restriction upon free movement of the meninges, and this effect will be pronounced if the patient slumps into a generally flexed posture.

(iii) *Neck flexion in lying* (Brudzinski's test[20])
The effect of traction exerted in this way upon the neural canal structures extends caudally as far as the thoracic and lumbar regions and for this reason it is perhaps a more valuable examination procedure for these regions than for the cervical region in that aggravation of low back, pelvic girdle or leg pain by this manoeuvre is a useful indication that the source of pain lies wholly or partly in the spine and neural canal rather than in more peripheral tissues.

(iv) It is sometimes necessary to apply the *combined effects* of (i) (ii) and (iii) when guides for action in treatment are not clearly afforded by any one of these tests performed alone. Thus it may be necessary to flex the patient's neck while raising the straight leg with foot at 90°, or further, to apply these tensions while the patient sits slumped.[130]

(v) *Knee-bending with hip extension*, passively performed with the patient prone and pelvis stabilised, may exacerbate 'root' pain of 3rd, and perhaps the 2nd and 4th, lumbar segment origin, since the femoral nerve lies in front of the hip joint and this test tends to disturb the sensitised root (if there be such) by traction. The range of movement available in the hip after the knee has been flexed is very small, and consequently forward pelvic tilting is difficult to prevent (Figs. 6.13, 6.14).

N.B. It is most important to bear in mind that these manoeuvres also put stress on joints, and responses can thus be equivocal when joints also are in an irritable state. For example, the *femoral nerve stretch test* applies compression to the knee and hip joints, torsion to the sacro-iliac joint with a forward-tilting effect upon the pelvis and thus also a disturbance of lumbar joints.

That this test may provoke low back, buttock, groin or anterior or posterior thigh pain should not be taken, willy nilly, as evidence of provoking the effects of trespass upon the cauda equina and/or spinal nerve roots by disc changes.[83]

Trespass may also be due to facet-joint arthrosis and ligamentum flavum thickening, and the test may merely be constricting a developmentally narrow canal. It is a prime example of the equivocality, in themselves, of positive signs (p. 42).

Similarly, besides its well-appreciated traction effects on the sciatic nerve and lumbo-sacral roots, the *straight-leg-raising test* also tends to move, because of the lumbar-spine-flexion effect via the pelvis, *joints* which may be irritable, the joints between the vertebral bodies and also the synovial facet joints. The pelvis is tilted backwards in the sagittal plane, and also upwards in the frontal plane, i.e. a lateral tilt upwards on the tested side. The pelvis is also slightly rotated towards the untested side, all of these effects occurring towards the end of range in the normal person. Hence, while standardised and precisely performed manoeuvres are necessary, standardised conclusions are unwise, and the examiner is never relieved of the obligation to *assess*, to weigh the value of what are frequently equivocal responses to standard tests.

Hazlett[80] observes that in 45 patients with a femoral distribution of symptoms and signs, the femoral nerve stretch test' was not particularly useful to diagnose irritative lesions of the upper lumber nerve roots, because of difficulties in controlling spinal motion on extension of the hip.

Hirsch, Ingelmark and Miller[84] have shown that lumbar and posterior thigh pain can be produced by irritant injections into the region of facet joints, and Mooney and Robertson[142] have demonstrated that facet-joint changes will painfully reduce straight-leg-raising. Anaesthetic block of the facet-joint restores normal straight-leg-raising within five minutes. The notion that a reduced straight-leg-raising is pathognomonic of lower lumbar disc protrusion could bear some inspection; in 40 per cent of patients who experienced pain relief (with interruption of the pain-muscle spasm cycle by denervation of the facet-joints with a thermistor probe under fluoroscopic control) a marked improvement in the straight-leg-raising test also occurred.

Where a limited straight-leg-raising *is* due to root involvement, this need not be due to 'a disc lesion', implying trespass. More than 30 years ago, Friberg and Hult found symptoms of sciatica without detectable herniation of lumbar discs.[56]

Fahrni[50] describes three patients with the classical symptoms and signs of disc protrusion, and consistently positive myelographic findings. *No disc protrusion was found at operation* but the nerve root was densely adherent to the disc. Full and lasting relief was obtained by surgical release of the root, leaving the disc intact. It is very probable that there need not be any involvement of roots or dura for straight-leg-raising to be limited. The limitation imposed can be due purely to an irritative joint lesion, i.e. involving disc or facet joint or ligament, or all three, not physically affecting neural tissue yet producing a greater or lesser degree of hamstring spasm. Where straight-leg-raising is limited by only $10°$–$20°$, the pain is possibly caused by beginning of tension in a root which is abnormally sensitive from causes intrinsic to the root itself, and not inevitably accompanied by any trespass of neighbouring tissues.

(vi) An additional, *active* straight-leg-raising test, seeking the'Hoover' sign[3] may assist in deciding between willingness and unwillingness of the patient to co-operate fully in the objective part of the examination. Normally, when the supine patient is asked to elevate one limb, the heel of the opposite foot is pressed to the couch. With the examiner's palm under the heel, the degree of downward heel pressure should be much the same for either limb in a normal subject. When a weak or painful-side limb is elevated, the opposite and normal-side heel is pressed harder into the examiner's palm than when the normal side limb is raised. Should no downward pressure be exerted by the normal heel, the patient is probably not attempting to raise the supposed painful and/or weak contralateral limb. The test should not be regarded as conclusive in itself, but can at times assist in assessment of clinical features.

(vii) *Tests of vertebrobasilar arterial sufficiency.* These are not really diagnostic tests, as is sometimes asserted, since a positive result does not necessarily provide a diagnosis, only the important information that certain postures and movements are likely to be reducing flow somewhere in the vertebrobasilar arterial system, and therefore these postures should be avoided during treatment.[70]

Precisely *where, and how,* the circulation is restricted by these tests in any one individual, whether this is a normal effect and has been so for that person throughout life and exactly what relationship a positive result has to the presenting symptoms, are not necessarily revealed by these tests alone.

There is angiographic evidence that head rotation, in normal people, may transiently impair blood flow in the *ipsilateral* vertebral artery in its course between the 6th and 7th cervical vertebrae, and in the *contralateral* vertebral artery as it passes through the foramen transversarium of atlas.

Frequently the vertebral arteries are of markedly unequal calibre, and in only eight per cent of individuals are the arteries of equal size.[16]

This, in itself, is enough to confound facile 'rule-of-thumb' interpretations of the precise cause of positive responses. It is the combination of cervical spondylosis, arthrosis, atheroma of vertebral arteries and developmental narrowness of one or more vessels, together with the great variability of central nervous system arterial supply between individuals, which is so productive of symptoms believed due to ischaemia—these may include a brief attack of 'giddiness', a feeling of impending syncope, diplopia or even a drop attack, when the patient suddenly falls to the ground without losing consciousness.

In a series of patients with atheromatous arterial changes, Biemond[11] observed that rotation with extension produced nystagmus, dysarthria and a transient abnormality of plantar responses.

Another factor is that of listing, dysequilibrium, giddiness or 'vertigo' being induced alone by extremes of stress, or abnormal relationships, of the cranio-vertebral complex of joints[70, 184] and the presence of this may compound findings suspicious of vertebrobasilar insufficiency.

Attributing responses to effects produced by certain movements, and combined movements, is not an exact science.

Thus while these tests do sift the wheat from the chaff so far as lines of physical treatment, and contraindications, are concerned, they do so only in a blunderbuss fashion, and it is a time-wasting mistake to introduce further roughly similar tests (e.g. those of Romberg and Hautant, and the Underberger stepping test) in the hope that clarification will follow, since most of the latter are tests for sensory ataxia, dorsal column integrity and vestibular mechanisms, which are not our immediate clinical concern in this context. An orderly concentration on one aspect at a time is wise, since some of the tests are similar to attempts to provoke pain by combined (quadrant) testing *movements* (p. 39) which we are not concerned with here. Vascular function is tested more by combined *postures* (Figs. 6.15–6.17).

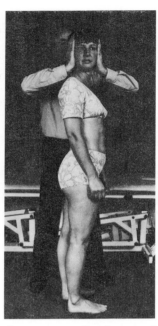

Fig. 6.15 *Standing posture test.* Stand to rear of the standing patient and stabilise the head by a palm over each ear. Under direction previously given, the patient shifts feet so that the trunk (with neck) is fully rotated to one side, and is maintained there for 30 seconds. Repeat to opposite side, the head remaining stabilised throughout. It is not conclusive if impending syncope is *not* revealed by this test, since there is also the factor of extension combined, which must also be investigated.

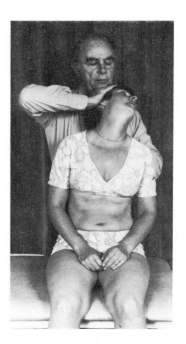

Fig. 6.16 *Sitting posture test.* Stand behind the sitting patient, and while using both hands to comfortably support the head and neck into full extension and then full rotation. Which side is first rotated towards does not matter, so long as the extension/rotation posture is gently maintained for some 30 seconds. Be ready to support the patient if the test is positive.

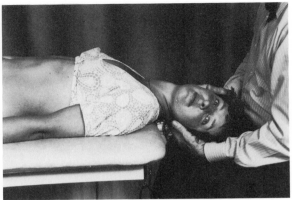

Fig. 6.17 *Lying posture test.* Sit at the head of the lying patient, whose shoulders should extend beyond the edge of the support. Both hands positively but gently support the head which is moved into full extension and then rotated, being held there for 30 seconds; repeat to opposite side. On the beginnings of a positive response, smoothly and quickly return the head to neutral posture.

(viii) *Vertebral percussion test:* When it has been established that an ache is most likely to be arising from a thoracic or lumbar joint problem, and examination with careful palpation has failed to localise the vertebral level(s) responsible, gentle percussion of the spine can assist in revealing it. The patient stands with the spine flexed or sits leaning forward with elbows supported on knees, and the therapist gently and successively taps the spinous processes with a patellar hammer, noting at which level(s) the response exceeds that of the mild discomfort of the test.

OBJECTIVE EXAMINATION—PALPATION

It is of interest to observe skilled clinicians carefully percussing the thorax over the lung fields, confident of their ability to gather valuable clinical information by this classical and important method of examination.

In discussing the clinical value of palpation is respiratory disease, a standard text of past years (*The Practice of Medicine*[162]) asserts: '...we must recognise that error is increased by carelessness, haste and indifferent techniques, and may be reduced by a careful routine and the skill born of long practice and experience. Secondly, we must remember that it is in the borderland separating slight abnormality from normality that mistakes are most easily made.'

It would be difficult to express more clearly the factors important in *all* examination by palpation, particularly the tactile search for tissue-tension abnormalities in the vertebral structures.

The daily occurrence of orthopaedic surgeons and rheumatologists carefully palpating a synovial sheath at the wrist, or the structures of an ankle, the first carpo-metacarpal joint, an elbow or a knee, and recording their findings about effusion, synovial thickening or crepitus, exostosis, the prevalence or absence of ligamentous laxity, patello-femoral crepitus or pain on approximation, and the 'clonks' or 'thuds' of an intra-articular derangement, is regarded not as unusual but proper to the discharge of professional responsibilities.

Assessing movement-abnormalities at vertebral segments, or arthrotic knee-joints, for example, employs criteria which are common to both, since there are at present no other. The manipulatively-minded worker is as earth-bound as his colleagues of other disciplines; his clinical ways and means are no more than the ways and means existing, yet by constant attention to what his fingers are telling him, and by practice, he has developed an examination method which employs the criteria in a more localised and specific way, not now to a large peripheral joint but to a vertebral mobility-segment.

Conclusions about the *nature* of the abnormality palpated, and its significance in relation to symptoms, are a matter for experienced assessment and therefore arguable, but of its *presence* there can be no doubt.

Procedure

A joint, with its immediate peri-articular tissues and surrounding muscle tissue, has not been adequately examined unless it has been investigated by localised passive movement and palpation, because these methods obtain information not available by any other means.

Palpation is used to test:

a. the state of the skin, with superficial and deep soft tissues

b. the state of peri-articular tissues (palpation of the *still* joint)

c. the characteristics of segmental vertebral *movement*.

Note that in (c) the range of movement examined may therefore be:

(i) that of regional and segmental *accessory* joint movement (Fig. 11.3), which by definition cannot be produced voluntarily, and

(ii) that of the *voluntary*, or physiological movement (Fig. 7.38) between two vertebrae (see below).

Skin, soft tissues and subcutaneous bony points

The temperature, texture and dryness or excessive moisture of the skin are noted. Abnormalities such as
— dysaesthesia (diminished sensibility)
— hyperaesthesia (unpleasantly increased sensibility)
— anaesthesia (loss of sensibility)
   are sought.

Swelling may be palpated and its nature discerned, e.g. it may be soft and fluctuant, or thickened and indurated. The texture, i.e. pliability and soft resilience of muscle bellies is noted, as is the presence and distribution of postural spasm. Undue tenderness of superficial bony points, and of superficial tissues including interspinous connective tissue, is sought. Body areas which are normally tender should be borne in mind.

Peri-articular palpation provides information of possible abnormalities of joint relationship, in the more superficial joints (this refers to a degree of fixation in an asymmetrical position — not 'subluxation', e.g. as stated by Coutts[31] '. . . a pathological fixation in a position within a normal range of motion.'), undue tenderness of deep periarticular tissues, deep thickening and the presence of undue bony prominence. The latter may be anomalies of bone structure which are of no clinical significance, or degenerative exostosis.

Accessory movement (regional and segmental)

(i) Flat-handed pressure, applied vertically downward upon the thoracic and lumbar *regions* of a prone patient, is an important objective test. It elicits much useful information, helpful in the assessment of what is normal from patient to patient, and when abnormality may be present (see Assessment in examination p. 107).

Passive tests of *segmental* accessory movement are performed by applying thumb-tips or pads, singly or more usually together, against vertebral bony prominences. Carefully-graded pressures are applied in various directions. Fingers should rest but be spread so as to stabilise the more active thumbs. The lumbar region in heavy patients may require some of the pressures to be applied via the pisiform of the operator's hand, reinforced and stabilised by the other.

Gentle longitudinal distraction and compression movements may also be manually applied to the cervical region, while the amount of distraction occurring at a mobile segment is palpated. Distraction may also be applied mechanically, via a cervical harness and pulley system.

Thumb pressures used are:
— postero-anterior central pressures on spinous processes
— posterio-anterior unilateral pressures over the joints between adjacent articular processes
— transverse pressures against the sides of spinous processes
— postero-anterior unilateral pressures on the angles of the ribs.

For fullest information, the main direction of testing movements are altered, in that central pressures may be angulated slightly cranially or caudally, transverse pressures may be likewise angulated, and unilateral pressures given a cranial, caudal, medial or lateral bias, sometimes in combination.

During this important stage of examination, most of the criteria (see p. 38) for testing active movements of vertebral regions are reapplied, because fullest information about the segmental localisation of a joint problem, and the way it is clinically manifesting itself, can only be gained by careful and orderly passive tests and palpation.

N.B. A suggested routine for palpation of accessory movement is included with the tabulated 'Examination procedures' for vertebral regions.

(ii) Passive tests of the available *functional or physiological* movement (PP-MT) between two vertebrae are performed when necessary.

By this examination method the three degrees of freedom — or available range in the sagittal, frontal and horizontal planes — which the spine can traverse by voluntary movement, are passively and rhythmically reproduced by the examiner; adjacent bony points are palpated in turn and their changing relationship is the basis for comparisons, and for assessment of segmental mobility. Translation movement and accessory ranges along the axis of the column, approximation and distraction, are also tested on occasions.

Technique is described on page 87.

7

Regional examination procedures

A basic 'drill' for the temporomandibular joint, vertebral regions and associated limb girdles is given below, each followed by a suggested palpation routine. These will frequently need elaboration to elicit special information, and should therefore be regarded as minimum essential testing procedure. Since pain is very frequently referred from proximal to distal, and since joints which are situated in areas to which pain of spinal origin is commonly referred often develop secondary dysfunction, which contributes to the total picture of signs and symptoms, all examinations should invariably proceed from the spine to the distal body parts, in an orderly sequence.

Some comment on clinical background is given where appropriate.

THE TEMPOROMANDIBULAR JOINT

Movements of the mandible are *coupled* by the bilateral articulation, in which the bearing surfaces are avascular fibrous tissue and not hyaline cartilage.

This unique articulation is best conceived as a hinge-joint with a moveable socket, provided by interposition of the tough fibrous disc between bone and mandibular condyle. The disc normally becomes frayed and thinned after 40. By reason of the attachments of some masticatory muscles (Temporalis, Medial Pterygoid, Masseter) at a distance from the fulcrum of movement, teeth, rather than the articular surfaces, sustain very powerful forces — not always in the patient's best interests; for example, the tension developed during unconscious teeth-grinding while asleep (bruxism) can well exceed the muscular effort when chewing a tough piece of steak, and muscles become fatigued, tending also to contracture.

In a normal jaw, most of the bite-force is taken by the teeth — unlike the hip, the jaw joints are poor at bearing compressive stress.[9] Lost or incorrectly-filled teeth, or an abnormal relationship on closing (mal-occlusion), or repetitive strong clenching, throws undue strain on the articulation which can become bruised and sore, often on one side.

Because the spinal tract of the fifth cranial nerve (Fig. 7.1) (descending to the level of C3 segment

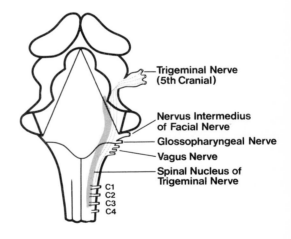

Fig. 7.1 Posterior aspect of brain stem and schematic view of floor of 4th ventricle. Note the extent to which the spinal tract of the 5th cranial nerve descends in the upper cervical spinal cord (see text).

before becoming continuous with the substantia gelatinosa) receives all nociceptive and thermal afferent inputs from:

5th cranial nerve
7th cranial (facial) nervus intermedius fibres
IXth cranial nerve (glossopharyngeal)
Xth cranial nerve (vagus)
C1
C2 } dorsal nerve roots
C3

and because afferent neurones also travel in the motor root of the fifth cranial nerve,[187] it should not be surprising that nociceptive traffic from anywhere in the districts served by these nerves may produce facilitatory effects underlying the clinical manifestation of combined musculo-skeletal neck and jaw problems. It is also important to remember that the temporomandibular joint may be strained in the extension phase of an acceleration ('whiplash') injury of the neck.[34] Temporomandibular joint conditions, with interrelated abnormalities of dental occlusion, very often co-exist with upper cervical joint problems and cervical postural defects; no examination of the cranio-vertebral region is complete without a thorough check of the jaw joints[163] and associated musculature, and conversely the cervical structures, particularly the state of the soft tissues from cranium to upper thorax, should always be comprehensively examined when approaching what may present solely as temporo-mandibular pain and dysfunction.

Such is the biomechanical interdependence of the whole axial skeleton and soft tissues, an associated consideration of pelvic and whole vertebral posture during examination is not as irrelevant as it may seem.[70] Any combination of the following twenty one features may occur:

— drug-resistant headache
— head pain, in known jaw-clinchers
— pain in or around the ear, and zygomatic and maxillary pain (atypical facial neuralgia)
— scalp 'soreness'
— unilateral burning neck pain
— throat soreness, and pain on swallowing
— upper trapezius pain spreading to acromio-clavicular region
— ear symptoms, including subjective hearing loss, ear 'fullness' and tinnitus
— tender or painful teeth
— tender muscles of mastication
— spasm of masticatory muscles (trismus)
— unilateral spasm of posterior neck muscles and spasm of one or both sternomastoids
— abnormal posture of head, neck and yoke region — the head is often ante-positioned[163]
— pain on jaw movement (chewing, yawning, laughing) which may be sharp and episodic, or a 'gnawing' soreness which persists after pain provocation
— limitation of movement
— deviation, or aberrant movement, on jaw opening and closing
— grating, grinding and milder degrees of crepitus
— clicking, popping or snapping on jaw movement
— phonation difficulties, swallowing difficulties
— facial, and mandibular, asymmetry
— mild dysequilibrium[57]

A recent retrospective survey[5] of 12 patients with temporomandibular joint problems revealed that all had headache, 11 reported neckache and 7 mentioned ear pain. 'Dizziness' was mentioned by 8 patients. Mandibular deviation on sagittal movement was observed in 8 patients.

The association between so-called 'tension' headaches, and tenderness of the masticatory muscles, is well-recognised.

ROUTINE TEMPOROMANDIBULAR JOINT EXAMINATION

Orthodontic tests for unilateral or bilateral over-closure, abnormal teeth approximation after phonation tests, possible sphenoid displacement maintained by mal-occlusion, and mal-occlusion itself, are not described since this is the province of orthodontists, to whom patients with suspected mal-occlusion should be referred.[61, 174, 93]

1. History ('Listen')	*Patient's occupation:-*	— Stressful, producing jaw clenching? — Seamstress, using teeth to break thread, for example?
	Pain	— Where? Ear, temporal area, maxilla, jaw, throat, neck, shoulder, upper pectoral? — Typical migraine distribution? Eyes? Unilateral? — Which side? Bilateral? Worst side? — *nature?* Scalp soreness? Gnawing ache? Shooting? Local 'catch' pain? — *pattern of provocation and relief?* When? Continuous? Only on movement? Which movements? Biting, chewing, yawning, laughing, teeth cleaning? Rising a.m.? Carrying shopping?
	Other symptoms	— Feelings of muscular/emotional tension? Teeth feel loose? Tendency to clench jaws? Lack of free movement? Difficult movement? Feeling of deviation or asymmetry on movement? — Evident jaw grating, grinding (crepitus), clicking, popping, 'jumping' in jaw socket? — 'Neck stiffness'? Yoke area restriction? — Orbital, facial, labial, lingual or occipital paraesthesiae? Feelings of retro-orbital pressure? — Hearing acuity? 'Fullness' or 'stuffiness' of ears? — Tinnitus? Speech difficulties (dysphonia)? — Swallowing difficulties (dysphagia)? Dysequilibrium? — Giddiness, vertigo, listing? Difficulties of concentration and remembering?
	Medical background	— Dental history? Dentures? Missing teeth? — History of trauma, physical violence, road traffic accident? General health? Weight loss recently? — Other illnesses? Operations? X-rayed? On systemic steroids or anti-coagulants?
2. Observation ('Look') (see p. 33)		— Facial asymmetry? Eye, ear or nostril higher than opposite? Eye sunken on one side? — Developmentally small mandible (micrognathia) or large mandible (macrognathia)? Carriage of head, neck and yoke area? Head and neck ante-ositioned? — obvious postural spasm of trapezii, sternomastoid? — jaw clenched? Kypho-lordotic cervico-thoracic junction? — flat interscapular area? *NB.* Check pelvic levels and whole spinal posture. Observe symmetry of lip closure. Note respiration—habitually mouth or nasal? Lingual position? Note phonation

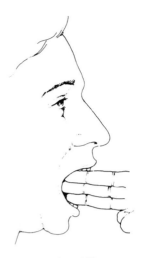

Fig. 7.2 Normal mouth opening ability.

3. Function ('Test')		Complete the neck and forequarter examination first, *then* turn to the temporomandibular joint.
	Active movements	*Mandibular movements.* Opening (Figure 7.2) and closing. Note incisor distance on opening wide (35–40 mm on average): watch for deviation or asymmetry of movement, also during lateral movement to either side, and protrusion and retraction. Note ranges of movement, and nature and degree of limitation, if any; with overpressure to confirm apparently normal movement. — If painful, which movement? Where does it hurt? Note presence of audible fine or coarse crepitus, popping, clicking or clonking, and if unilateral determine which side.
	Muscles	Give manual resistance, i.e. 'static' resisted contractions, to musculature performing opening, closing, lateral movement, protrusion and retraction. *N.B.* Pain provoked by these movements does not necessarily inculpate the muscle or its attachments (see p. 41).
	Passive movements	Aside from over-pressure during active ranges, i.e. passive 'end-feel' tests of physiological or voluntary movements (PP–MT), it is necessary to passively test the accessory movements (PA–MT) which are not possible actively, and these are approximation, distraction, anterior, posterior, and latero-medial movement (Fig. 7.4). — are they painful? Hypomobile? Hypermobile?

4. Palpation
('Feel')

Feel for tenderness over the temporalis muscle (anterior, middle and posterior fibres), masseter and medial pterygoid; at attachments and muscle bellies. (Intra-oral palpation of the lateral pterygoid muscle and its attachments is more an act of faith than a fact.)[93]

Palpate bilaterally over joint and in auditory meatus (Fig. 7.3) as patient opens and closes jaw. Palpable clicks on opening? On closing, too? Get patient to close strongly.

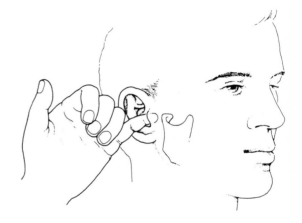

Fig. 7.3 Palpating movement of the temporomandibular joint by insertion of the fifth finger-tip in the patient's ear. (Figs. 7.2 and 7.3 reproduced from Beresford-Jones R 1981 Migraine: the dental involvement. Country Publications, Carlisle, with permission)

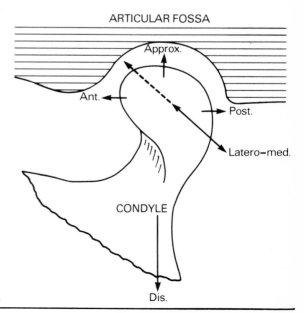

Fig. 7.4 Scheme of passive accessory-movement testing (PA-MT) for the left temporomandibular joint.

Ant.	anterior
Post.	posterior
Approx.	approximation
Dis.	distraction
Lateromed.	lateromedial.

ARTICULAR FOSSA

Approx.

Ant.

Post.

Latero–med.

CONDYLE

Dis.

5. Record	Write a readable account of findings, asterisk salient signs and symptoms.
6. Assess	Can we help the patient by physical treatment, and where should we place the first emphasis — treating pain or treating dysfunction? Should the patient be referred to an orthodontist? Do we need to treat the upper cervical spine, too?

ROUTINE EXAMINATION OF NECK AND FOREQUARTER

1. History
('Listen')

a. What is patient's usual daily activity (work and play)?

b. Details of
present pain
— site and boundaries — radiation to arm? Hand?
— headache? Which part of cranium? Face pain?
— *nature* — deep or surface — shooting?
— improving or worsening?
— area of worst pain?

c. *Behaviour of pain*
related to time, posture
and activity
— constant, episodic or occasional?
— what aggravates?
— what eases?
— any functional restrictions, because of pain?
— night pain?
— rising a.m.? Day/evening pain?
— time dependent or stress dependent?

d. *Other symptoms*
— paraesthesiae? Where? Which fingers? (Any fullness, puffiness, numbness?) Dizziness? Dysequilibrium? Visual symptoms?
— what aggravates/eases?
— any symptoms in legs?

e. X-rayed? Drugs? Systemic steroids? History of Rheumatoid Arthritis? Anticoagulants? General health?

f. *Onset of this,* and previous attacks (after *all* details of *present* symptoms understood). Previous treatment, and result of that treatment?

N.B. Now *plan* which spinal and peripheral joints need *more* than routine examination (e.g. thoracic joints, shoulder, elbow or wrist, lower limbs (c.f. cervical myelopathy)).

2. Observation
('Look')

Patient sitting
Head and neck posture — shoulder levels?
Spasm — asymmetry — any other contour change, especially around deltoid?
Initial palpation
— feel muscle bellies for presence of consistency changes and postural spasm. Palpate eyebrow tissues.

Patient rests forehead on operator's chest
Palpate
— sub-occipital region
— lateral mass of atlas near mastoid process
— paraspinal region, over neural arches.

N.B. If applicable, tests for vertebro-basilar insufficiency, in standing and sitting (p. 48), must be carried out. The similar test, in lying (see below), should be included as standard drill in all cases (Figs. 6.15–6.17).

3. Function ('Test')	*Patient sitting*	

	Ext. ⎫	Limitations and *reasons* for limitation, i.e.? pain?
	LSF ⎪	stiffness? spasm. Always give overpressure to clear,
	RSF ⎬ *Watch for:*	if apparently normal. Repeat if necessary for
	Flex. ⎪	asymmetrical movement, deviation; watch for level
	LR ⎪	affected —painful/painless when prevented?
	RR ⎭	Employ quadrant movements and compression

Employ quadrant movements and compression (localising effect to cranio-vertebral, mid-cervical or cervico-thoracic as applicable) if need be, to clarify. Seek regions of muscle tightness.

Muscle power
(resisted isometric
contractions)

— tuck chin in ⎫ —C1 and C2
— push chin up ⎭
— press head and neck laterally   —C3

Peripheral joints
Temp/mand. joint   — check if face pain (see p. 54)
Clavicular joints   — test accessory movement
Shoulder girdle   — elevation (active) then *resist* (for C3–4)
Shoulder joint   — elevation through flexion and through abduction (active)
                          — passive overpressure to clear
Elbow/forearm   — check
Wrist and hand   — check

Patient lying supine
Gently hold head fully extended and rotated for 30 seconds either side, to see if headache aggravated or incipient syncope produced.
Cervical root tension test[46]
a. With elbow straight and arm very slightly extended, passively abduct arm to point of pain-provocation
b. retreat a trace, then externally rotate limb gently until pain is again elicited
c. retreat a trace, then supinate forearm while holding arm steady
d. carefully flex elbow, without other movement added.
Provocation of pain, which may be elicited earlier in proportion to the degree of neck flexion, suggests the presence of cervical root trespass.

Muscle power (resisted isometric contractions)	Shdr. Abd	Deltoid	(C5)
	Elb. Flex.	Biceps	(C6)
	Elb. Ext.	Triceps	(C7)
	Wrist Ext. or Flex.		(C7)
	Thumb Ext.	EPL	(C8)
		EPB	
		APL	

	Hand	Intrinsics	(T1)	
Reflexes	Jaw jerk	V cranial nerve		
	Biceps	C5	C6	test six
	Brachioradialis	C6	C5	successive
	Triceps	C7		times

Sensation   Stroking test along dermatomes and sensibility to pin-prick if applicable.

---

4. Palpation
('Feel')

a. Find abnormality (see separate drill)
b. Decide whether abnormality is significant (sometimes is not)
N.B. Passive physiological-movement test (PP–MT) is only included if necessary.

---

5. Record

Write a readable account of findings; asterisk salient signs and symptoms.

---

6. Assess

Where to place the first emphasis on treatment

Palpation of cervical spine
Patient lying supine
Feel, with testing pressures: anterior aspects of transverse processes, acromio- and sterno-clavicular joints, and upper three ribs.
Forehead rest, prone lying

General palpation:	Sweep fingers lightly, paravertebrally, occiput to upper thoracic region.
Seek:	— general information of state of soft tissue — sensitivity of sub-occipital tissues to pinching and skin rolling — tenderness 2 fingers' breadth lateral to sub-occipital mid-line — frank thickening of deep sub-occipital tissues
Segmental palpation:	Feeling: Allow thumb-tips to sink in gently—the harder you press the less you feel. Try to make thumbs more perceptive; visualise the structures you are palpating.
Seek abnormalities:	Thickening—undue tenderness–undue bony prominences—apparent bony asymmetry.
Moving the joint:	By thumb-tip pressure against vertebral prominences, increase movement progressively, Grade I–IV; only palpate in depth if indicated.
Seek abnormalities:	Irritability—elicited spasm—diminished or increased accessory movement–provocation of pain and/or paraesthesiae locally and/or distally.

Postero-anterior central pressures	— C2–T3
Postero-anterior unilateral pressures	— C1–T3
Postero-anterior unilateral pressures	— Ribs 1–2–3 (plus other levels if indicated earlier in examination)
Transverse pressures	— C2–T3

For fullest information: — alter direction of palpation movement:
      — cephalad   — towards head
      — caudad   — towards feet
      — more medially
      — more laterally.

If applicable: — passive physiological-movement test (PP–MT) of active intervertebral range of each segment.

THE SHOULDER AND SHOULDER GIRDLE

The shoulder complex comprises five joints:

1. The shoulder (gleno-humeral) joint. As opposed to the hip-joint whose dynamic *stabilisation* is of functional importance, the shoulder joint is characterised by its *mobility* and *instability,* which reflect its function.

2. The extra-capsular joint, which comprises the inferior surface of the acromion process and acromio-clavicular joint above, the greater tuberosity of the humerus and superior rotator cuff tendons below and the interposed sub-acromial or sub-deltoid bursa. It is appropriate to conceive the bursa as the synovial membrane of this unique articulation, which has no capsule, of course.

3. The very mobile soft-tissue scapulo-thoracic joint, between scapula and sub-scapularis behind and the ribs, their muscular coverings and loose areolar tissue in front. This enjoys great freedom of movement.

4,5. The acromio-clavicular and sterno-clavicular joints.

When examining the neck and upper limb, never leave out a check of the scapular and clavicular joints; conversely, never examine the clavicular and scapular joints without a full examination of neck, upper thorax and upper limb.

Since the simple everyday act of raising the arm to full elevation, through either flexion or abduction, imposes movement, tension, compression, gliding and rotational stress on, among other structures
— the cervical and upper thoracic spine
— the upper rib joints
— the sterno-clavicular, acromic-clavicular, shoulder (gleno-humeral) and scapulo-thoracic joints and requires the actions of a great many muscles as fixators, prime movers, antagonists and synergists, pain and movement-limitation during upper limb use can be due to changes in, among other tissues, one or other of the clavicular joints, or to painful scapulo-thoracic movement. This will very often be apparent, or suspected, during the basic routine forequarter examination (p. 63) and shoulder-joint examination which should nevertheless be fully completed before turning to more detailed examination of the acromio-clavicular, sterno-clavicular and scapulo-thoracic joints.

Articular signs often crop up in regions unmentioned by the patient, e.g. weakness of serratus anterior, and will dictate the need for clarification.

N.B. Because it is examination of the shoulder (gleno-humeral joint) which so often reveals the need to examine the clavicular and scapulo-thoracic joints more thoroughly, the shoulder-joint is taken first.

While it is sometimes suggested that identification of shoulder lesions is merely an exercise in applied anatomy,[33] equally experienced clinicians regard shoulder problems as perhaps the most difficult of all musculo-skeletal lesions to evaluate.[26]

ROUTINE EXAMINATION OF SHOULDER

1. History
('Listen')

a. What is patient's usual daily activity (work and play)?

b. Pain — extent and nature of present pain? Any head, neck, scapular, thoracic or axillary pain?
— radiates to elbow, hand or fingers? which aspect of arms? Which fingers?

c. *Behaviour of pain* related to time, posture and activity
— constant, episodic or occasional?
— what aggravates, what eases?
— pain at rest, or only on movement?
— which movements? Of neck? Of shoulders? Of shoulder girdle?
— how much pain is caused?
— how long after movement does pain persist? (i.e. assess degree of joint irritability)
— pain at night? Can sleep on that side?
— other functional restrictions by pain?

d. *Other symptoms*
— any paraesthesiae, numbness, vascular changes?
— which fingers?
— any 'deadness'/'heaviness' of arm? What provokes these? Audible or perceptible crepitus on movement?
— general health?

e. *Onset* of this attack, and of previous attacks, if any.

N.B. Plan examination of more distal joints, e.g. elbow, wrist, hand, if needed.

2. Observation
('Look')

Patient sitting
Posture, shoulder levels, abnormalities of contour and attitude (e.g. around head of humerus), clavicular levels, scapular and upper rib symmetry, postural spasm.

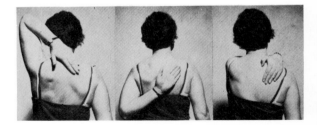

Fig. 7.5 To demonstrate the normal functional range of the shoulder and shoulder girdle joints, i.e. the ability to place fingers on opposite scapula by the three movements of elevation with elbow flexion, internal rotation and elbow flexion and protraction. A patient may exhibit this ability, yet be in pain from a covert gleno-humeral joint lesion which is only revealed on careful passive tests (see Fig. 7.6). (Reproduced from Apley A G 1973 A system of orthopaedics and fractures 4th ed. Butterworth, London, by kind permission of Author and Publishers.)

3. Function	*Patient sitting*
('Test)'	a. Routine examination of neck and clavicular joints, with active movements of shoulder *girdle,* protraction, retraction, elevation, depression, circumduction then detailed examination of:

b. Shoulder

Active, then
passive:

— elevation forwards
— elevation sideways
        (abd.)
— flexion/extension
        at 90°
— external rotation arm
at side with forearm at 90°
flexion.
— internal rotation back
of hand moving up
between scapulae
Fig. 7.5

Note these factors:
— willingness to move?
— quality of movements?
— scapulo-humeral rhythm?
— range limited?
— by how much?
— what appears to limit it?
  — pain primarily?
  — spasm primarily?
  — both?
  — inert tissue-resistance primarily?
  — muscle weakness?

Pain
— when does it begin?
— how quickly does it increase?
— where is it felt?
— when is it felt ('arc' of pain)?
— is it provocation of presenting pain?
— does it increase without limiting the movement?
— how severe is it?
— how soon does it settle?

Seek: regions of muscle tightness.

Patient lying and side-lying
c. *Neurological test* of reflexes, sensation and distal muscle (C8–T1)
d. Passive test of 1st. rib, clavicular and gleno-humeral joints:

1st rib   — accessory gliding
Clavicular   — accessory gliding repeated
Gleno-humeral   — abduction
                     — external rotation
                     (as for active test,
                     and also at 90°
                     abduction)
                     — internal rotation
                     (lying on unaffected
                     side)
                     — flexion/extension
                     at 90°
                     — elevation

Carefully recheck the factors noted during active movements

e. Resisted contractions
with shoulder held still
in neutral and elbow
bent to 90°

Shoulder: Abductors
              Adductors
              Ext. rotators
              Int. rotators
              Flexors
              Extensors
Elbow: Flexors
              Extensors
              Supinators of
              forearm

N.B.
1. Local pain elicited by these tests *may* indicate that muscle attachments are contributing to the symptoms.
2. Do not include these tests if the patient is in a lot of pain, but complete the examination as soon as practicable.

---

4. Palpation
('Feel')

Patient lying

N.B. Brachial plexus tension tests already completed in Neck and Forequarter examination. (p. 59)

Complete the passive test by examination of accessory glenohumeral joint movement (a-p, p-a, lateral, caudad, cephalad, compression) and 'quadrant' test and 'locking' position (Fig. 7.6) (i.e. combined movement) if applicable

How does the humeral head move in the glenoid?
Is accessory range reduced?
Compare with opposite arm

Palpate also for local tenderness, swelling, temperature.

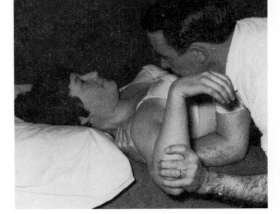

Fig. 7.6 By stabilising the scapula with his near hand and carrying the patient's slightly extended arm, flexed at the elbow, into some 90° or more abduction, a point is reached when further abduction, without some protraction, is not possible. This 'locked' position may cause discomfort, but should not be painful. If it is, there is a joint abnormality requiring careful mobilisation treatment.[129]

5. **Record**	Write a readable account of findings. Asterisk salient signs and symptoms.
6. **Assess**	Where to place the first emphasis in treatment, and general treatment approach.
	N.B. Recall tendency for conditions of heart, liver and diaphragm to refer pain to shoulder and arm.

ROUTINE EXAMINATION OF THE SHOULDER GIRDLE (CLAVICULAR AND SCAPULAR JOINTS)

1. History ('Listen')	As for examination of shoulder
2. Observation ('Look')	As for examination of shoulder. Eyes level with C7 vertebra (Fig. 7.7)

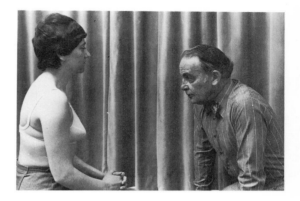

Fig. 7.7 Observe clavicular contours and attitude from the same horizontal level.

Patient sitting
Give particular attention to the *prominences* at the medial and lateral clavicular joints, i.e. the abnormalities of *contour,* also of upper ribs anteriorly. There is a particularly frequent abnormality of *attitude* often missed, i.e. a slightly forward carriage of the whole affected side shoulder girdle. That shoulder lies in advance of the other, the subclavicular hollow is deeper, the scapula is further forward around the chest wall, and later objective tests of soft tissue extensibility will clearly show that the pectoral musculature and its fascial investments unilaterally are a bit shortened.
This finding is so constant in shoulder and shoulder girdle problems that it may well be more cause than effect in many.

Look for a characteristic 'step-up' silhouette, on para-sagittal view, from the superior surface of the acromion to the superior surface of the lateral end of clavicle, and also take a lateral view of acromio-clavicular relationships.
Observe contour and attitude of scapulae from behind, i.e. distance of medial borders from median plane, levels of inferior angles, contour of medial borders.
Observe contours from above, with patient on low stool.

3. Function
('Test')

a. *Active movement.* Repeat all *shoulder-joint* movements, now observed from behind:

— elevation forwards
— elevation sideways
— flexion/extension at 90° abduction
— external/internal rotation

} Note particularly scapular rotation for bilateral asymmetry, and scapulo-humeral rhythm

Palpate both acromio-clavicular joints repetition of these movements (Fig. 7.8). Crepitus?

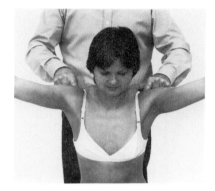

Fig. 7.8 Palpating the acromio-clavicular joints during active elevation.

Emphasise over-pressure to horizontal flexion and extension movements (Fig. 7.9 (a) + (b)).

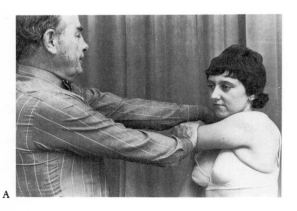
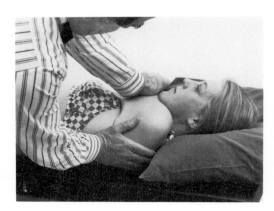

A

B

Fig. 7.9 Overpressure to the active movement of protraction (A) in sitting, and (B) in lying.

Repeat all *shoulder-girdle* movements:

— elevation
— depression
— protraction
— retraction
— circumduction

} Standing in front, observe range and symmetry. Give over-pressure where feasible, particularly to protraction (Fig. 7.10) thereby compressing clavicular joint surfaces

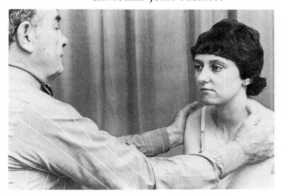

Fig. 7.10 Compressing all four clavicular joints by manually approximating the patient's shoulders.

Palpate sterno-clavicular joint during repetition of those movements (Fig. 7.11). Crepitus? Abnormal excursion?

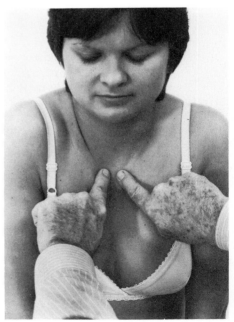

Fig. 7.11 Palpating the sterno-clavicular joints during active shoulder girdle elevation.

b. *Resisted movements* of shoulder girdle with trunk stabilised (Fig. 7.12).
— compare sides.
— (resisted movements for shoulder joints and rotator cuff musculature have been completed). (p. 65)
— observe possible scapular 'shift' during resisted pushing forward.

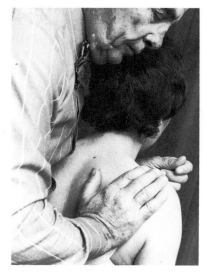

Fig. 7.12 Stabilising the patient's torso with his left arm and trunk, the therapist tests the power of the shoulder girdle retractor muscles, by giving resistance to dorsal aspect of scapula.

c. *Passive movement*
— compare amounts of scapular distraction during extension at medially-rotated shoulder joint and palpate soft tissues at medial scapular border (Fig. 7.13)

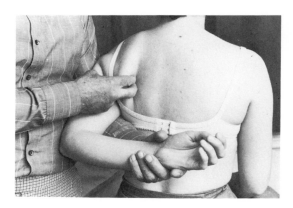

Fig. 7.13 Palpation of soft tissues at medial border of scapula, with the patient's arm in extension and medial rotation.

— stabilise scapula and mobilise lateral, then medial, end of clavicle by anterior pressures (Fig. 7.14)

— repeat for acromio-clavicular joint with clasped hands (Fig. 7.15)

N.B. This does not 'compress' the joint.

— caudal pressures, acromion and clavicle

— palpate acromio-clavicular joint (Fig. 7.16) Swelling? Thickening? Tenderness?

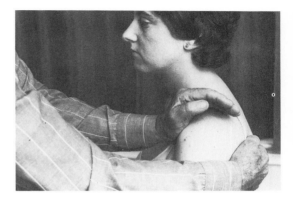

Fig. 7.14 Testing antero-posterior gliding range of the lateral end of clavicle; the acromion is stabilised by the therapist's right hand on the scapula.

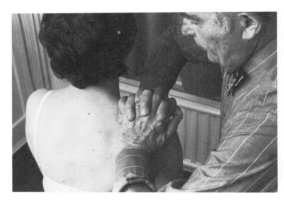

Fig. 7.15 Some therapists prefer this method of testing accessory a-p gliding range of clavicle on acromion.

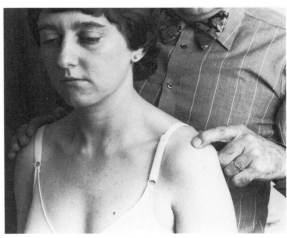

Fig. 7.16 Palpating the superior aspect of the acromio-clavicular joint.

Patient side-lying on unaffected side
d. *Passive movement*
Scapular

— distraction (Fig. 7.17)
— if preferred, repeat
palpation in side-lying
— retraction
— protraction
— elevation
— depression
— medial and lateral
rotation (Fig. 7.18)

Excessive movement?
Reduced movement?
Tethered by
contracture?
Painful?   Where?

Acromio-clavicular joint
— coraco-clavicular pressure and gliding (Fig. 7.19)

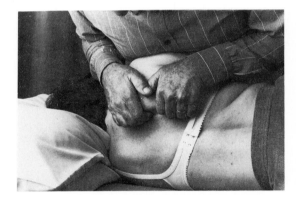

Fig. 7.17 Testing for the normal degree of scapular distraction from the postero-lateral chest wall.

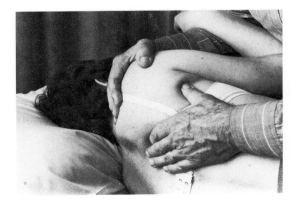

Fig. 7.18 By changing the grasp, the medial and lateral range of passive rotation can be tested.

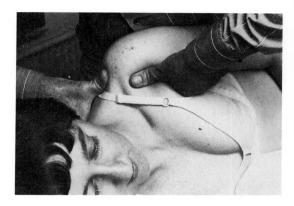

Fig. 7.19 By supinating the left forearm and stabilising the coracoid process with thumb pressure, the postero-anterior gliding range, of clavicle on acromion, can be tested. The therapist's right thumb applies movement to the posterior aspect of the lateral end of clavicle.

Patient lying
e. *Passive movement*

Repeat a–p glide *acromio-clavicular* joint
Test *sterno-clavicular* joint movement:

— antero-posterior
— caudal
— cranial
— during passive elevation (Fig. 7.20)
— with clavicle grasp
Distract sterno-clavicular joint (Fig. 7.21)
Distract acromio-clavicular joint (Fig. 7.22)

Excessive movement?
Reduced movement?
Tethered by contracture?
Painful?
Where?

Seek muscle tightness, e.g.
— scaleni (Fig. 7.23)
— pectoralis minor
— pectoralis major

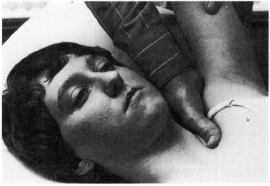

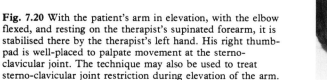

Fig. 7.20 With the patient's arm in elevation, with the elbow flexed, and resting on the therapist's supinated forearm, it is stabilised there by the therapist's left hand. His right thumb-pad is well-placed to palpate movement at the sterno-clavicular joint. The technique may also be used to treat sterno-clavicular joint restriction during elevation of the arm.

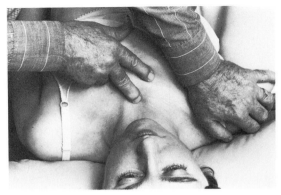

Fig. 7.21 Distraction of the sterno-clavicular joint. Index and middle fingers rest on first costal cartilage and manubrium sterni, respectively, while the distracting pressure is applied with heel of opposite hand resting on the anterior concavity of lateral end of clavicle.

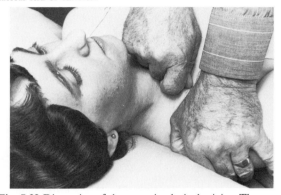

Fig. 7.22 Distraction of the acromio-clavicular joint. The clavicle is grasped between finger and thumb, while distraction pressure is applied, distal to the joint, over the acromion process. Placing of the distraction hand requires some care. In both of these distraction techniques, the therapist stands on the opposite side and leans over the patient.

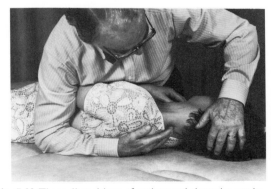

Fig. 7.23 These dispositions of patient and therapist can be used for palpation of muscle tightness, in the scaleni and other muscle groups, and also for post-isometric relaxation treatment techniques, for upper rib fixation or tethering by hypertonicity of muscle.

ROUTINE EXAMINATION OF THORACIC SPINE

1. History
('Listen')

a. What is patient's usual daily activity (work and play)?

b. Details of *present* pain
— site and boundaries? — radiation? — rib areas, breast, sternum, abdomen? — Upper limb? — Neck? — *nature* — aching or stabbing?
— getting better or worse?
— where worst?

c. *Behaviour of pain* related to time, posture and activity
— constant, episodic or occasional?
— what aggravates?
— what eases?
— neck movements?
— arm movements?
— trunk movements?
— coughing and deep breath?

d. *Other symptoms*
— paraesthesiae in arms, in legs?
— any weakness in arms, in legs?

e. X-rayed? Recently on systemic steroids? Gastrectomy? (Latter two because of possible osteoporosis, when ribs are especially vulnerable). Anticoagulants? Rheumatoid Arthritis? General health?

f. *Onset* of this and previous attacks? How treated? Result of treatment?

2. Observation
('Look')

Patient sitting (after checking pelvic levels and leg lengths in standing)

Posture:
(especially increased a-p curves, e.g. localised or generalised 'dowager's hump')
Patient crosses forearms in front of body — inspect for rib asymmetry, prominence of Trapezius on one side, carriage of scapulae
Often useful to feel for rib prominence by flat-handed sweep over postero-lateral surface of hemithorax.

3. Function
('Test')

Patient sitting

Neck
Usual tests (see 'Neck examination')
Try to clarify effects of neck and arm movements on thoracic pain

Upper limbs
Examine cursorily if no symptoms there (*N.B.* Elevation of arms extends thoracic spine)

Thoracic spine (patient places palms on opposite shoulders)

Slump (sag sit)	Watch for limitation.
Ext. (not from hips)	Give overpressure to clear if apparently painless and full range.
LSF	
RSF	
LR	Watch for asymmetrical movement.
RR	

Deep breath and cough (Check chest expansion)
Seek regions of muscle tightness.

Patient lying supine
Passive neck flexion, then straight-leg-raising, then active neck flexion *with* each straight-leg-raise to clear.
N.B. Neurological test of lower limbs. (Do not leave this out.)
Sacro-iliac joint: approximation and gapping of ilia.

---

4. Palpation
('Feel')

While patient is supine, palpate costo-chondral junctions and xiphoid and symmetry of ribs and intercostal spaces.
Patient prone with arms to side
a. Find abnormality (see separate drill)
b. Decide whether abnormality is significant (sometimes is not).

---

5. Record

Write a readable account of findings; asterisk salient signs and symptoms.

---

6. Assess

Where to place the first emphasis on treatment.

Palpation of thoracic spine (Upper thoracic area included in Cervical spine examination)
Prone lying —arms to side, head to one side

General palpation:	— sweep flat hand, paravertebrally, for state of skin texture and moisture — thumbs across Sacrospinalis for spasm — fingers longitudinally in paravertebral sulcus, for undue prominence and line of spinous processes — flat-handed vertical pressure
Segmental palpation:	Feeling: allow thumb-tips to sink in gently —the harder you press the less you feel. Try to make thumbs more perceptive; visualise the structures you are palpating.
Seek abnormalities:	Thickening —undue tenderness —undue bony prominences
Moving the joint:	By thumb-tip pressure against vertebral prominences, increase movement progressively, Grade I–IV; only palpate in depth if indicated
Seek abnormalities:	Irritability —elicited spasm —diminished or increased accessory movement —provocation of pain and/or paraesthesiae locally and/or distally
Postero-anterior central pressures	— T1–T12
Postero-anterior unilateral pressures	— T1–T12
Transverse pressures	— T1–T12
For fullest information:	— alter direction of palpation movement: — cephalad —towards head — caudad —towards feet — more medially — more laterally
If applicable:	— passive physiological-movement test (PP–MT) of active intervertebral range of each segment.

ROUTINE EXAMINATION OF BACK AND HINDQUARTERS

1. History ('Listen')	a. What is patient's usual daily activity (work and play)?

1. History
('Listen')

a. What is patient's usual daily activity (work and play)?

b. Details of *present* pain — site and boundaries? —radiation to buttock, thigh, leg, foot, toes?
— *nature*—deep or surface?
— improving or worsening?
— area of worst pain?

c. *Behaviour of pain* related to time, posture and activity — constant, episodic or occasional?
— what aggravates?
— what eases?
— effect of sitting and rising from?
— effect of stooping and rising from?
— night pain? Rising a.m. (stiffness or pain)?
— day pain? Evening pain?
— time-dependent or stress-dependent?
— other functional restrictions by pain (e.g. cough or sneeze)?
— standing? Walking?

d. *Other symptoms* — paraesthesiae? Where?
— which toes? 'Saddle' area?
— micturition?
— weakness in legs?

e. X-rayed? Drugs? Systemic steroids? Anticoagulants? General health?

f. *Onset* of this, and of previous attacks (after *all* details of *present* symptoms understood). Previous treatment, and result of that treatment?

N.B. Now *plan* which spinal and peripheral joints need *more* than routine examination (e.g. sacro-iliac, hip, knee, ankle).

---

2. Observation
('Look')

Pelvic and shoulder levels —spinal posture —iliac crest levels —leg lengths — postural spasm —swelling —other contour changes. (*N.B.* see also Examination of sacro-iliac joint). (Figs, 7.24 and 7.25)

---

3. Function
('Test')

Patient standing (feet a little apart and parallel)

Ext. ⎫
LSF ⎪
RSF ⎬ *Watch* for: limitation and reasons for limitation, i.e. ? pain, ? stiffness, ? spasm
Flex. ⎭

Overpressure to clear. Corner extension movements and compression, if need. Asymmetrical movement? (repeat if necessary, and watch for level affected) Deviation? Painful or painless when corrected?

Seek regions of muscle tightness.

Muscle power: Toe standing for calf (S1–2). Repeat six times consecutively for each side.

Patient sitting (knees together and arms folded)
(Compare sitting posture to standing posture)

R. Rot. ⎫
L. Rot. ⎬ *Watch* for: abnormalities as in standing

Patient lying supine
Passive neck flexion — iliac gapping and approximation — hip and knee flexion and rotation — straight-leg-raising — straight-leg-raising with neck flexion. Test straight-leg raising with hip slightly adducted, and in neutral rotation, and with foot held at 90°.

Functional test:	Neck rest crook lying with feet fixed: trunk raise forward.
Muscle power:	Psoas L1–2
(resisted isometric	Quad. L3
contractions)	TA L4
	EHL L5
	Tib. Post. L5
Reflexes:	Knee jerk (L3–4) six times, and plantar response Gt. toe jerk (L5) Test for ankle clonus
Sensation	Stroking test, and sensibility to pin-prick if applicable.

Palpate for adominal wall tenderness.

Patient lying prone

Reflexes:	Ankle jerk (S1). Test tendon jerk six times
Muscle power:	Ham. S2
	Glut. S1
Femoral nerve stretch test:	Prone knee bending, with hip extension (stabilise pelvis)
Functional test:	Feet fixed: head and shoulder raise.

---

4. Palpation
('Feel')

a. Find abnormality (see separate drill)
b. Decide whether abnormality is significant (sometimes is not)
N.B. Passive physiological-movement test (PP-MT) if necessary, in appropriate positions.

---

5. Record

Write a readable account of findings; asterisk salient signs and symptoms.

---

6. Assess

Where to place the first emphasis on treatment.

Palpation of lumbar spine
Patient in prone lying (arms to side, head to one side)

General palpation:	— sweep flat hand, for skin state — thumbs across Sacrospinalis, for spasm — fingers longitudinally in paravertebral sulcus, for undue prominence and line of spinous processes — flat-handed vertical pressure.
Segmental palpation:	Feeling: allow thumb-tips to sink in gently — the harder you press the less you feel. Try to make thumbs more perceptive; visualise the structures you are palpating.
Seek abnormalities:	Thickening — undue tenderness — undue bony prominences

Moving the joint:	By thumb-tip pressure against vertebral prominences, increase movement progressively, Grade I–IV; only palpate in depth if indicated.
Seek abnormalities:	Irritability—elicited spasm—diminished or increased accessory movement—provocation of pain and/or paraesthesiae locally and/or distally
Postero-anterior central pressure	—L1–L5
Postero-anterior unilateral pressure	—L1–L5
Transverse pressure	—L1–L5
Whole of sacro-iliac sulcus	
Tip of coccyx	
Use pisiform pressure technique if indicated.	
For fullest information:	—alter direction of palpation movement: —cephalad—towards head —caudad—towards feet —more medially —more laterally
If applicable:	—passive test of physiological interverbral movement (PP–MT) of each segment.

THE SACRO-ILIAC JOINT[68]

The comprehensive examination of this joint should be regarded as an expanded section of the 'Routine examination of back and hindquarters' (q.v.). The sacro-iliac joint should not be examined comprehensively until the lumbar spine, hip and lower limb examinations, including neurological tests, have been completed.

This self-discipline is necessary because of our ubiquitious tendency to jump to conclusions about supposed sacro-iliac joint conditions as the cause of the patient's low back pain and/or sciatica. A good rule of thumb might be: 'Deformity or asymmetry does not always mean pathology'.

Examination

Because the joint lies in an area to which pain is very frequently referred from the lumbar spine and occasionally from the hip, it is desirable to exclude lumbar lesions, lumbosacral conditions, conditions of one or both hips and serious disease of the sacro-iliac joint before admitting the probability of a benign sacro-iliac condition as responsible for the symptoms reported and likely to respond to the appropriate manual techniques. This is desirable,

but not always possible. Following thorough examination, one must sometimes proceed initially on a basis of greatest likelihood, thereafter depending upon continuing assessment of the results of treatment to provide more guidance.

The distribution of pain can be important, yet its segmental significance is not always easy to clarify because:

1. Dermatomes are neurophysiological entities, whose boundaries can fluctuate with the levels of facilitation at cord segments
2. Patients vary considerably in their patterns of pain reference or projection from similar, common joint abnormalities
3. Pain may be referred to sclerotome areas, which differ from dermatomes.

Proceeding in a logical sequence of comprehensive tests for the suspected joints, we ask: 'What does it look like?' and 'What is the X-ray appearance?' but most importantly: 'Which applied compressions or tensions and other stresses aggravate or reproduce the symptoms reported by the patient?'

Examination techniques

It is good practice to try to restrict testing procedures on the lying patient to either the lumbar spine or the sacro-iliac joint, and not test both together. This is difficult (e.g. the ilio-lumbar ligament present problems) but it is worth attempting at all times. The number of tests is legion. Some so-called 'tests' do not merit description while others induce quite gross movement in the lumbar spine and are much too unspecific; a few are seemingly based on the idea that rotatory movement of the ilium, around an axis at S2 level, is the only important movement occurring at the sacro-iliac joint. Yet others are so subjective that description of them is an irrelevance.

Observation

While the cervical spine and the craniovertebral joints are important in disturbances of vertebral *mobility*, the lumbo-pelvo-hip region is more important in disturbance of *posture*; a careful analysis of pelvic posture is necessary (Figs 7.24, 7.25).

Feeling and looking simultaneously can cause confusion; when clinically testing for symmetry, it is wiser to localise thumbs or fingers on bony points without also visualising the area, and then to observe the levels being palpated. Whether the thumbs are settled upwards or downwards onto bony points is unimportant. One should resist the tendency to find what one would like to find.

A method of detecting movement abnormalities, in the standing patient, is that of palpating the changing relationship of bony points of the sacrum and posterior ilium when the patient flexes the hip and knee of the unsupported side. This test, included in the teaching on post-registration manipulation courses in the UK since 1970, is illustrated in Figure 7.26.

The fact that the ischial tuberosity moves laterally during hip flexion, while the PSIS moves downward during the same movement, is a clear indication that normal movement of the ilium, at the sacroiliac joint, is other than simple rotation.

Piedallau's sign[158]: With the patient sitting on a hard flat surface, one posterior superior iliac spine, more frequently on the painful side, is lower than its fellow. On forward flexion, the position is reversed, the previously lower bony point now becomes the higher of the two.

Maigne[126] explains it as being due to muscular contracture; Piedallu asserts that the 'blocked' joint moves solidly as one, while the sacrum on the painless side is free to move through its small range with the lumbar spine. Whatever the explanation, the sign is that of an unmistakable movement abnormality with a torsional component.

Neurological tests

The presence of lumbo-sacral nerve root and/or cauda equina involvement, due to the consequences of spondylotic changes and/or other pathology, should be accepted if:

1. There are manifest neurological signs currently associated with the episode being treated.
2. Coughing and sneezing produce a smart exacerbation of the pain, more especially in the limb
3. Brudzinski's neck flexion sign is positive in that it aggravates haunch and limb pain.
4. Bilateral jugular vein compression also aggravates the pain within a short interval, often almost immediately.

A sacro-iliac condition can of course co-exist.

Patients with sacro-iliac problems often report paraesthesiae in the absence of neurological signs, which appear to stimulate the consequences of lumbo-sacral root involvement; also a diminished ankle jerk and some residual muscle weakness may be the 'tombstone' of a past discogenic episode and may have no connection with a current sacro-iliac condition. Straight-leg-raising is not an exclusively neurological test; besides its tendency to disturb lumbar joints in various ways it also applies stress to the sacro-iliac joints, and this can at times be used as a differentiation method. If straight-leg-raising on one side is restricted to 70° by a jab of haunch and leg pain, and the contralateral leg can be raised to a painless 90°, then raising both legs together to a painless 90° indicates that reduced range on the affected side is due to unilateral torsional stress on that sacro-iliac joint. This test does not preclude a possible co-existing lumbar problem, it only indicates the cause of straight-leg-raising restriction, yet this is clearly helpful when assessing. Exacerbation of 'sciatic' pain, by forcible foot dorsiflexion near the end of a painfully-limited straight-leg-raising range is not always a reliable indication that the extra pain is due to further sciatic nerve stretch;

foot dorsiflexion will often produce calf pain at 60° to 70° on a normal leg, and simple calf tenderness often accompanies purely sacro-iliac conditions, being exacerbated by the dorsiflexion test.

Iliac gapping and approximation test

The importance of these tests is their usefulness in excluding joint irritability, hypermobility and serious disease. They should never be left out, yet they are frequently negative in the presence of benign sacro-iliac problems, which are confirmed by other tests, and which can be relieved by mobilisation or manipulation techniques applied specifically to the joint.

Hip extension

When there is hypomobility in one sacroiliac joint, an additional test may serve to confirm it. The therapist stands level with the pelvis and leans over the prone patient to stabilise the sacrum with the palm of one hand, while the other hand passively extends the hip with an above-knee grasp. The leg on the hypomobility side feels heavier and cannot be extended as much as its fellow.

Prone knee-bending hip-extension test
(Figs. 6.13 and 6.14)

When pelvic asymmetry, in patients with equal leg lengths, accompanies unilateral sacro-iliac joint pain, e.g. on the right, the right pubic ramus and anterior superior iliac spines will often be a little forward and higher, respectively, than the same bony points on the left; similarly, the right posterior superior iliac spine will be a little lower than on the left. The prone knee-bending hip-extension range on the right side is often restricted, sometimes painfully, since the attachments of rectus femoris on that side have been drawn slightly apart. That the range is not invariably restricted or painful is a reminder the 'backward rotation' of one ilium is not the only form in which pelvic asymmetry can present; confident pronouncements about 'a posterior innominate' as the cause of the patient's pain are not always justified, because the painful side is occasionally on the left in the example quoted, and at times there appears to have occurred a slight bodily shift of one ilium, with little 'rotation'. The clinical states of this mysterious joint have not yet been satisfactorily clarified and are by no means understood. Attempts to 'clarify' problems by dogmatic assertions serve only to cloud the issue and to retard real understanding. For example, the objective evidence, of palpable asymmetry of the posterior margins of the ilium on the side of pain, is not always most manifest at the posterior superior iliac spine, but equally manifest along the whole length of the posterior margin; thus it is apparent that the asymmetry can be more of a slight shift in relationships rather than a pure 'rotation', which is plainly not possible at such a joint. Whether this 'asymmetry' has anything to do with what the patient reports by way of symptoms is a matter for experienced assessment.

Palpation

The joint can be palpated in one locality only, i.e. at its inferior extent in the region of the posterior inferior iliac spine. Acute unilateral tenderness here is very common in painful sacro-iliac conditions, and when well localised (as opposed to a general referred tenderness of the whole buttock) is a useful confirmatory sign. When palpating for movement abnormalities in the sacro-iliac sulcus, it is impossible to feel 'movement in the joint'; what one senses is a rhythmic, shifting relationship of adjacent bony prominences. After a little practice, changes in tension and 'springiness' of the sacro-tuberous ligaments are surprisingly easy to feel through the gluteal mass, although gluteal tenderness must be taken into account before admitting the value of this test in individual cases and assessing the differences in tension, if any.

A change in joint relationships, which tends to approximate the sacral and tuberous attachments of the ligament, will slightly reduce the tension on one side, and vice versa, provided such a change has occurred. We have already noted that pain from the joint need not be accompanied by asymmetry.

Palpation of pubic tubercles

By placing palmar surface of finger-tips at the umbilical region of the supine patient, it is possible to test pubic tubercle symmetry with the heel of the hand. By also accentuating first thenar and then hypothenar pressure, tenderness of superior rami of pubes can also be determined by this single considerate test.

Sacral apex pressure test

This is one of the most valuable tests because it is the most localised and specific, when applied on the prone patient. On a firm surface, the pelvis rests on a 'tripod' of two anterior superior spines and the pubis. Sacral apex pressure tends to shear the sacral joints and the lumbo-sacral joint on the stabilised ilia. While apex tenderness alone is inconclusive, exacerbation of the unilateral sacral pain complained of is strong supportive evidence of a sacro-iliac problem. The fact that lumbo-sacral 'shearing' may also be referring pain to the sacro-iliac joint must be borne in mind—one is never relieved of the obligation to assess.

Radiography

Not surprisingly, a patient with unremarkable X-ray appearances may be in considerable pain from a sacroiliac lesion. Continental radiologists have developed the technique of sacroiliac radiography in the craniocaudal axis. The tube is positioned above the patient who leans the trunk forward a little while sitting on the cassette.[70] The view gives better detail of the bony joint surfaces, particularly of the ventral aspect at the level of the pelvic brim; the cirumscribed opacities seen in orthodox views can be shown to be intra- or extraosseous.

In osteitis condensans ilii, the thickness of the involved ilium can be shown. Whether it will become possible to radiographically show subtle yet painful changes in joint relationship remains to be seen. Figure 4.59 on page 476 of the 36th edition of *Gray's Anatomy* beautifully depicts a right-sided so-called 'posterior innominate' sacroiliac lesion in a female patient!

A SUGGESTED EXAMINATION DRILL MAY BE TABULATED AS FOLLOWS: OBSERVATION — TESTING MOVEMENTS — PALPATION:

(Patient stands feet almost together and parallel)
Symmetry of general spinal contours?
Stands with pelvic rotation?
Buttock contour? Level of gluteal folds?
Asymmetry of gluteal cleft?
Level of iliac crests, and tubercle of crests?
Swollen appearance over one or other joint?
PSIS levels from behind? ASIS levels in front?
(Figs. 7.24 and 7.25)
Lateral pelvic tilt? Real or apparent leg shortening?

Standing hip and knee flexion tests (Fig. 7.26)

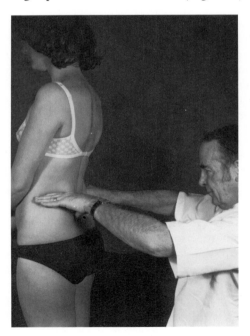

Fig. 7.24 Observing iliac crest levels, and symmetry of bony points, from behind.

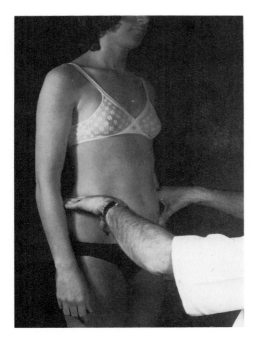

Fig. 7.25 Observing iliac crest levels, and symmetry of bony points, from the front.

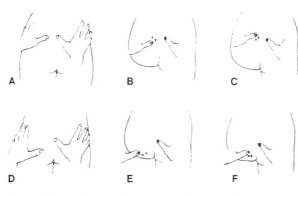

Fig. 7.26 Tests for sacroiliac fixation. To test the left side (upper part of joint A to C) (A) Place thumb of right hand over spinous process S2 and thumb of left hand over the posterior superior iliac spine. (B) and (C) Instruct patient to flex the hip and knee to 90° and observe movement of the thumb. In the normal joint the thumb will move caudally. In the abnormally fixed joint the thumb will move cephalad. (Lower part of joint D to F.) (D) Place right thumb over last sacral spinous process and left thumb over ischial tuberosity. Again instruct the patient to flex the hip and knee to 90°. (E) In the normal joint the left thumb will move laterally. (F) In the abnormally fixed joint the thumb will remain stationary or move cephalad. (Reproduced from Kirkaldy-Willis WH, Hill RJ 1979 A more precise diagnosis for low back pain, Spine 4: 2: 102, by kind permission of the authors and publisher.)

(Patient bends forward)

Skyline view of gluteal mass from in front of patient
Reobserve and repalpate PSIS for asymmetry (Piedallu's sign) (Figs. 6.2 and 6.3 p. 35)

(Patient sits erect on hard level surface, and then bends forward)

Repeat observations and palpation of bony points from behind, in both positions—lateral pelvic tilt still present or previous lateral tilt in standing now eradicated?
Many patients have anomalies of bony points; interpret findings conservatively.
When testing, compare sides and seek unequal movement, loss of movement, tissue contracture, hypermobility, undue tenderness, irritability.
Before using thigh as a lever, check that there is no hip joint involvement.

(Patient lies supine)

Check for leg lengths and 'set' of the pelvis, with patient lying straight (see p. 36).

Examine hips:

Compare tension, by passive stretch of:
Abductors, and ilio-tibial band
Adductors, i.e. abduction of flexed limb, foot alongside opposite knee (Patrische test)
Ilio-psoas, i.e. with opposite hip fully flexed to allow passive extension of affected side
Passive flexion-adduction test. Hurt in groin or buttock? End-feel?
Add pressure down length of femur, with opposite ASIS stabilised in this position. Hurt?
External and internal rotation. Limited?
Static isometric contractions of hip abductors and adductors. Painful?

Examine sacro-iliac joint:

Iliac gapping and approximation tests with flat hard pillow under patient's lumbar spine
Palpate in sacro-iliac sulcus of same side while repetitively flexing, and then flex-adducting, hip. Movement abnormalities?
Straight-leg-raising—either leg, then both together.

Palpation:

Baer's point (iliacus spasm and tenderness). Compare sides.
Adductor insertion, for undue tenderness.
Anterior acetabular region.
Configuration of symphysis pubis, and undue tenderness there.

(Patient lies prone, with arms to side)

Skyline view of gluteal mass.
Check leg lengths in extension and in knee flexion (see p. 36)

Examine hips:

Compare tension of rectus femoris, e.g. press heel to buttock with pelvis stabilised, then gently extend hip. Limited? Hurt?
Passively lift relaxed limb.

Examine sacro-iliac joint:

Flex far knee to 90° and medially rotate far hip repetitively; with pelvis stabilised by operator's chest, palpate near sacro-iliac sulcus. Movement abnormalities? (Fig. 7.27)
Rock sacrum by repetive pressures to its apex (at sacro-coccygeal joint), compare movements at sulci. Does it hurt at sacro-iliac joint? (Fig. 7.28)
Stress sacrum upwards and ilium downwards and vice versa. Painful? (Fig. 7.29)

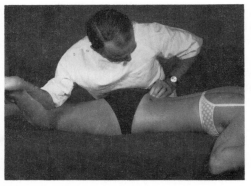

Fig. 7.27 By stabilising the patient's near buttock with his abdomen, and palpating the left sacro-iliac sulcus with his cranial hand, the small amount of sacro-iliac gapping movement can be felt as the opposite thigh is repetitively internally rotated, by the therapist's caudal hand and forearm.

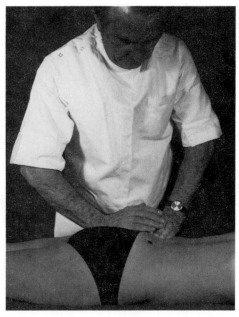

Fig. 7.28 The 'tripod' test. Since the three-point contact, of pubis and anterior ends of ilia, with the surface of the plinth will stabilise the pelvis, repetitive downward pressures on the sacral apex will induce a small degree of movement of sacrum on ilia. By palpating in the sulcus, a value judgement between sides can be made.
N.B. Discrepancies between sides do not necessarily imply the presence of 'abnormality'.

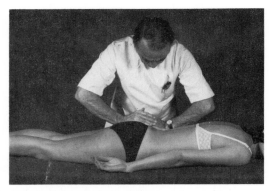

Fig. 7.29 Applying cranio-caudal and caudo-cranial pressures to the components of the sacro-iliac joint. This test does not often reveal much which cannot be revealed by the tests already described; nevertheless, it is sometimes of real value.

Palpation:

Relative depth of sulci
Undue tenderness medial to PIIS
Symmetry of sacro-tuberous and sacro-spinous ligaments through gluteal mass (which may itself be tender).

Discussion

Plainly, indications for treatment will become more marked in an almost direct relationship to the number of factors which are accurately assessed. The more comprehensive the examination, the more likely appropriate treatment will be found, as the weight of emphasis gradually mounts up during examination. Therefore it is of first importance to be thorough and comprehensive, and to place more reliance on observable facts than on an over-imaginative interpretation of them.

Nevertheless, the vagaries of referred pain can cause great difficulty, and it is wise to remember that combined sacro-iliac and symphysis pubis conditions tend to refer pain to haunch, groin and antero-medial thigh; also that it is not rare for a sacro-iliac problem to be accompanied by abnormalities at the third and higher lumbar segments.

EXAMINATION OF HIP

The comprehensive examination of this joint should be regarded as an expanded section of 'Routine examination of back and hindquarters' (q.v.).

Some of the tests here are included in that routine. Nevertheless, exclusion of problems at the lumbar spine and sacro-iliac joint, and neurological tests of the lower limbs, should accompany the more detailed hip examination set out below.

Pain in the hip region need not arise from the hip joint, and that due to a hip condition is not necessarily felt in that area.

Comparative anatomy

Arm. The shoulder is a mobile, unstable, multi-jointed tool for handling, manipulating tools, waving, gesticulating—functionally, its *instability* and *mobility* are of paramount importance; therefore, when examining the joint it is quite appropriate, after active tests, to put the emphasis on careful passive movement with the patient in supine, side-lying or prone.

Hip. The hip is a weight-bearing support, a stabilised column upon which the superincumbent weight is dynamically balanced—functionally, *the dymamic stabilisation of the joint during weight-bearing* is of paramount importance; therefore, the joint should not be examined quite like a shoulder, and a degree of emphasis in examination now shifts to static, dynamic and functional tests *while weight-bearing*. The degree of pain and disablement will govern the severity of these tests, of course, and careful passive tests remain important, as in all joints.[72]

1. History ('Listen')	a. What is patient's usual activity (work and play)?	
	b. Details of *present* pain	—extent and nature?
		—any back, buttock, trochanter, groin, thigh/leg pain?
		—what aspect of limb? Which toes?
	c. *Behaviour of pain* related to time, posture and activity (Assess degree of joint irritability)	—continuous, episodic or occasional?
		—pain at rest, or only on movement?
		—what movement? Of back? Of hip-joint?
		—how much pain is caused?
		—how long after movement does pain persist?
		—pain at night? Can sleep on that side?
		—other functional restrictions by pain? Standing? walking? stairs? driving? dressing?
		—how far can patient walk comfortably?
	d. *Other symptoms*	—paraesthesiae? Numbness? Blanching or flushing due to vascular changes? Which toes?
		—any 'deadness'/'heaviness' of limb? What provokes this?

e. X-rayed recently? Drugs? Systemic steroids? Anticoagulants? History of Rheumatoid Arthritis? General health?

f. *Onset* of this, and previous attacks? Previous treatment? Result of treatment, if any?

   N.B. Now *plan* which more distal joints need *more* than routine examination, e.g. tibio-fibular, knee, ankle joint, foot.

---

2. Observation
('Look')

Patient standing
Changes of contour — swelling? — wasting?
Changes of attitude — stance?

---

3. Function
('Test')

Patient standing
Observe:

— standing from sitting
— walking
— standing and flexing alternate knee to chest, and extending, abducting and rotating non-weight-bearing leg
— hopping lightly on one leg
— wide stride standing
— stepping up on stool on either leg
— full squat position from standing

Equilibrium test:

— patient stands on one leg, with eyes closed, and is lightly supported by one hand. Check stabilisation efficiency of each hip when vision is denied.

Patient lying supine
Passive test:

of all ranges compared with other limb, with overpressure and assessment of 'end-feel' (i.e. assess nature of limiting factor, if any), especially of combined ranges, e.g. flexion-adduction (Fig. 7.30).

Fig. 7.30 The passive flexion-adduction test of the hip-joint.

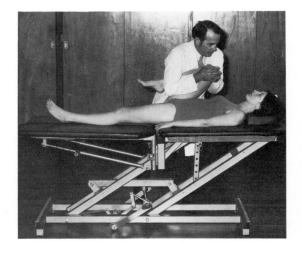

	Test compression and distraction
	Seek regions of muscle tightness
Muscle power:	resisted isometric contraction

Flexors ⎫
Abductors ⎪
Abductors ⎬ of hip
Extensors ⎪
External rotators ⎪
Internal rotators ⎭

Palpation:	Baer's point (flexor spasm)
	Swelling
	Wasting
	Tenderness anteriorly and laterally over bursae
	Temperature

Patient lying prone
Press heel to buttock with pelvis stabilised—extend hip-joint

Muscle power:	resisted isometric contraction
	Hamstrings, as knee flexors and knee rotators
Palpation:	— ischial tuberosities and posterior trochanter area
	— bulk of gluteus maximus when statically contracted.

---

4. Record Write a readable account of findings. Asterisk salient signs and symptoms.

---

5. Assess Where to place the first emphasis in treatment, and general treatment approach.

PASSIVE PHYSIOLOGICAL-MOVEMENT TESTS (PP-MT)

Because examination of intervertebral movement may employ both *accessory*-movement tests and *physiological*-movement tests, it is necessary to distinguish clearly between them, and for this reason the following procedures are named as above.

Descriptions of examination procedures are best used as companions to practical teaching sessions, because the method cannot be adequately learned from a text; familiarity with the nature and extent of movement at the different segments takes some time to acquire.

There are many ways of perceiving movement, and the techniques described are somewhat basic; they can be developed as the therapist gains skill. Some therapists test each segment in both weight-bearing and non-weight-bearing positions.

The examiner should adopt a procedure which comes most easily to hand and is methodical; apart from modification to suit a particular patient's physique, it is better to stick to the method chosen—the same tests should be done in the same way every time.

Procedure

Any *apparent* positional abnormalities should be noted first (Fig. 7.31) (in this connection, transverse processes are more important than spinous processes); tests for segmental mobility are then applied. No more pressure than is needed to adequately detect the ranges of movement should be used. It is important not to 'waggle' but to produce precise, rhythmic movements of fair amplitude and regular frequency.

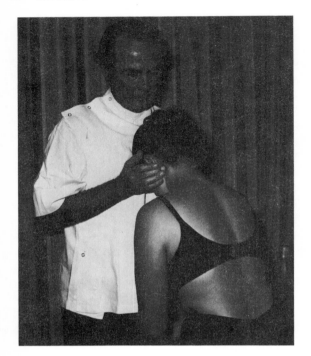

Fig. 7.31 Assessing occipito-atlantal joint relationship, by simultaneous palpation of the mastoid process and lateral mass of atlas on each side. 'Abnormalities' are not necessarily clinically significant.

C0–C1

Patient lies supine with head on a flat pillow (Fig. 7.32).
Therapist stands at head with patient's vertex in contact with his abdomen

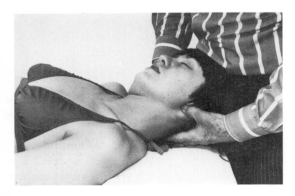

Fig. 7.32. Passive physiological-movement test (PP-MT) of side flexion of C0–C1 segment. It is important to isolate movement to the cranio-vertebral junction.

Side-flexion:

Support occiput with fingers of left hand while left thumb-tip rests between lateral mass of C1 and mastoid process. Place right hand as required for efficient support of patient's head.

Repetitively side-flex cranio-vertebral junction to right side as thumb perceives amount of gapping between C1 and mastoid on the left. Isolate movement to upper C. *only*.

Repeat to opposite side after changing grasp.

Rotation:

Stand a little clear of head and rotate it away from palpating thumb. Repeat to opposite side, with changed grasp (Fig. 7.33).

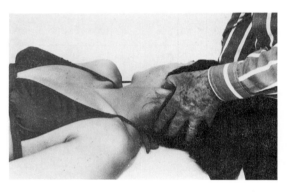

Fig. 7.33 Passive physiological-movement test (PP-MT) of the small degree of rotation between the atlas and the occiput. The neck itself should be held in the neutral position so far as sagittal movement is concerned.

Flexion:

Rest patient's occiput on small block and place palm (fingers caudally) on patient's forehead. Press forehead caudally so that chin is repetitively depressed by movement at cranio-vertebral junction. Palpate, with finger or thumb, the left and then the right basiocciput at the joint as the head flexes (Fig. 7.34).

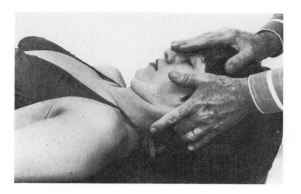

Fig. 7.34 Passive physiological-movement test (PP-MT) of the range of flexion at the cranio-vertebral junction (C0–C1).

Extension:

Remove block, and with patient's vertex in therapist's abdomen, together with each forefinger against the joint on that side, repetively extend the patient's head at the cranio-vertebral junction by flexion of therapist's knees (Fig. 7.35).

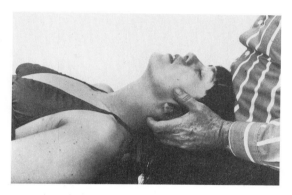

Fig. 7.35 Passive physiological-movement test (PP-MT) of the extension range at the cranio-vertebral junction (C0–C1). The point of contact between patient's vertex and therapist's abdomen moves through an arc, the axis of which is the cranio-vertebral joint. This necessitates considerable movement of the therapist's trunk, hips and knees.

C1–C2

Patient lies supine. Therapist stands at head (Fig. 7.36).

Rotation with side-flexion:

Support head with palm of left hand, while the index or middle finger is rested on the tip of C2 spinous process. The right hand rests as convenient on

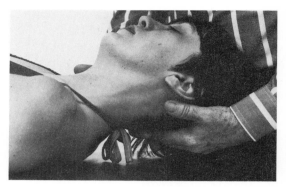

Fig. 7.36 Passive physiological-movement test (PP-MT) of rotation-with-side-flexion of the atlanto-axial joint (C1–C2) with the patient supine.

the right side of the patient's head, and help to guide the testing movement. With the left palpating fingertip kept in the mid-line, the patient's head is side-flexed to left and right; the degree of offset of the spinous process of C2 to the opposite side is a measure of both side-flexion and rotation range, since these two degrees of freedom are inter-dependent. (For alternative method see below).

Flexion:

Support head with palm under occiput, and pads of middle fingers resting on the postero-lateral aspect of the C1–2 joint; check that it is not C2–3. Flex head repetitively and compare movement.

Extension:

Extend head, keeping movement confined to upper cervical region only.

An alternative method of testing rotation and rotation-with-side-flexion is as follows: Patient sits on a low stool or plinth. Therapist stands at side (Fig. 7.37).

Rotation:

Palpate or grip spinous process of C2 with finger and thumb of one hand, and with the other hand placed on the vertex spin head about 30° from side to side. Perceive degree of head rotation at which C2 begins to move.

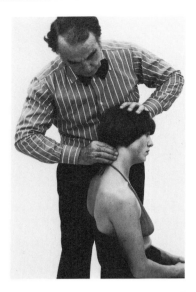

Fig. 7.37 Passive physiological-movement test (PP-MT). Alternative method of examining the physiological range of combined side-flexion and rotation of the atlanto-axial joint (C1–C2) with the patient sitting.

Rotation with side-flexion:

Head is side-flexed and degree of side-swing of C2 spinous process to the opposite side is assessed.

C2–C6

Patient lies supine on high plinth.

Flexion (Fig. 7.38):

Therapist sits or crouches at patient's head, supports occiput with one palm (fingers towards patient's vertex) and repetitively flexes neck while edge of

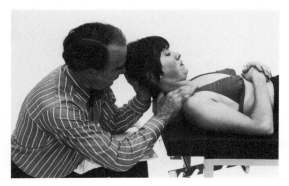

Fig. 7.38 Passive physiological-movement testing (PP-MT) of flexion, between segments C2–C6.

opposite thumb palpates gapping between successive spinous processes from above downwards.

Flexion is gradually increased for the lower segments.

Extension (Fig. 7.39):

The therapist stands at patient's head and supports occiput with the non-palpating hand. With palm of the palpating hand conveniently placed, the therapist places index or middle finger (or one reinforcing the other) over the junction of adjacent vertebral arches, and pushes the neck into extension. The therapist's trunk is somewhat involved in the movement. Repeat on opposite side.

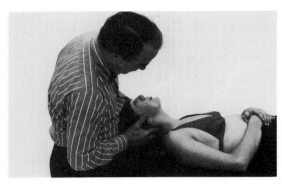

Fig. 7.39 Passive physiological-movement testing (PP-MT) of extension at cervical segments between C2 and C6.

Side-flexion (Fig. 7.40):

The therapist places the right foot a pace out and forward; otherwise the starting position is virtually the same. Side-flexion is palpated during bending

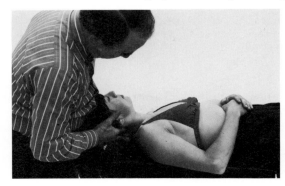

Fig. 7.40 Passive physiological-movement testing (PP-MT) of right side-flexion, between segments C2–C6.

the patient's neck towards the right by some movements of the therapist's body. Movement is gradually increased for the lower segments. Change starting position and repeat to opposite side.

Rotation (Fig. 7.41):

The therapist stands facing the side of the patient's head and cups the occiput in the fingers of the cranial hand, with palm near to the patient's ear.

The palm of the caudal hand is placed over the patient's far zygoma and cheek, while the pad of middle finger rests postero-laterally on the far vertebral arches.

Rotation movement is perceived by a reciprocating action of both hands, turning the head towards the therapist.

Repeat to opposite side.

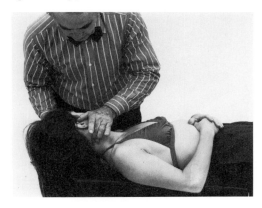

Fig. 7.41 Passive physiological-movement testing (PP-MT) of left rotation, between segments C2–C6. The therapist's hands rotate the neck with a reciprocal action.

C6–T3

All of the movements of this region are examined with the patient in side-lying and the therapist facing the patient, resting his sternum on the deltoid area of the uppermost folded arm to provide some stabilisation of the patient's trunk (Fig. 7.42).

The therapist's cranial forearm supports the patient's head, with fingers curling round the patient's lower neck — the medial fingers are more active in grasping, while the therapist's cranial forearm and trunk take part in the movements.

Avoid stress on the patient's neck.

Flexion, extension, rotation and side-flexion are all tested in this position, while one finger of the caudal hand palpates movement between adjacent spinous processes.

Side-flexion and rotation are repeated to the opposite side.

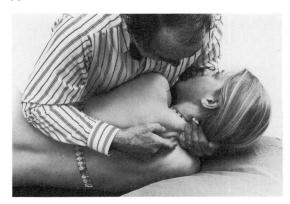

Fig. 7.42 Passive physiological-movement testing (PP-MT) of rotation, between segments C6–T3. This disposition of patient and therapist is used for all tests of this kind, for this region.

T3–T10

Flexion:

Patient sits sideways at end of plinth in 'neck rest' position with elbows together, i.e. adducted (Fig. 7.43).

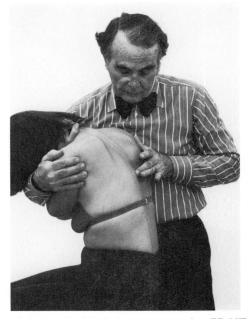

Fig. 7.43 Passive physiological-movement testing (PP-MT) of flexion between segments T3-T10.

Therapist stands at side, reaching *over* the patient's forearms to grasp the opposite upper arm and hold the patient's trunk against his own.

Movement is palpated between the spinous processes with the free hand, while the therapist repetitively flexes the patient's trunk by dipping his own in a side-flexion movement.

Extension:

Patient as above, with elbows still adducted but now raised forward (Fig. 7.44).

Therapist as above, but now reaching *under* patient's arms to place hand on lateral aspect of opposite scapula. Both patient's and therapist's trunk are rhythmically moved to produce extension as the spinous processes are palpated from above downwards.

N.B. In the two tests above it is important that the therapist moves his trunk as one with the patient's trunk.

Side-flexion

Patient in 'neck rest' position as before.

Therapist stands at side, reaching across the patient's upper pectorals and under the opposite axilla to grasp as in extension testing. The patient then rests both arms on the therapist's forearm (Fig. 7.45).

The palm of the therapist's free hand is placed on the near hemithorax, with index or middle finger against the near side of adjoining spinous processes. The patient's trunk is repetitively side-flexed, by a reciprocating movement of both hands. Movement is palpated either as gapping or approximation of the bony points.

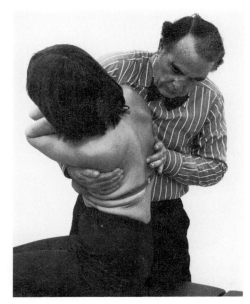

Fig. 7.45 Passive physiological-movement testing (PP-MT) of side-flexion between segments T3–T10.

Rotation:

Patient is in crook-side-lying with arms folded and adducted (Fig. 7.46). The therapist sits in the 'crook' of the patient (or stands facing the head) and stabilises the pelvis by placing his near axilla on the patient's upper trochanter. The therapist's outer hand is placed over the patient's upper arm, and movement is produced by rhythmically pushing the trunk away from the therapist into rotation. The therapist's free forearm lies parallel with and against the trunk, assisting in stabilisation of its lower part as the middle finger, reinforced by the index, is placed

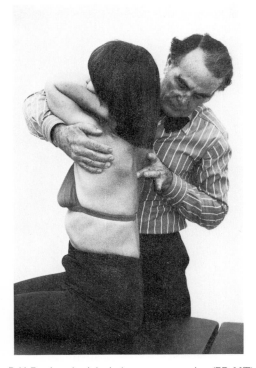

Fig. 7.44 Passive physiological-movement testing (PP-MT) of extension, between segments T3–T10.

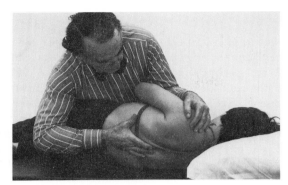

Fig. 7.46 Passive physiological-movement testing (PP-MT) of rotation, between segments T3–T10.

from below upwards on the sides of adjacent spinous processes. The finger-pad fixes the lower spinous process while the tip perceives rotation movement of the upper process.

Combined movements:

More information, about the physiological movement of a segment, is gained if the normal *combinations* of movement (p. 12) are passively tested, i.e. the combination of extension, left side flexion and right rotation (Fig. 7.47), or flexion, right rotation and right side flexion (Fig. 7.48).

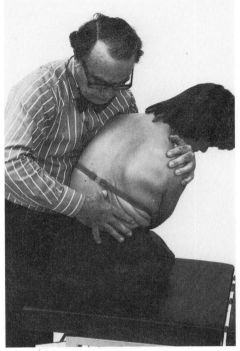

Fig. 7.48 Passive physiological-movement testing (PP-MT) of combined flexion, right side-flexion and right rotation, of segments T3–T10.

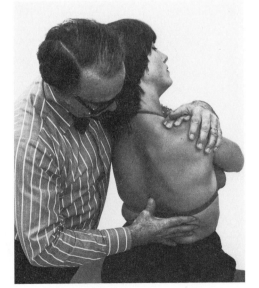

Fig. 7.47 Passive physiological-movement testing (PP-MT) of combined extension, left side-flexion and right rotation, of segments T3–T10.

T10–S1

(A small flat pillow under the patient's loin will keep the lumbar spine in neutral position).

Flexion:

The patient lies on side with knees and hips bent. The therapist, in walk-standing facing the patient's head, supports the patient's shins across his lower abdomen by clasping the lower bent knee with his outer hand (Fig. 7.49). The index or middle finger of inner hand rests between adjacent spinous processes, and perceives the amount of movement as the patient's knees are rhythmically moved towards his head by the therapist's pelvis in a forward and backward rocking movement.

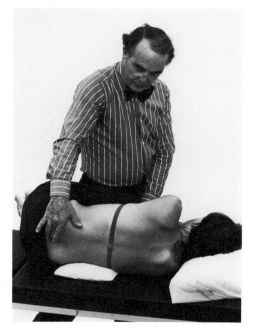

Fig. 7.49 Passive physiological-movement testing (PP-MT) of flexion, between segments T10–S1.

Extension:

The operator turns to face the patient, maintaining the shin-lower abdomen contact, and also changes his grasp so that the caudal hand now supports the patient's underneath leg (Fig. 7.50).

The therapist's cranial hand now palpates movement between adjacent spinous processes, as extension is rhythmically produced by movement of the therapist's trunk.

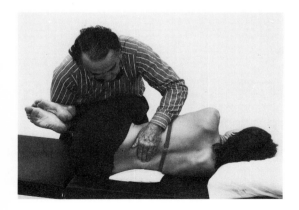

Fig. 7.50 Passive physiological-movement testing (PP-MT) of extension, between segments T10–S1.

Side-flexion:

The flat pillow is removed and the therapist, facing the patient, applies his caudal arm round the whole of the patient's upper rump (Fig. 7.51). By a rhythmical side-sway of his own trunk towards the patient's head, the therapist produces a side-flexion movement which can be palpated either as gapping or approximation by a finger of the cranial hand. Repeat to opposite side.

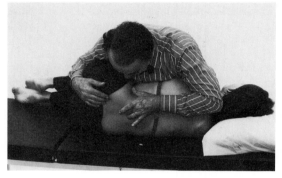

Fig. 7.51 Passive physiological-movement testing (PP-MT) of side-flexion, between segments T10–S1.

Rotation:

The flat pillow is replaced and the therapist places the palm of his caudal hand on the patient's upper trochanter. By leaning his cranial-side axilla on the patient's upper ribs, his forearm lies along the lower thoracic spine and a re-inforced finger can rest against adjacent spinous processes. (Fig 7.52)

Rotation is perceived as the patient's pelvis is rocked backwards and forwards.

It is not always necessary to repeat on the opposite side, but this should be done at first.

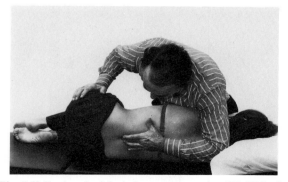

Fig. 7.52 Passive physiological-movement testing (PP-MT) of rotation, between segments T10–S1.

Sacro-iliac joint

Positions of the patient, and techniques for examining movements of the sacro-iliac joint, are described with the basic examination drill (on page 82).

Notes

It will be apparent that more than one starting position is employed in testing most of the spinal regions, and when a complete vertebral examination is done, less time is taken up if a sequence of sitting, lying and side-lying is adopted, and findings at the different levels recorded out of numerical order.

8

Recording examination

A systematic and accurate record of examination facilitates quick reference during treatment to *salient* findings, which should be noted especially (see listed Examination Procedures).

Methods of setting out information are varied to suit requirements; shorthand symbols save time and are desirable so long as their meaning is agreed.

Findings should be written on a Vertebral Examination Recording Sheet, ending with comments on initial assessment and treatment approach selected. Comprehensive examination of peripheral joints can be recorded on a separate sheet.

The author has formulated a layout for recording the initial vertebral examination findings (Figs. 8.1, 8.2, 8.3, 8.4) which is being adopted, with minor changes, both at home and abroad; there is need for similar method of recording examination of peripheral joints, and head pain.

A specimen Recording Chart is set out with one side devoted to subjective examination and the other to objective examination, with remarks on initial-assessment and the first choice of treatment.

The format is suitable for recording basic information gathered from any vertebral district.

While the example given is that of the examination and treatment of a lumbar joint problem, the panel 'Other tests' in Figure 8.2 could be replaced by a panel Figure 8.4 for all associated peripheral joints, or by the right hand column only when a separate format is intended exclusively for neck and thoracic joint conditions. This is my own recording practice, since one needs room for even the briefest comment on findings in peripheral joints.

Separate forms are required for head pain (including the temporomandibular joint), upper limb and lower limb. It may well be that therapists of the future will employ an electronic method of recording examination, in which the totality of single and combined examination movements, and their effects, are electronically systemised, and thus incorporated into something resembling the modern pocket calculator which could display the salient factors. Certainly, the detailed written account of a comprehensive vertebral and associated peripheral joint examination requires considerable organisation of method.

Recording palpation findings

The nature of the range-limiting factor, together with the degree of limitation invariably decide the grade employed in treatment, and frequently also the positioning of the patient's joint and the particular technique; thus when recording palpation and passive movement findings it is necessary to record not only the point of encounter on the expected normal range but also the nature of the limiting factor (see Palpation in Assessment, p. 104).

During examination, it is probably easiest to note the former as being in the 'early', 'middle' or 'late' part of the expected normal range.

In summary:

(i) Palpation findings during *examination and initial assessment* are expressed as factors encountered during the 'E', 'M' or 'L' part of the expected normal range, these being conveniently recorded on a spinal chart alongside the segment concerned.

(ii) The *treatment* grade employed refers to the *available* range (see p. 127).

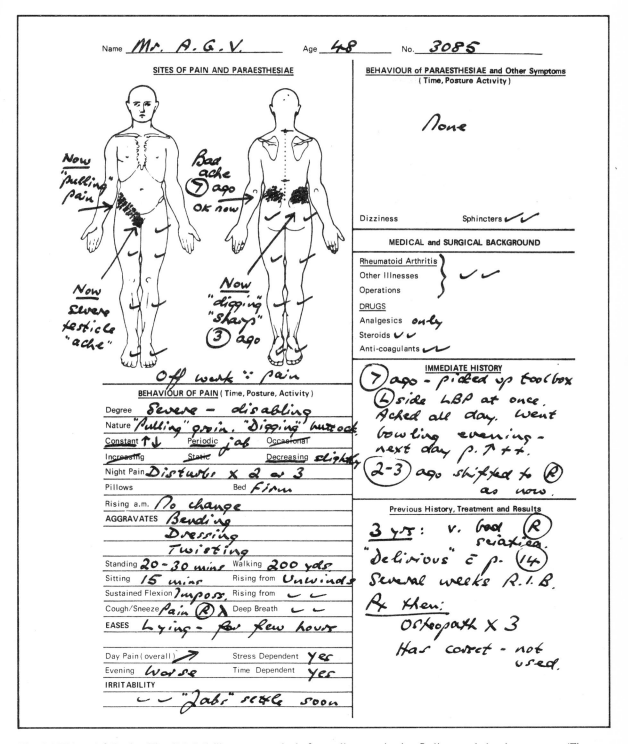

Fig. 8.1 This and following Figs (8.2–8.6) illustrate a method of recording examination findings, and also the treatment (Fig. 8.3). Figure 8.1 shows subjective findings.

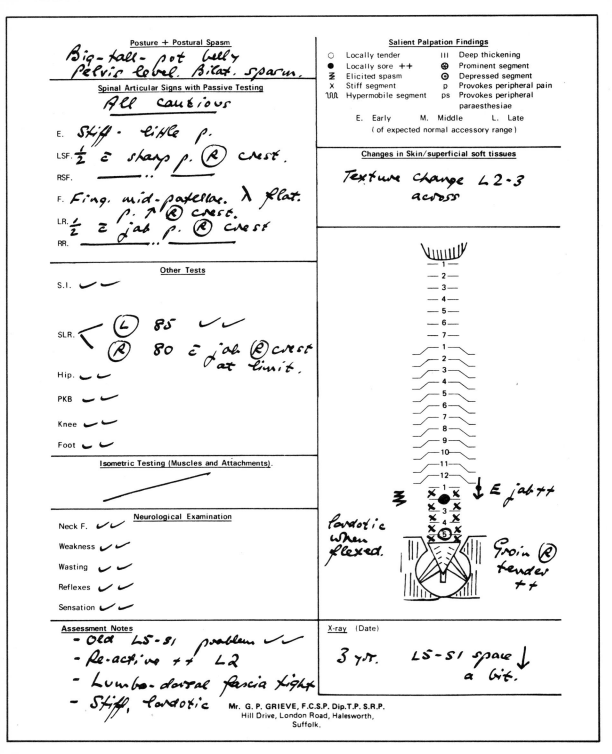

Fig. 8.2 Objective findings, and assessment notes concerning the same patient.

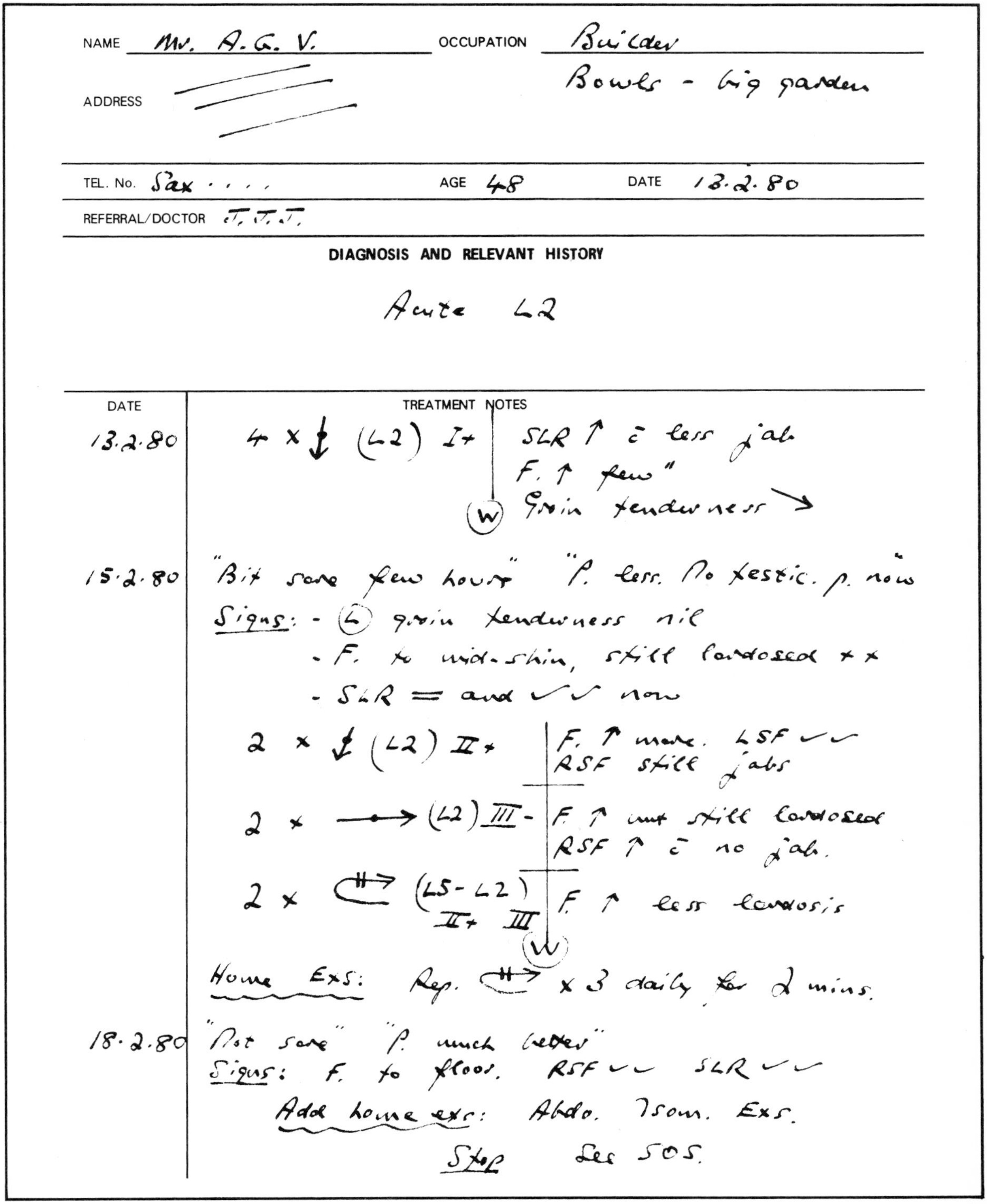

NAME *Mr. A. G. V.*   OCCUPATION *Builder*

Bowls – big garden

ADDRESS ~~~~~~~

TEL. No. *Sax . . . .*   AGE *48*   DATE *13.2.80*

REFERRAL/DOCTOR *J. J. J.*

DIAGNOSIS AND RELEVANT HISTORY

Acute L2

DATE	TREATMENT NOTES
13.2.80	4 × ↓ (L2) I+ SLR ↑ c̄ less jab F. ↑ few" (W) groin tenderness →

15.2.80	"Bit sore few hours" "P. less. No testic. p. now
	Signs: – (L) groin tenderness nil
	  – F. to mid-shin, still lordosed ××
	  – SLR = and ✓✓ now
	2 × ↓ (L2) II+ F. ↑ more. LSF ✓✓ / RSF still jabs
	2 × ⟶ (L2) III– F. ↑ more still lordosed / RSF ↑ c̄ no jab.
	2 × ⤴ (L5–L2) II+ III F. ↑ less lordosis
	(W)
	Home Exs: Rep. ⤴ × 3 daily for 2 mins.

18.2.80	"Not sore" "P. much better"
	Signs: F. to floor. RSF ✓✓ SLR ✓✓
	     Add home exs: Abdo. Isom. Exs.
	         Stop See SOS.

Fig. 8.3 Notes of treatment procedures and result.

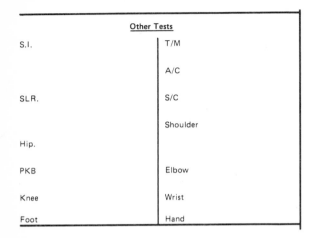

Other Tests	
S.I.	T/M
	A/C
SLR.	S/C
	Shoulder
Hip.	
PKB	Elbow
Knee	Wrist
Foot	Hand

Fig. 8.4 An alternative panel for 'other tests'

Here are two examples of recording *salient* findings, and in the first (Fig. 8.5) the patient has reported left occipital and left scapular pain. Left postero-anterior testing pressures ( ) over the lateral mass of the atlas reveal that early (E) in the expected normal accessory range, local soreness ( ) precludes further testing of movement and the feel of the movement suggests that the joint is stiff (X). It also feels thickened (III) although the precise cause of the 'thickening' is not yet revealed.

Similar testing pressures over the transverse process of the axis elicit a mild voluntary muscle guarding response in the middle (M) of the expected normal accessory range, of that testing movement. Over the angle of the 3rd left rib, marked soreness is revealed during the middle (M) range of the expected movement. What has been recorded, therefore, are the essential findings for guidance in selection of the initial treatment techniques. The examiner will certainly have uncovered much more information, of less immediate importance, than is illustrated; whether this also is recorded is a matter of preference.

When learning this or any other system of notation it is best to record *everything*, because the student is quickly confronted by the need to be precise and tidy.

In the second example (Fig. 8.6) the patient reports a symmetrical interscapular pain, worst in the median plane, and the prime cause for seeking help. Postero-anterior central vertebral pressures reveal that segments T1–T2, T2–T3 and T6–T7 are stiff (X), also that there is tenderness of bony points at T3, T6 and T7. Pressures on T4 and T5 spinous processes reveal marked soreness ( ) early (E) in the expected normal accessory range, and elicited spasm ( ). Because of this, it is not possible to assess whether the segments T3–T4 and T5–T6 are also stiff, yet on careful movement of spinous processes T4 and T5 the 'feel' suggests a sogginess which is uncharacteristic of mid-thoracic segments. Thus hypermobility, but not necessarily instability, is suspected there; careful passive physiological-movement testing (PP–MT) reveals that T3–T4 and T5–T6 are moving satisfactorily but that the T4–T5 segment is indeed hypermobile. Since pain is the dominant feature, sufficient important information has been recorded to allow selection of initial treatment techniques and also their grading.

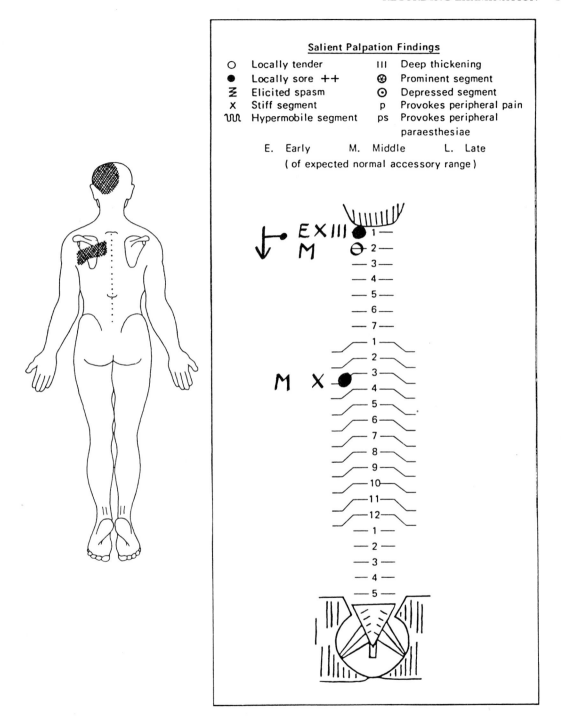

Fig. 8.5 Record of palpation findings in a patient with left hemi-occipital and left hemi-thoracic pain.

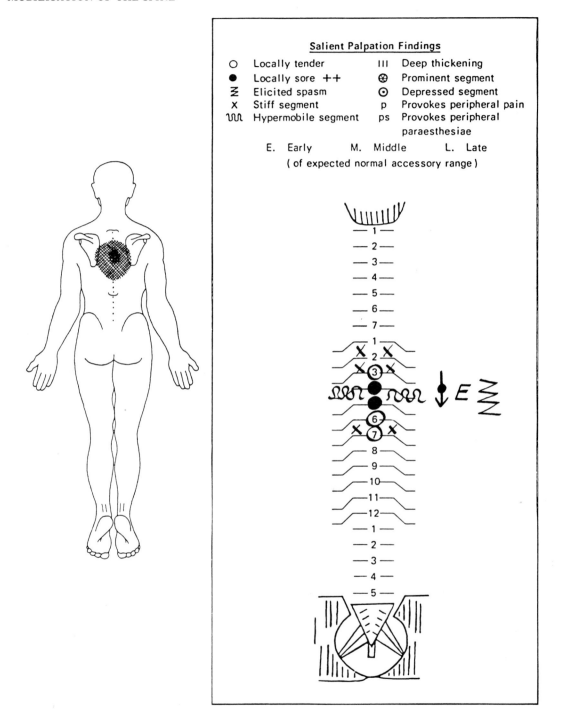

Fig. 8.6 Record of palpation findings in a patient with posterior central and spreading mid-thoracic pain.

9

Assessment in examination

Depending upon the patient's pain, temperament and degree of anxiety, and the complexity of the joint and soft tissue changes, descriptions of symptoms and their behaviour related to time, posture and activity amount at times to the therapist being handed a tangled ball of wool. Examination and assessment must unravel the tangle, clarifying the priorities and relative importance of the signs elicited.

The purpose of examination is to fully and clearly grasp *how* the patient is troubled, and then to seek a physical basis for these symptoms, in terms of objective signs. These provide initial guides for action in treatment, but a degree of judgement is necessary, and therefore assessment—of the patient; of the relationship between the symptoms reported and the signs of disturbed function; of priorities, when two or more aspects need attention—is equally important, so that the first choice of treatment method is closely related to the findings.

This may not be easy when patients are treated in groups, or when specific treatment prescriptions must be followed precisely, but an endeavour always to relate treatment and its results to examination findings and assessment is repaid by a better understanding of the behaviour of degenerative joint disease.

Some mention of assessment during examination has already been made in preceding pages.

History

There is considerable variation in the way patients describe their symptoms and functional difficulties; some make less of their troubles than others, and may find difficulty in recalling the important time-sequence of developing symptoms. The therapist must assess how complete, fulsome or sketchy an account is being given.

Pain intensity is not always proportional to objective findings; also a patient's response to pain may appear average, low or high. Accounts of pain intensity will vary with the patient's temperament. It is important to note that the site of a previous and painful limb injury will be disproportionately painful if referred pain of vertebral degenerative disease later invades that limb. The central nervous system appears to retain a memory for previously well-trodden neurone pathways, and pain at the old site is easily rekindled in later years.

Observation

Patients' functional difficulties can be noted when they are undressing, reaching to demonstrate painful areas, reaching for shoes, getting onto the plinth, and moving on it. Sometimes their agility belies the difficulties reported.

Objective tests

Logical treatment depends upon finding signs which are reasonably compatible with history and symptoms presented by the patient. A thickened and stiff spinal segment may be the 'tombstone' of a past episode, and not directly responsible for the pain currently troubling the patient; also it is unlikely that paraesthesiae of the three middle fingers, with a weak triceps muscle, would arise from a tender and irritable C2–C3 segment, although a lower cervical lesion may co-exist of course.

For example, pain in the upper medial pectoral area can arise from the sternoclavicular joint, pain more laterally may be referred from the cervical region and/or shoulder joint, and lower paramedian pectoral pain can be referred forward from upper thoracic segments.

Objective tests by active and passive movement, and careful palpation of all joints and associated tissues likely to be giving rise to the pain, will help to clarify the cause by a process of exclusion.

Again, the distinction between (a) muscular aches in the region of the vertebral joint problems, (b) the pain referred into more distal limb muscles from the vertebral lesion, and (c) pain also referred distally from a coexisting limb girdle joint problem, is not always easy, but is an important part of clinical assessment. For example, during assessment of the priorities of treatment of the ubiquitous neck/shoulder problems, a helpful guide may be:

1. Where (i) the cervical and upper half of the thoracic spine and the clavicular joints show no significant clinical abnormality, and (ii) the pain of a single resisted shoulder movement is dominant among the clinical features, and (iii) there is clearly no restriction of shoulder mobility on active and passive careful testing (although the movement which stretches the tendon concerned may be painful) attention localised to the rotator cuff tendon appears indicated.

2. If (i) there are clinical abnormalities of the lower cervical and upper thoracic spine, (ii) restricted shoulder movement is more dominant in the clinical features, and (iii) more than one resisted movement is painful, there might be clear indications for giving attention to both vertebral and peripheral joints, with the first priority being the spine.

In general terms, the amount of pain referred distally into a limb from spinal problems is an index of difficulty (the further distal, the more difficult) in applying quickly successful treatment.

PALPATION IN ASSESSMENT

Schmorl and Junghann's[167] concept of the 'mobility segment' is a great advance in the way we think about the vertebral column and its benign or more serious abnormalities, and it is suggested that 'no vertebra is an island'; we may usefully add to this 'and no mobility segment'.

It is wise to note the functional interdependence of the spinal regions (see p. 7). We are not dealing with a simple perpendicular arrangement of bony segments bound together by straps of ligament, but a dynamic body axis in which no localised abnormality can exist without sooner or later affecting more distant segments and ultimately the whole spine. Just as one cannot passively move a vertebra without moving all soft tissues attached to it, so no event, anywhere in the spine, remains completely isolated.

Because:

1. few musculoskeletal testing procedures are unequivocal (pp. 42, 46)
2. of the vagaries of referred pain, referred tenderness and spasm of muscles in areas to which pain is referred
3. there is so much overlap of dermatomes, and a fluctuation of their boundaries according to the state of facilitation at cord segments
4. sclerotome boundaries transgress axial lines, and correspond only very roughly with dermatomes
5. the innervation of vertebral structures may be derived from cord segments two, three or more distant
6. patterns of innervation may vary by prefixation and postfixation of plexuses

the greatest weight of assessment, when endeavouring to localise the segmental level of vertebral joint abnormalities, rests on what is found by palpation, and passive tests of intervertebral movement.

Many workers (i) use physiological-movement testing infrequently and place much more reliance on careful segmental examination of *accessory movement*, noting the effects of the variety of testing movements employed and which of these either reproduce or aggravate symptoms reported by the patient, and to what degree. In this way, having previously noted the history of pain behaviour during everyday functional occupations, and its behaviour and changing distribution during the regional spinal movements (single and combined) of active tests, the examiner seeks the fullest grasp of the relationships overall, that the subjective and objective effects of segmental treatment techniques may be wholly observed during subsequent assessments.

Other workers (ii) regard passive testing of *voluntary movements* (single or in combinations) as standard examination procedure, and therefore the routine mechanical basis for assessment of joint problems.

Palpation includes feeling the state of the skin surface, the superficial and deep soft tissues including muscles and attachments, the configuration of superficial and deep bony prominences, and the deeper periarticular connective tissues —*while the joints remain still.*

For appreciation of the characteristics of vertebral *movement,* methods include passive tests of: regional accessory movement; segmental accessory movement; functional or physiological movement.

The examiner should always bear in mind that palpable asymmetry of segmental contour, attitude and movements are not necessarily abnormalities — *findings must invariably be assessed in terms of their relation to the symptoms reported and signs previously observed.*

1. Palpation with joints at rest

a. *Undue tenderness.* Tenderness can be very misleading, e.g. the first rib, the clavicle and the midthoracic spinous processes in young women are naturally tender, and of no significance when this tenderness is unaccompanied by other signs or symptoms. Tenderness as such does not necessarily indicate abnormality unless, in relation to neighbouring structures of the same region, it is marked — and is accompanied by symptoms and signs reasonably associated with the marked tenderness of that structure.

Tenderness just medial to the posterior inferior iliac spine in suspected sacroiliac joint problems, for example, is of less significance when the whole of the gluteal mass is tender (probably referred tenderness) but decidedly of significance when (i) accurately localised and (ii) this positive finding is buttressed by negative findings elsewhere.

The problems of assessment are compounded by referred tenderness as well as referred pain (see p. 26) and this factor should be borne in mind.

b. *Postural spasm,* i.e. hypertonus of vertebral muscle in the static postures of sitting, standing and lying, is not as a rule localised but tends to be regional. It can be palpated in the sternomastoid and trapezius muscles, axilla-boundary muscles and the sacrospinalis, for example.

When a vertebral region is obviously fixed by postural spasm, which remains largely unchanged whether the patient is standing, sitting or lying, its

cause is likely to be a lesion whose degree of irritability is not gravity-dependent. Rarely, this may be gross facet-locking by overriding, or an apophyseal fracture, conditions requiring inpatient attention, but far more often it appears due to a localised soft tissue derangement, which can be freed by manual mobilisation.

The important point is that traction, or distractive techniques, are less likely to help in this case than in lesions whose postural fixation by spasm immediately disappears with the patient lying down. In these cases, where the degree of irritability and postural spasm is plainly gravity-dependent, distractive techniques are very likely to help, whether applied manually or mechanically, and may be the sole type of mobilisation needed.

It is wise to remember that the muscles of an area to which pain is being referred may be in a degree of postural spasm, and also that 'spasm' may be the natural expression of the patient's anxious temperament, in which case its *distribution* and degree, relative to the musculature as a whole, is the important assessment factor.

In addition to the sensory changes which accompany joint problems, there is the facilitated motor response which has been well demonstrated by Denslow.[38] Stoddard[169] observes that: 'Segmental motor reflex thresholds were determined by measuring in kilograms the amount of pressure applied to the spinous process of each segment which just evokes contraction of the paravertebral muscles at that segmental level. Muscular contractions were detected and evaluated by electromyographic recordings.' Vertebral segments showing movement abnormalities invariably required weaker stimuli than did those with normal movements.

c. *Undue bony prominence.* Complete anatomical symmetry of paired structures probably does not exist; close observation of the body contours, and palpation of the vertebral column, in a large group of healthy young people tends to confirm this impression. Cervical spinous processes are asymmetrically bifid, the lateral masses of most atlases show asymmetry, and thoracic spinous processes are very often deviated from the 'mid-line'. Less so do asymmetry of rib angles and of vertebral body laminae in the thoracic region occur, and asymmetry of the lumbar laminae is not frequent.

For this reason, undue prominence of a single rib

angle or vertebral lamina is more often than not of significance; this does not mean to say that malalignment or subluxation is thought to be present; only that there may be a degree of fixation at some point on the normal range of movement, and that in one or more of the joints of that vertebral segment or costovertebral region there are soft-tissue changes hindering free movement. When these findings exist in the absence of other signs, and there are no symptoms, treatment is certainly not merited on account of the asymmetry, unless there is a clear case for regarding the abnormality as part of an interdependent clinical entity incorporating the changes at that segment and causing symptoms in other vertebral regions. Neither is localised treatment likely to be profitable when localised changes of contour and attitude are clearly the result of long-standing adaptive shortening, although it is often of help to the patient if the mobility, and thus tissue-fluid exchange, of soft tissues are improved *adjacent* to the site of fibrotic contracture.

In general, it is wise to conservatively interpret 'undue prominence', or asymmetry of the bony structures of normal anatomy, and to be slow in ascribing vertebrogenic pain to their presence alone. The easily felt exostosis of degenerated cervical facet-joints is another matter, and this may well be significant when assessing the segmental level of joint changes giving rise to pain.

d. *Thickening*. Not surprisingly, thickening is very frequently localised over the site of painful joint problems, even though the joint itself cannot be directly palpated. It is probable indurated oedema, at times combined with a degree of capsular and ligamentous thickening due to fibrosis, although on occasions one may also be palpating the belly of small intersegmental muscles in a degree of postural spasm. Further intensification of the spasm will be produced by palpation which is too aggressive or rough, and these findings are common in the suboccipital region and at the cervicothoracic junction. When not accompanied by symptoms, painless thickening combined with a degree of movement restriction should be left alone, but see (c) above.

2. Palpation of accessory movement

a. *Diminished/increased accessory movement.* Per-

ception of diminished or increased accessory movement by manual testing requires (i) an appreciation of the wide variations of body type and normal regional range of movement, and (ii) a familiarity with the normal accessory ranges of each segment.

A normal vertebral *region* may feel generally: hard and springy; soft and yielding; soft and springy; tight, tough and unyielding.

Further, comparisons between the normal amplitude of anteroposterior *accessory* movement, e.g. of C2, C6 and C7, in the order of millimetres, can with attention and a little practice be made quite readily, and the differences would be as follows:

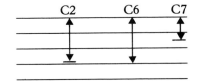

MOVEMENT

Vertebral segmental accessory movement may be *restricted*, as is often detected in tests of antereposterior gliding between proximal and distal rows or a carpus, for example, or it may be *increased*, as is frequently detected during anteroposterior gliding tests for cruciate ligament laxity at the knee, and in applying passive abduction/adduction strains of the same joint when testing for instability.

(i) If segmental accessory movement is *limited* the examiner must then ask: What is the amount of limitation? What is the nature of the limitation? Is it pain, primarily, evidenced by voluntary muscle guarding? Is it irritability, evidenced by eliciting involuntary and well-localised spasm very early in the small range of movement? Is it not so much pain, or irritability, but moderately painful restriction (felt as resistance to free movement) imposed by connective tissue thickening? Is it virtually painless and old-established fibrotic contracture? In what way, if any, are these findings related to the symptoms reported by the patient?

(ii) If segmental accessory movement is *increased*, are the testing movements painful, or painless? By how much is the movement increased? Does the increase arouse suspicion of an unstable segment?

When assessing examination findings during this fundamentally important procedure one is doing no more and no less than in exactly similar assessments being carried out by professional colleagues many hundreds of times on the same day during examination of shoulders, hips and knee joints. The findings are, as in all clinical assessments, incorporated into the larger context of the patient, the symptoms, and the unique combination of all factors so that formulation of precise individual needs may be made and treatment planned.

b. *Elicited spasm*, e.g. that provoked in response to testing movements of a reactive irritable joint, is sometimes very localised indeed, and one needs to know on which side, and to which vertebral level, it is most localised, and particularly whether the response is elicited in the early, middle or late part of the available accessory-movement range. A knowledge of what the normal regional and segmental accessory movement should be, from spine to spine, is presupposed, and the point on the range at which spasm is provoked allows an assessment of the grade to employ for the initial mobilising technique, i.e. the degree of irritability is a fundamental factor governing the grade of mobilisation.

c. *Provocation of pain and/or paraesthesiae locally and/or distally.* This provides vital information and is a valuable localising sign. As in testing voluntary movements (p. 38) the therapist seeks to reproduce or aggravate the patient's symptoms, or at least find evidence of abnormality which could be underlying them. For example, the patient's response to a regional flat-handed pressure (p. 51) may vary in that:

(i) if local guarding spasm is immediately elicited, and pressures either side of the locality do not elicit spasm, the presence of a vertebral lesion is generally confirmed, and more detailed segmental tests are indicated

(ii) if a brisk guarding response involving the whole thoracolumbar spine is elicited, pathology of a more serious nature may be present, and further tests of movement should not be made until the suitability of physical treatment has been confirmed

(iii) a slightly delayed response may indicate a wish to impress the examining therapist.

Similarly, if repetitive gentle pressure localised to the 6th thoracic spinous process provokes the submammary pain of the patient's complaint, and pressure on T5 and T7 produces slight local pain only, the joints and associated tissues likely to be responsible are those related to T6. When postero-anterior movement applied to the spinous process of L5 aggravates or provokes pins and needles in the forefoot of a sciatic limb, and the same movement applied to the fourth and third segment does not, (a) it is very likely that there is already a degree of trespass upon the root by related structures, and (b) treatment techniques should be carefully chosen so as not to further provoke the irritable root; likewise if postero-anterior unilateral pressure on the C5–C6 facet-joint provokes paraesthesiae in the forefinger of the same side.

Further, if the same kind of testing movement on C2 inferior articular process reproduces the hemicranial pain of the patient's complaint, while testing other segments on the same and opposite sides does not, it is perhaps reasonable to assume that the lesion responsible is associated with the C2–C3 segment on the side palpated, since this is the segment moved most by that particular pressure, and to treat initially on that basis. The same applies to posterior axillary and upper arm pain on palpating the second or third rib angle on the same side.

Further, if simultaneous transverse vertebral pressure in opposite directions, on the spines of two adjacent vertebrae of the painful region, provoke or aggravate the patient's pain, and no other combination of transverse pressures does this, or to such a degree, it is reasonable to assume that the segment responsible has been localised (Fig. 9.1). Postero-anterior unilateral pressures then assist localisation. In contrast to this when, in the absence of neurological signs, the uni- or bilateral upper limb 'glove paraesthesiae' diagnosed as of vertebral joint origin, are provoked by central pressure on T345 segments, this cannot be due to a C5678 somatic root involvement (other than possibly a spread of excitation by facilitation to those cord segments) but is more likely to be due to mediation via the autonomic neurones accompanying somatic nerves to the limb. Here, mobilisation of those segments by this same technique is a reasonable procedure to begin with, and it will often relieve the paraesthesiae, whatever the true explanation of the phenomenon may be.

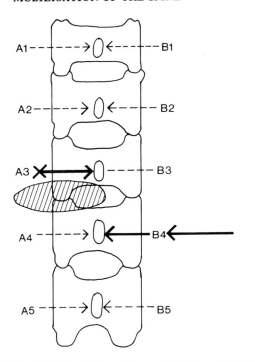

Fig. 9.1 Stabilisation of the middle vertebral spine by pressure A3, with simultaneous movement to the opposite side of the subjacent spine by pressure B4, is the only combination of pressures which provoke or aggravate the patient's pain. Frequently, transverse pressure B4 alone, in the direction indicated, and posteroanterior unilateral presure between A3 and A4 is enough.

d. *Crepitus.* This is more evident on active movement and often reported in the cervical region, occasionally at the sacroiliac joint, by patients who are anxious that the 'noisy' movement might be ominous evidence of 'the crippling disease of arthritis'. During examination by passive movement, it is sometimes felt during cervical rotation in extension, but more usually the simple act of lying down reduces crepitus-on-movement considerably.

It is probably due to the approximation and rubbing together of roughened facet-joint planes, is more subdued during rotation in flexion, and is seldom encountered in the thoracic and lumbar regions, other than the scapulo-thoracic crepitus which very frequently accompanies 'the scapulo-thoracic syndrome'. It is, however, occasionally encountered in the lax sacroiliac joints of young mothers, and indicates the need for external support.

3. Palpation during functional or physiological movement

Functional mobility varies with posture; it may not be the same in standing as it is in sitting, or lying, and may also vary with the time of day, there being less mobility early in the forenoon and in the evening, and rather more in the middle hours, as a rule.

The functional range of a vertebral 'mobility-segment', i.e. movement between two bony points of adjacent vertebrae, is difficult to detect at first, and requires long, constant and attentive practice. Movement of a typical cervical segment is perhaps the hardest to assess. Assessments of segmental mobility must take into account the different general nature of spinal movements from person to person, e.g. lax and loose jointed; tight jointed.

Movement is assessed as:

4 — Hypermobile
3 — *Normal*
2 — Reduced
1 — Trace
0 — Ankylosed.

These are assessments of mobility, and not diagnosis of the cause, for example, of what is assessed as 'ankylosis' at a segment.

Fused vertebrae are not rare in the cervical spine, or transitional vertebrae in the lumbrosacral region; further, the degree of postural gap palpated between two spinous processes in any vertebral region is not a reliable indication of the mobility of that segment. The sole criterion is the amount of movement, since assessments of postural bony-point relationship would already have been made prior to these procedures.

Technique is described on page 87.

Examples of assessment in examination

The innervation of spinal structures is especially rich and is often derived from spinal cord segments unusually remote from the innervated structure. Filaments of mixed somatic and autonomic nerves, after being formed from paravertebral plexuses outside the intervertebral foramen enter it and wander up and down the neural canal before terminating. This wandering is particularly marked in the cervical and upper thoracic spine, but occurs in other regions too.

Because of this diversity and richness of innervation, the nature and volume of the afferent impulse traffic from vertebral receptors is also rich. The upper cervical spine is especially important in this respect (see p. 88). Voluntary movement is only as good as reflexogenic efficiency, and these arthrokinetic reflexes are disturbed by changes in joints which are degenerating, as evidenced by abnormalities of movement.

Therefore, when transverse vertebral pressure to the left, for example, on C2 spinous process provokes the upper left-sided neck pain and suboccipital pain of the patient's complaint, we have provoked it by disturbing at least *two* 'mobility segments', i.e. C1–C2 and C2–C3. We have disturbed, in asymmetrical ways, soft tissues at those two levels on the patient's right and the patient's left. We have also disturbed the attachments of muscle bellies which may span several segments, connective tissue structures spanning neighbouring regions and, in the foramen transversarium, the vertebral artery with its sympathetic plexus destined for distribution to intracranial structures.

The muscles will include scalenus medius, the inter-transversarii, semispinalis cervicis, longus colli, rectus capitis posterior, rectus capitis anterior and lateralis, and obliquus capitis inferior.

Connective tissue structures will include joint capsules, the apical ligament, alar ligaments, accessory atlantoaxial ligaments, anterior and posterior longitudinal ligaments and the ligamentum nuchae.

We canot ignore the structural, functional and neural interdependence of the vertebral column; it is a constant factor underlying clinical presentation (see p. 114), and further, a constant factor to be borne in mind when examining, assessing, choosing techniques and formulating plans of treatment.

After other tests we seek by palpation irritability, elicited spasm, diminished or increased accessory movement, provocation of pain and paraesthesiae — we are trying to reproduce the symptoms reported by the patient, and if we can do that we have usually localised the focus of the abnormality. We have found the segment(s) responsible, although we may not understand precisely *how* they are responsible.

Here are two examples of palpation findings. In Figure 9.2 a patient complaining only of *left* occipital

pain is found to have a prominent, thickened and very tender *right* lateral mass of atlas, movement of which aggravates the pain, with much less tenderness at C2 and C3 on the same side, slight tenderness at C1, C2 and C3 on the *opposite, left side,* and at C2 and C3 centrally. Had we palpated down the *left side first*, and accepted without question that the stiff, thickened and slightly tender C2 and C3 segments were responsible for the left-sided occipital pain, even though testing did not provoke this, we might not have discovered that the left-sided headache was provoked or reproduced only by unilateral movement of C1 on the *right*. If localised right-sided movement of C1 provokes the left-sided occipital headache, and left-sided movement of C2 and C3 does not, then the important segment to initially mobilise is C1 on the right, not C2/3 on the left. The left-sided stiffness at C2/3 is something of a red herring in this particular clinical presentation, and we are likely to get the patient out of pain sooner by attending to the movement *which accurately reproduces the pain*, than by working on the assumption that the C2/3 stiffness ought to be responsible for the symptoms. We have listened to whàt the joints are telling us, and we have assessed which are the treatment priorities.

To complete the full treatment of that patient one should attend to the stiffened C2/3 segment on the left, after the greatest progress in relieving the patient's headache has been achieved, yet the stiffness may be very old and virtually irreversible; consequently vigorous mobilisation or manipulation may only hurt the patient without profit, and the decision must then rest on whether a painless functional range of upper cervical movement has been rendered possible, as evidenced by repalpation and active tests with overpressure. If these show that further improvement in ranges of movement can be achieved by mobilising C2/3 on the left, the treatment is indicated, but when to stop is as important as when to start (see p. 181).

Referring once more to the example given, had we not been able to provoke the left occipital pain by moving C1 on the right, it would have been proper to accept the left-sided stiffness of C2–C3 as the cause and to begin treatment there, subsequently being guided by assessment of effects.

In the second example (Fig. 9.3), the slight tenderness at C123 on the right side is of no great

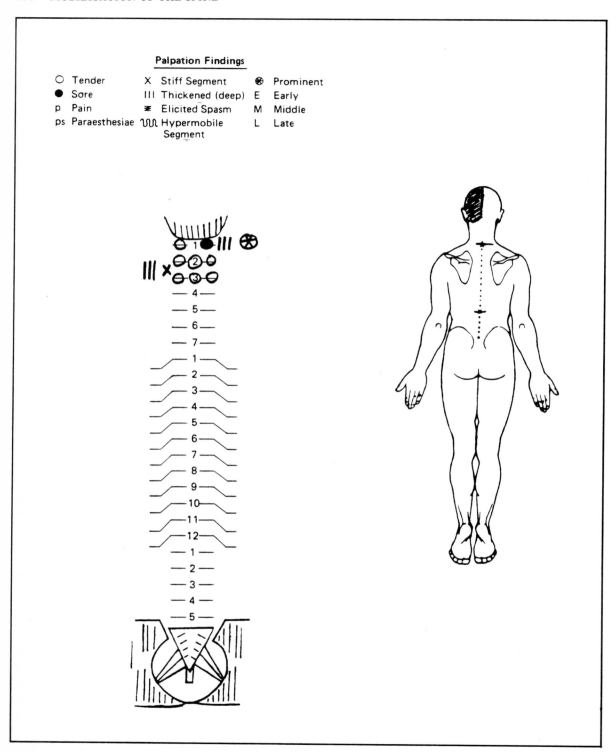

Fig. 9.2. Chart of palpation findings in a patient with headache (see text).

significance, because we find that unilateral movement of the thickened, tender and prominent C2–C3 segments on the left immediately reproduce the left hemicranial pain, whereas right unilateral movement does not. It is clearly indicated to mobilise C2–C3 on the left, in the appropriate grade. Thus, when assessing the segmental locality of the changes underlying clinical features, our first priority is, 'How can we reproduce them?', and if, despite a careful search, we are unable to do this, we should then proceed on the basis of, 'Which segmental changes have we found which are most likely to be responsible?', and the search for these may require testing physiological ranges, too.

Mention has been made of slightly altering the direction of vertebral pressure techniques, when examining, i.e. a little caudally, cranially, medially or laterally.

When examining the consequence of degenerative joint disease, we come upon the clearest and most potent expression of the abnormality existing by subtle changes in how we apply the localised testing movements; adding a little bias in one direction or another often makes all the difference between a fairly relaxed, inert patient allowing testing movement to continue, and the sharp response of involuntary muscle guarding to protect a highly reactive joint, *which is most sensitive to that movement with that bias*.

We may now conceive the view that we do not treat 'mechanical joint problems' so much as *movement abnormalities, highly individualised from patient to patient* —radiological appearances and theories of biomechanics notwithstanding (see p. 9).

The more attentive, searching and subtle is examination, the more comprehensive our grasp of how they are uniquely presenting. This does not mean we know any more about 'why?', only that we have a better insight into what we are trying to deal with, using treatment methods which themselves are based on movements of one kind, or degree, and another.

When looking for the site of what frequently transpires to be 'reversible diminished movement due to soft tissue changes' (p. 120) expressed as 'limitation', 'restriction' or 'blocking', we must be able to distinguish between hypomobility and hypermobility. Aside from considerations of why it

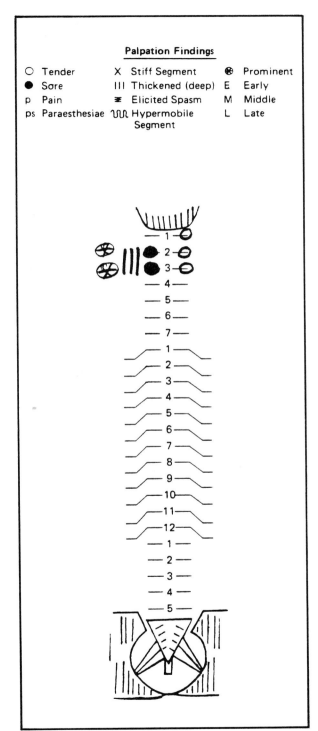

Fig. 9.3 Chart palpation findings in a patient with headache (see text).

is so, tenderness and pain may arise from both a hypermobile and a hypomobile segment. The latter we try to reverse, the former is certainly not a case for grade V manipulation techniques, although we can significantly reduce pain and irritability by gentle, repetitive mobilisation which is kept well within the normal movement range of adjacent segments.

In a small proportion of cases, the testing of *accessory* movements may be insufficient to fully elucidate the nature of a joint problem, and it is necessary to palpate each segment while passively performing the normal active movements of rotation, side-flexion, flexion and extension (p. 87–95) —we are not now concerned with accessory movements, and these tests may sometimes be necessary to clarify questions of whether restricted or increased movement of vertebral segments is essentially the change which underlies the clinical features.

Again, in middle-aged men reporting a lumbar ache, there is clearly reason to assume that these symptoms *do* arise from the vertebral joints, yet there seems to be no great tenderness, no elicited spasm, no hypermobility and no undue thickening or prominence, and physiological movement tests are occasionally necessary to clarify the site of diminished movement. These tests are usually more necessary at or near the junctional regions of the spine than the segments between (see p. 113). We should observe that workers of much academic and clinical experience naturally tend to rely on examination methods to which they have become accustomed and by which they work to the best effect.

When testing vertebral segments, different abnormalities can be detected by a sense of tissue-tension, or 'end-feel', and they can be classified as types (see below) familiar to all experienced workers, whatever may be their preferred palpation methods. The differences can be apparent to one worker employing accessory-movement tests only for the majority of patients, because he is experienced in interpreting findings in this particular way. Another will assess the type of 'end-feel' by the routine use of passive physiological-movement tests only, or combinations of them, sometimes reserving the moment of greatest attention to the 'feel' of movement limitation after positioning the segment for a particular technique and just prior to performing the final manipulative thrust.

Yet another will place the greatest reliance on the particular pattern and degree of voluntary movement restriction, employing palpation routinely but in a general way and not necessarily deriving precise treatment indications from palpation.

The latter may tend as a rule to employ regional manipulations (see p. 143) as the main therapeutic basis.

Perceiving the nature of factors limiting movement

Distinguishing between *types* of movement limitation is easy when handling normal mobile peripheral joints, e.g. the abrupt stop when testing full extension of elbow or knee is quite different to the squashy feel of soft-tissue approximation when the same joints are flexed to their limit.

As MacConaill[119] has shown, flexed joints are 'loose-packed' and movement is limited by soft-tissue contact, whereas extension movements are limited by 'close-packing', when the female surface is in most complete congruence with the male surface, the capsule and ligaments are in maximal tension and it is difficult, although not impossible, to separate the bones by traction.[179] A moment's examination of the close-packed humeroulnar joint in fullest extension reveals that a measure of accessory abduction and adduction range can still be passively produced, without releasing the degree of extension —the limit of extreme movement is always something of a moveable feast (see pp. 37, 40) and this ability to accurately assess, by observation and by feeling, what is normal and abnormal in peripheral joint movement is served basically by applied anatomical knowledge, the assessment becoming more accurate with clinical experience; this too applies to the vertebral joints.

a. *On giving overpressure at the extremes of voluntary movement of spinal regions.* The 'end-feel' in normal young subjects is mostly that of soft-tissue tension, i.e. the combined resistance in varying degrees of muscle with its attachment-tissues, fascial planes, ligaments, joint capsules and the annulus fibrosus of discs. We know, for example, that the main limiting factors in sagittal lumbar movement is the annulus, although other soft tissues are put on tension; rotation and side-flexion of the three regions, with flexion of the lumbar and thoracic regions, have an elastic resistance to manual attempts to increase range, and the precise end-of-range is difficult to pinpoint; however, comparison between sides allows assessment, and range abnormalities can readily be perceived on over-pressure, if not by simple observation beforehand, or both.

That cervical and thoracic extension are limited by bone-to-bone contact (or cartilage-covered bone contact, in the normal) and not especially by soft-tissue tension, cannot fully be perceived manually because all one can feel is a somewhat harder and less elastic stop to the movement, although a degree of elastic resilience remaining is easily detected.

Gently forcing cervical extension produces unpleasant discomfort before a solid limitation, if a normal subject allows this degree of questing. Cervical flexion is limited by approximation of mandible and sternum compressing the soft tissue between, yet movement can be continued for a few degrees as the posterior vertebral tissues are stretched by the "beer-handle' effect of pressing downwards on the occiput.

Craniovertebral extension is limited by the posterior edge of the atlantal facets engaging the condylar fossae of the occiput; the same movement is limited at the cervicothoracic junction by the inferior articular processes of C7 engaging horizontal grooves below and behind the superior facets of T1. Thoracic extension is limited by contact of inferior articular processes with the laminae below, and by contact of the spinous processes.

At the thoracolumbar junctional region, a 'mortise' effect is produced in full extension by engagement of the articular facets of T11 and T12 (sometimes T12 and L1) and this is one of the few articular mechanisms in the body where a practically solid bony-contact lock occurs at the extreme of movement.[34]

Practically all other so-called bone-to-bone locks, with the exception of dental occlusion and lumbar rotation in neutral or extension, occur to a degree only.

b. *When testing vertebral accessory-movement ranges by rhythmic pressures against the bony prominences available to palpation*, with the patient lying prone in a neutral position, the anatomical and functional criteria governing *voluntary-movement*

assessments do not apply on a one-to-one basis at each segment. (See Figs. 2.5, 2.6 p. 10.)

For example, (i) the 35°–45° range of rotation at C1–C2 is not reflected in the degree of movement palpable on postero-anterior pressure on the C2 spinous process—the odontoid prevents this—and to appreciate the limit of available range of rotation it is necessary to turn the patient's head through 90°, and feel how far short of this amplitude the spine of C2 has moved. Nevertheless, should voluntary cervical rotation to one side be limited to 30° or less, by pain arising from changes at the C1–C2 segment of that side, this will be very accurately reflected in the ease with which involuntary spasm and voluntary muscle guarding are provoked on applying unilateral pressures to C1 on the painful side, and transverse pressures to the spine of C2 towards the painful side, with the patient lying in the neutral position.

Again, (ii) in the presence of pain referred forward to the pectoral region and breast which is arising from thoracic joint changes at interscapular levels, cursory examination of voluntary thoracic movement does not invariably reveal positive signs, neither does overpressure at the limit of the customary regional movements always reveal abnormality.

Limitation at individual segments is sometimes concealed from detection during observation of regional movements, only to be revealed on searchng tests of *combined movements* (see p. 93), or more surely on careful and systematic palpation at segments T345.

Further, (iii) stiffness spanning three mobility segments between L1 and L4 is often detectable by careful observation of the patient's back during active tests, but not invariably so, yet after active tests which may be somewhat inconclusive, a flat-handed downward pressure on the lumbar region declares the probability at once, and segmental palpation confirms it.

IMPORTANCE OF JUNCTIONAL REGIONS

With a step-by-step process of exclusion, beginning with the history and proceeding through observation, active-movement tests, regional and then segmental palpation, the essential purpose of examination is to precisely localise the source of symptoms reported. Assessment of the *presentation* of the movement abnormality, i.e. how it is manifesting itself, then provides the guide for action, even though we may not be able to know all we would like about its true nature.

Self-education in the accurate localisation of spinal joint problems is probably the most important single aspect for the beginner to develop following training courses; one learns the importance of going like a dog after a cat for the *precise level* of vertebral involvement. Sooner or later, however, depending upon the 'mileage' of patients treated, it will become evident that the interdependence of the vertebral column is asserting itself in various ways, e.g.

1. Postero-anterior unilateral movement of T1 or the first rib provoking the unilateral hemicranial pain reported by the patient
2. Cervical rotation and side-flexion restrictions disappearing on mobilisation of T1
3. Lumbar side-flexion improving on mobilisation of the sacroiliac joint of that side
4. The frequency with which patients report with concurrent upper cervical and lumbosacral joint problems
5. The frequency with which the so-called carpal tunnel syndrome is accompanied by ipsilateral joint problems at the upper ribs and/or low cervical spine
6. The even greater frequency with which unilateral occipito-atlantal joint problems co-exist with lesions of the third rib on the same side
7. The combined presentation of L3–4, or L4–5, lesions with ipsilateral sacro-iliac dysfunction. Lumbar mobilisation relieves the lumbar articular signs and limited ipsilateral straight-leg-raising, but techniques localised to the sacro-iliac joint are necessary to relieve the haunch pain provoked by extremes of hip movement, even though internal hip rotation is freer than the normal side when tested in the neutral position. Internal rotation at 90° flexion is painful at the end of range and a bit limited, as are flexion and combined flexion/adduction.

There are many further examples of this phenomenon, simple explanations of which are always attractive; one could analyse (1) on the basis of scalenus muscle spasm, since the scalenus medius

has partial attachment to C2 above and to the first rib below, and analyse (4) on the basis that should the foundation of a structure be disturbed its most superincumbent parts are likely to be affected most. Since the craniovertebral articulation is a prime organ of equilibration, the analogy is a reasonable one, whatever the biomechanical and neurophysiological mechanisms may prove to be when comprehensive analysis ultimately becomes possible.

The analogy does not take into account, of course, whether the craniovertebral abnormality might have developed first, with subsequent effects upon more distant but interdependent segments.

Further to (1) above, Frykholm[59] describes the observation that many patients with brachialgia, due to a cervical rib, have also suffered from cervical migraine, which was relieved by adequate decompression of the brachial plexus.

While the treatment of the segments giving rise to pain remains the priority, a careful check of the junctional regions and subsequent attention to any movement abnormalities found can be worthwhile, since the more comprehensive the examination and the treatment, the less do the problems seem to recur.

Lewit[111] stresses the fact that 'we always have to restore the function of a chain of disturbances and it is next to impossible to be certain which link of this chain is the most important in each individual case.' Thus, the further we progress in this work, the more apparent becomes the vital issue of *assessment*, as each problem is unique.

PROGNOSIS

Examination findings allow an assessment of the length of treatment likely to be required. Aches and pains of moderate intensity localised to vertebral and paravertebral regions, with little or no reference to limbs and no neurological involvement, may often be significantly reduced by treatment counted in days rather than in weeks.

Experience with manipulative treatment shows that it is rarely sufficient to mobilise the affected joint on one occasion only. The number of treatments required varies enormously from patient to patient.[13]

The need for periodic medical treatment of diseases with episodic exacerbations, like chronic bronchitis for example, is unquestioned, yet the similar need for periodic attention to a like disease, which also has existence in time as well as space, i.e. vertebral degenerative joint disease, is seemingly not understood as plainly as it should be. For some, it seems that manipulation means getting everything tidied up with one expertly applied manipulative thrust, and anything other than this is not properly manipulative treatment.

This is not true. Progress is likely to be slow in the following situations:

1. When there is a localised distal area of objective numbness
2. When there is marked muscle wasting, as a consequence of degenerative joint disease
3. When there is severe limb pain, or when the worst pain is more distal than proximal
4. When pain is sufficiently severe to produce facial distortion
5. When neurological deficit indicates involvement of the following nerve roots (in order of difficulty): L3, S1, S2. Patients with neurological signs from L4 and L5 are easier to relieve
6. Where postural spasm is maintaining:
   a. a lumbar spine deviation towards the painful side, or
   b. marked lordosis on attempted flexion, or
   c. a flattening of the lumbar curve, or
   d. a frank lumbar kyphosis.
7. When extension is grossly limited, and either produces or exacerbates arm or leg pain
8. When straight-leg-raising is severely restricted unilaterally and especially bilaterally
9. If palpation at a single vertebral level elicits brisk protective spasm over a much wider area
10. Where symptoms are felt locally *and* referred, from one acutely tender spinous process
11. Long-standing cases
12. Result of recent trauma
13. Moderate or severe whiplash injury during last three to four years
14. Juniors and adolescents.

The nature of pain is a further factor in duration of treatment. A generalised ache or a restrictive nuisance is more quickly relieved than is a throbbing intense pain, or a shooting, stabbing pain.

N.B. It is uncommon for spinal joint problems to be single and where multiple problems require careful analysis and appropriate treatment, relief cannot be achieved by the facile production of a single joint 'click'.

Some other common fallacies are:

1. That the obese patient is more prone to discogenic lumbar joint problems, and to recurrences, than is the slimmer person.
2. That postural asymmetry of the pelvic joints must *necessarily* be responsible, sooner or later, for low back pain; it is more than likely, but not inevitable.
3. That in suitable cases a corrective heel raise, for patients well over 40 who have chronic lumbar pain due to a laterally tilted pelvis, cannot quickly relieve intractable symptoms; the prognosis need not be gloomy in these cases, simply because the patient is mature.
4. That joint conditions of sudden onset are invariably easier to relieve than those of insidious onset; this is by no means true.
5. That the longer a joint problem has existed, the more difficult it will be to relieve. This is not always true.
6. That restricted straight-leg-raising indicates discogenic trespass upon a root of the lumbosacral plexus, and that the prognosis is therefore that of neurological involvement.
7. That provocation of the unilateral midlumbar and anterior thigh pain by the 'femoral nerve stretch test' is corroboration of an irritative lesion of a root of the femoral nerve, and justifies a like prognosis.

A retrospective analysis of 146 patients with 'whiplash' injuries, after 5 years, indicated that there was a statistically significant correlation between poor treatment results and the following findings soon after injury:

(i) Numbness or pain, or both, in an upper limb
(ii) A sharp reversal of cervical lordosis visible on X-ray
(iii) Restricted motion at one segment on 'bending' films
(iv) The need for a collar for more than three months
(v) The need to resume physiotherapy more than once because of a recurrence of symptoms.[86]

While low back pain accompanied by listing or deviation, but without limb pain or neurological symptoms and signs, can significantly be improved in under four days,[125]a previous history of more than three similar episodes, a gradual onset of symptoms, delay in reporting symptoms and pain radiation beyond the knee all suggest a long or relapsing course.

NEOPLASMS

The recognition of neoplastic disease, earlier rather than later, depends more on awareness, vigilance and suspicion rather than a set of rules. One must *always* be thinking of it, all the time and every time. Whenever it is confirmed, tracking back on the clinical features, or lack of them, may sometimes reveal where history-taking or physical examination might have been more attentive or more comprehensive.

The factors which may provide warning of the possibility of neoplastic disease could be summarised as follows:

1. Occipital pain which is aggravated on neck-flexion but which is not accompanied by vertebral movement-limitation and in which palpable signs of upper vertebral involvement are absent.
2. The 'globally' rigid cervical spine with all movements greatly reduced, in the absence of trauma and other factors significant enough to warrant the clinical articular signs.
3. The combination of shoulder girdle pain, neurological signs in the distribution of C8–T1 and Horner's syndrome.
4. Thoracic pain which is accompanied by lower limb pain and/or a bizarre distribution of unpleasant paraesthesiae in lower limbs (Fig. 9.4). This may be discogenic or neoplastic. The majority of vertebral neoplasms occur in the thoracic spine, and pain in the body wall together with bizarre limb symptoms should alert the therapist at once.
5. Severe intractable pain accompanying muscle spasm and vertebral deformity in young people. Sciatic scoliosis is not invariably a simple joint problem.

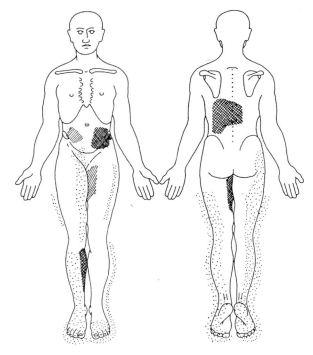

Fig. 9.4 The bizarre distribution of pain in thorax, abdomen and in both legs, and extensive extra-segmental bilateral paraesthesiae of an unpleasant kind, in lower limbs, is strongly suggestive of a neoplasm in the thoracic region. Presentation is not always as florid, so one must be awake at all times, with a high index of suspicion.

6. Disturbing or more severe and inexorable pain at night, in middle age or later, unrelieved by resting and uninfluenced by changing position of trunk or limbs.
7. Meralgia paraesthetica which is accompanied by intractable pain at night.
8. Backache in a patient with a known history of malignancy during the past two years.
9. Sciatic pain with bizarre extrasegmental sensory symptoms, and neurological deficit, but no backache.
10. Backache with pronounced loss of hip flexor power is always suspect.
11. The spontaneous onset of backache in late middle age, in the absence of a previous history of back pain, is more likely to be due to osteoporosis or malignant disease than to benign joint problems.

12. Pain which is severe enough to be uninfluenced by the usual analgesics, and requires morphia for more than 48 hours, is likely to indicate malignancy.
13. Persistent backache which is not quietened or reduced by rest, and not influenced by posture. The older the patient, the more is malignancy suspect.
14. Shock, vomiting and loss of spinal function following a trivial jolt or stress; the cause is likely to be pathological fracture.
15. Back pain with weakness, sphincter disturbance, malaise and pyrexia.
16. Back pain with marked difficulty in walking, in the presence of normal foot, ankle, knee and hip joint function.
17. The coexistence of back pain and ankle clonus, with a normal range of straight-leg-raising.

10

Principles of treatment

Although largely benign and eventually self-limiting, degenerative joint disease of the spine resembles chronic respiratory disease, in that its slow progression over many decades is marked by exacerbations which are frequently related to functional, environmental and other stresses; as in the management of chronic bronchitis, for example, treatment aims must be realistically assessed against the known natural history of the disease.

In clinical practice, the classical division between conservative and radical treatment becomes less important as the combined skills of the medical, surgical and paramedical team are applied to help the patient. Consequently, treatment methods are marshalled under the headings of general principles, one of which may be the guide for medical, physiotherapy, and surgical procedures. For example, in the management of three patients, *relief of pain* is the dominant reason for the three treatments of:

— medical prescription of analgesic drugs
— carefully graded manual mobilisation to the vertebral segment
— surgical removal of prolapsed disc material or overgrowth of bone for relief of severe root pain by decompression.

Again the principle of *stabilisation* of a vertebral segment may underlie:

— provision of a supportive collar for the neck
— exercises to strengthen the abdominal wall muscles in low back pain
— segmental strengthening of intrinsic muscle like rotatores and multifidus
— surgical fusion (arthrodesis) of an unstable segment.

Further, one method of treatment may meet different requirements; for instance, while support in the form of a stiff cervical collar may temporarily or semipermanently *stabilise* a painless but dangerously unstable segment, for which surgical fusion may not be feasible, for another patient the purpose of a soft collar is to *ease the pain of an irritable spinal segment by resting it* for a short period, or to provide support at times of particular stress such as long car rides, long sessions of embroidery, house decoration or cleaning windows.

AIMS OF TREATMENT

The primary treatment aim is restoration of normal painless joint range by:

1. Relief of pain and reduction of muscle spasm
2. Restoration of normal tissue-fluid exchange, soft-tissue pliability and extensibility, and normal joint mobility
3. Correction of muscle weakness or imbalance
4. The stabilisation of unstable segments
5. The restoration of adequate control of movement
6. Relief from chronic postural or occupational stress
7. Functional reablement of the patient
8. Prevention of recurrence
9. Restoration of confidence and the teaching of self-help.

The aims will assume differing orders of importance between individuals.

The following tabulated list, which is not exhaustive, is arranged as examples of method to indicate the variety of ways in which the principles of treatment may be applied.

Relief of pain

Injection of	*Surgical*
—local anaesthetic	Epidural injection
—hydrocortisone	Chymopapain injection
Oral analgesic and/or	Rhyzolysis:
anti-inflammatory drugs	(i) by stab injection
Heat—SWD	(ii) by radio-frequency
—MWD	Anaesthetic injection into
Ice	facet-joint spaces
Ultrasound	Disc fenestration
Ethyl chloride spray	Disc enucleation
Interferential therapy	Decompression
Rest	Fusion by arthrodesis
Support	
Massage, e.g. inhibitory pressures	
Connective tissue massage	
Mobilisation	
Stretching	
Post-isometric relaxation techniques	
Manipulation	
Traction	
Acupuncture	
Operant conditioning	
Electro-analgesia	
Counter-irritation	
Manual/mechanical vibration	

Movement

Active mobility exercises	*Surgical*
—regional	Joint manipulation under
—segmental	anaesthesia
Hydrotherapy	Nerve root stretch under
Massage	epidural and/or general
Mobilisation	anaesthesia
Stretching	
Post-isometric relaxation techniques	
Manipulation	
Traction	
—manual	
—mechanical	

Stabilisation

Support	*Surgical*
Muscle-strengthening exercises	Fusion
—regional	Sclerosant injection
—segmental	
Correction of muscle imbalance	

Postural correction

Passive stretching of contracted	*Surgical*
soft tissue	Cervicolordodesis[17]
Active exercises to stretch	
contracted tissues	
Re-education by postural exercises	
Correction of sleeping posture	
Persuasive correction of lateral	
spinal deviation	
Unilateral heel raise, for example	

Functional reablement

Restoration of confidence	*Surgical*
Job analysis	Postoperative rehabilitation
Ergonomic correction of	
—work posture	
—driving posture	
—lifting and handling	
Prophylactic advice	

Because the common vertebral (and peripheral) joint problems are, in the main, abnormalities of movement for one reason or another, it follows that treatments involving the application of movement would form the lynchpin of therapeutic methods, together with one or more associated treatments; it is for this reason that treatment by movement forms the bulk of the methods described in this text.

Common vertebral joint problems, and more especially low back pain, comprise by far the most costly ailment of modern society.

While there is a gratifying increase in recognition of the value of manipulative and allied procedures, *a much more important development is recognition of the potential of informed and experienced manipulative therapists working ethically as part of the medical team.*

Mooney and Cairns[143] emphasise this aspect:

We believe that there is a role for passive assisted joint mobilisation (manipulation?) by the therapist. There is every reason to expect that a joint unable to proceed through its full anatomic range is abnormal. If mobilisation by manual therapy can increase this range, the joint should benefit. If this is the only therapeutic manoeuvre it is a short-sighted one, but when incorporated into a progressive exercise program focused on improving function and enhancing strength and endurance, it has a useful role. Physical therapists functioning in a responsible medical environment offer the greatest potential for this manoeuvre to be pursued in an ethical setting wherein comparison of results with other methods can be challenged.

The pace and degree of degenerative changes in joints and their associated tissues differ widely from person to person, and in general terms the morphological changes of degeneration have little direct relationship to the amount of pain or functional disablement suffered by an individual at any particular time. Consequently, so far as physical treatment is concerned, a *working hypothesis* may be stated as a set of principles:

1. There is relatively little relationship between radiologically evident degenerative change and the symptoms reported by the patient.
2. There is a very close relationship between *loss of function, or abnormal function,* and signs and symptoms.
3. Loss of function is very frequently found at sites other than those of degenerative change as such.
4. Chronic degenerative changes will remain when normal function consistent with age is restored, and symptoms are partially or completely relieved.
5. Loss of function is, for the most part, manifested in terms of abnormalities of movement.
6. Treatment is directed, in the main, to *states of reversible diminished movement due to soft-tissue changes,* with their consequences; but also at times to mild degrees of hypermobility.
7. Methods are essentially regional and localised movement (including traction) begun and graded according to examination findings.
8. Syndromes of instability are treated by measures to stabilise vertebral segments.

GROUPING OF TECHNIQUES

Because every joint movement, whether active or passive, also affects the soft tissues; almost every soft tissue technique disturbs joints to a greater or lesser degree; the grouping of treatment methods is often governed by treatment rationale rather than by the actual nature of the movement, *there is no universally acceptable arrangement of the various categories.*

For commonly used procedures, descriptive terms and phrases may vary between groups of workers and from country to country, e.g. the word 'manipulation' may for one group refer specifically to localised thrust techniques of short amplitude and high velocity, while for another national group the word may be used mainly as a general term covering *any* manual or mechanically applied movement of body parts. Again, the one word may correctly be employed in either the general or the specific sense. The same applies to the word 'mobilisation', of course. Plainly, there are three main categories of this method:

Passive movement

Any movement mechanically or manually applied to a body part, with no voluntary muscular activity by the patient. Such treatment therefore includes:
1. Massage of soft tissue
2. Maintenance movement
3. Mobilisation
4. Manipulation
5. Persuasive, sustained correction of lateral spinal deviation
6. Stretching (A) —see also stretching (B) in 'Massage' on p. 122
7. Traction (see 'auto-traction' under active Movement)

Manually assisted or manually resisted active movements

1. Self-correction of spinal deviation by active exercises with hand placement to assist performance (p. 188)
2. Post-isometric relaxation techniques (p. 188).

Active movements

1. Regional or localised active exercises (p. 198)
2. Auto-traction for the cervical, thoracic and lumbar spines, by manual effort (p. 211)
3. Actively-imposed sustained or repetitive stretch of shortened soft tissues

---

That 'soft tissue' (see p. 121) appears under both passive and active movement categories illustrates the difficulties of classification, yet one is an imposed movement to relaxed tissues and the other is an active, sustained exercise.

11

Passive movement

Definitions are given below for terms used in this text:

1. *Massage:* Passive movement of soft tissues, usually manually but sometimes mechanically applied

2. *Maintenance movement:* Passive movement to preserve existing joint mobility, soft tissue extensibility, and kinaesthesis, where voluntary movement is not possible or is temporarily undesirable.

3. *Mobilisation:* The attempted restoration of full painless joint function by rhythmic, repetitive passive movements to the patient's tolerance, in voluntary and/or accessory range *and graded according to examination findings.* The patient is at all times able to stop the movement if so wished. This may affect a whole vertebral region or be localised so far as is possible to a single segment

4. *Manipulation:* An accurately localised, single, quick and decisive movement of small amplitude, following careful positioning of the patient. It is not necessarily energetic, and is completed before the patient can stop it. The manipulation may have a regional or a more localised effect, depending upon the technique of positioning the patient.

5. *Correction of lateral deviation:* Persuasive techniques in which the standing patient's pelvis is manually stabilised while sustained pressure is applied, in the coronal plane, to the patient's trunk via the therapist's trunk.

6. *Stretching (A):* Sustained or rhythmically intermittent force applied manually or mechanically to one aspect of a body part, to distract the attachments of shortened soft tissue. Both the therapist's hands are in firm contact with bony points providing attachments for the shortened tissue.

See Stretching (B) under 'Massage'.

7. *Traction:* Sustained or rhythmically intermittent force, manually or mechanically applied in the longitudinal axis of a body part, and thus to all aspects of it.

It may also be arranged so that the emphasis of distraction is to the posterior, anterior or unilateral aspect of an intervertebral joint.

In 1–7 there should be no voluntary muscular activity by the patient, although involuntary spasm (either postural or elicited by movement) is often present and may be the reason for treatment.

1. MASSAGE: MOBILISATION OF SOFT TISSUES

In the final analysis, all movement techniques whether mobilisation, stretching, manipulation or traction, are movements of the soft tissues, and the justification for a separate classification is to draw attention to the prime importance of including techniques which have the specific purpose of improving the vascularity and extensibility of the soft tissues.

Because:

(i) Normal muscle function is dependent upon normal joint movement
(ii) Impaired muscle function perpetuates and may cause deterioration in abnormal joints
(iii) Muscles cannot be restored to normal if the joints which they habitually move are not free to move

the treatment of joint disturbances should include measures which relax *muscle* and restore its normal vascularity and extensibility, while restoration of *normal painless joint range* remains the primary treatment aim. The classical use of massage, as a method of relieving pain, promoting relaxation and the reduction of muscle spasm, reducing swelling and improving circulation must be as old as pain itself, and is well described in many texts.

Similarly, the importance of deep transverse frictions and the technique of their application are described by their innovator, Dr James Cyriax.[32]

The following description of treatment methods for soft tissue is restricted to those which are commonly employed in the management of vertebral joint problems:

a. Stroking
b. Stretching (B)
c. Inhibitory pressure
d. Kneading
e. Vibration
f. Frictions
g. Connective tissue massage

a. *Stroking, or effleurage,* may be firmly and deeply applied with the greatest possible area of hand contact, to relieve fluid congestion of a body part, but is more usually employed as a method of inducing relaxation in a tense, anxious patient. A minute or two spent in slow, rhythmic stroking over a region of muscle spasm is often worthwhile, since it not only allows time for the patient to begin settling down but also gives the therapist an opportunity to become more familiar with the state and texture of the soft tissues.

b. *Stretching (B)* is applied either along the length of a muscle or transversely across its belly, and while the technique is called muscle stretching it will be plain that all musculoskeletal soft tissues are influenced by it in varying degrees. Distinguished from Stretching (A) because the therapist's hands, fingers and thumbs remain in contact with soft tissue only.

In longitudinal stretching techniques, the slow, deep finger, thumbpad or heel-of-hand traction movements are rhythmically applied with the body part disposed so that elongation of muscle and connective tissue is possible; when giving transverse stretching movements across muscle bellies, the same disposition of the patient is necessary.

c. *Inhibitory pressure.* With the patient com-

fortably disposed and the attachments of the hypertonic muscle(s) approximated, pressure is applied over the belly of the muscle by finger or thumbpad, thenar or hypothenar eminence. Pressure is slowly increased and as slowly relaxed, after a minute or so of sustained contact. Pressure may be repeated at the same locality or on an adjacent section of the muscle, and is continued until the palpable contraction is felt to relax, or it becomes plain that the hypertonicity will not respond to this particular technique.

d. *Kneading and petrissage* are not dissimilar in that both techniques are directed to improving the tissue-fluid exchange, vascularity and normal texture of subcutaneous and deep soft tissue. The various manipulations all have the quality of alternate traction, picking-up or squeezing and relaxing movements of a localised mass of tissue held between fingers and thumbs, or between hypothenar eminences; a muscle mass is treated by handling small sections of it at a time until the whole region has been treated (Fig. 11.1). The method may be combined with stretching (which is only a regional variant of kneading) or with inhibitory pressures, and an important effect is that of assisting muscular and general relaxation.

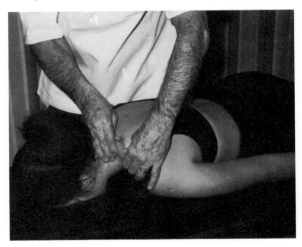

Fig. 11.1 Soft-tissue technique. Mobilising the soft tissues of trapezius.

e. *Vibrations* may be applied by fingertips, but effective technique is difficult to acquire and requires long practice; further, the method is less suitable for the large muscle masses of the trunk and limb girdles, and since a powered vibrator is much easier to use as well as being effective, it seems sensible to employ one.

f. *Frictions* may be applied transversely to the localised attachment points of muscle, tendon, aponeurosis and ligament, or in a firm fashion with thumbpad or heel of hand along an extensive bony attachment such as the iliac crest (Fig. 11.2).

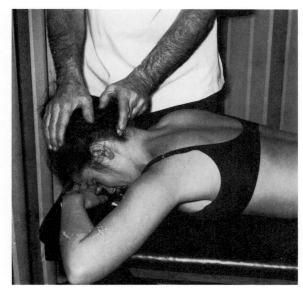

Fig. 11.2 Transverse friction to aponeurotic attachments of muscle at the nuchal line of the occiput.

g. *Connective tissue massage.* Superficial soft tissue manipulation, by rhythmic and carefully applied fingertip traction strokes, can achieve physiological and therapeutic effects which are difficult to explain[44], other than on the basis of somatic and visceral structures sharing a common segmental neurone pool in the spinal cord.

In this connection, it is important not to overlook the rich and varied innervation of the one structure which lies between us and our environment, i.e. the skin with its superficial connective tissues, together with its equally rich central nervous system connections.

Careful palpation of superficial structures reveals areas of tightness and hyperaesthesia which are often unknown to the patient, and which when appropriately treated by the stroking techniques can improve the blood supply of extremities and assist in the treatment of back pain.

The zones for treatment are based to a degree upon the topography of Head's Zones (p. 21).

N.B. The benefits of improved vascularity, tissue-fluid exchange and restoration of normal extensibility may well be an important factor in the therapeutic effects of treatments like regional mobilisation, specific mobilisation or rhythmic traction, although there is no absolute certainty that this is so.

2. MAINTENANCE MOVEMENTS

As previously defined, these movements sometimes have a place in re-education of postural abnormalities of the vertebral column, but for the most part find their best use in the management of inflammatory arthritis and neurological conditions.

3. MOBILISATION

These passive movements, techniques which are under the control of the patient, may be categorised as follows:

— regional mobilisation
— specific or localised mobilisation.

They have the quality of rhythmic repetition, and the patient can stop the movement at any time if so wished. They are graded from I to IV.

4. MANIPULATION

This is not under the patient's control because the movement is completed before the patient can prevent it; it may also be categorised as:

— regional manipulation Grade V
— localised manipulation, localised Grade V (locV)

In accordance with the grading system which applies to both groups of technique, it is convenient to consider the factors governing their use under the one heading of Manual Mobilisation Method.

Manual mobilisation method

Whatever may be the chosen *method of treatment* by persuasive passive movement to the patient's tolerance, there has been ample demonstration that it does not need to be applied in the plane of the facets, or at right angles to these planes, to be therapeutically effective. This does not mean to say that such movements should not be an integral part of any repertoire of mobilisation techniques; but only that they are certainly not the only effective way to treat patients. For example, one commonly used technique of postero-anterior vertebral pressures $\updownarrow$ applied by thumbpads or heel of hand to the spinous process of a cervical, thoracic or lumbar vertebra will plainly produce accessory movement of a dissimilar nature at each region because: the morphology of the vertebrae differs considerably; the orientation of facet-planes is different; the nature of connective-tissue attachments is not the same in each region (Fig. 11.3).

inclination of the direction of pressures, a full and precise biomechanical analysis of the small movement becomes difficult. When transverse vertebral pressures $\longrightarrow\!\!\bullet\!\!\longrightarrow$ are applied to spinous processes, equally complex movements are produced.

Whether either, or neither, of these techniques is ultimately employed in the successful relief of signs and symptoms would not depend upon something approaching a *diktat* in a textbook, but would depend upon the initial responses of the abnormal joint and its associated soft tissues, since each patient is unique.

Since these modest and economical ways of mobilising vertebral joints have been shown to occupy a most useful place in the range of available techniques, it follows that therapeutic effectiveness

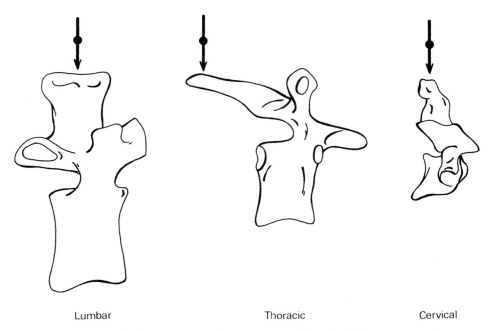

Lumbar   Thoracic   Cervical

Fig. 11.3 Posteroanterior central vertebral pressures on spinous processes will produce different segmental movements according to regional characteristics.

Notions of the vertebrae 'just going up and down' in response to these repetitive pressures plainly will not do, since a moment's consideration of vertebral anatomy indicates that the small movements are likely to be complex, and also to vary considerably between individuals.

As a little bias is added to the movement (see p. 51) by way of a caudal, cephalic, medial or lateral

does not derive solely from considerations of what is thought to be the 'correct' geometry of the direction of movement.

Expressed otherwise, the responses of each abnormal joint are more important than 'logical' and arbitrary rules of manipulative method.

A treatment method which seems appropriate to adopt is formulated on the basis of:

(i) Examination procedures in which the therapist *assumes nothing* but provides opportunities for the nature of the joint abnormality to fully declare itself, in terms of the 'range-pain-resistance' relationship (p. 129)

(ii) Giving the greatest weight to the unique individual combination, and degree, of the abnormal signs and symptoms, rather than to generalised diagnosis

(iii) Grading the degree of applied movement in accordance with detailed examination findings, and

(iv) Changing the technique and/or the grade of applied movement according to the changing nature of the joint abnormality during treatment

(v) Employing the least vigour which will achieve the desired effect.

This treatment approach is by no means the prerogative of any one school of manipulation, yet in the author's opinion Maitland[128] has developed it to the highest degree, and so far as applied movement under the control of the patient is concerned, the following observations on *grading* concern this particular method.

Grouping joint abnormalities

To have complete control of the treatment movements we apply, and also to apply them with the most effectiveness, we need to develop two things:

a. A precise *grading* of the mobilisation movements and manipulations used in treatment, and

b. A good understanding of the great variety of ways in which abnormal movement may present.

The nature and characteristics of the abnormal movement give us our indications for treatment, both in terms of the grade of movement to use initially, and subsequently the modifications needed as the signs and symptoms change during treatment.

So far as abnormalities of joints, and their effects, are concerned, patients can be placed into one of five main groups:

Group 1 There is plenty of pain from the joint, either at rest and/or on movement; it is very irritable, (i.e. undue reactiveness) and the pain and irritability limit the movement early in the range

Group 2 Resistance (either as contractile-tissue tension, i.e. spasm; or inert tissue-tension, i.e. adhesions and fibrosis; or tissue-compression) and *pain,* are *both* responsible (in varying combinations) for limiting the movement. This is a very large group

Group 3 *Resistance,* as inert-tissue tension or compression, is manifestly the range-limiting factor. It may hurt slightly to test the joint, and there may be a trace of spasm, but these latter two are negligible in the face of resistance as the movement-restriction factor

Group 4 There is a 'catch', or momentary 'twinge' of pain, either *during* a movement which is otherwise of full range and painless, or more often at the end of it. This group often show the twinge or catch of pain at the end of *combinations* of movement, such as combined extension and side-flexion of the neck, or combined abduction with extension of a shoulder

Group 5 comprises those patients in whom an accurate and confident diagnosis of *joint derangement,* often confirmed radiologically, can be made; we need not consider this group any further in this particular context.

Notice how the criteria for categorising these patients are the factors of abnormal movement. It is not the pathology which is of first importance, but the particular phase of the pathology the patient is in. Even then it is still not the pathology we give our main attention to, but how the abnormalities are manifested in terms of movement.

Examination and assessment must be accurate enough to elicit which group the patient falls into, and subsequent reassessment must be accurate enough to detect when the joint is moving from group to group. The joint abnormality may move from group to group in one treatment — it may not move from one group to another in a week of daily treatments.

Maitland[128] proposes a treatment method in which the careful testing movements of examination, and the precise passive movements employed in treatment, are kept totally under control throughout every clinical session.

Huxley said that science was nothing but trained and organised common sense. Since even professionally trained individuals frequently appear to organise 'common sense' according to taste, there is no satisfactory substitute for measurement; as the followers of Galileo were instructed: 'count what is countable, measure what is measurable, and make measurable that which is not.'[172] While this demands full concentration at all times and a high degree of attention to detail, the rewards are soundly-based, reliable assessments of the *effects* of treatment, and a steadily increasing grasp of what is clinically happening, to which, and why.

In passing, a thorough understanding of this clinical system is well worthwhile, since it is an excellent method of self-education in which one learns from the patient rather than the text-book.

Grades of movement in treatment:
mobilisation and manipulation

The *five* grades of passive movement are applicable, with suitable modifications, when needed, to disordered joints or joint complexes requiring treatment, e.g.

— the available excursion of physiological range of a single large peripheral joint (e.g. the shoulder or elbow joint)
— the available *physiological* range of a multi-joint articulation, e.g. rotation of the cervical spine
— the available *accessory* range of one joint, or segment, within a complex of joints, e.g. the cuboid, the axis, the 3rd lumbar vertebra or the 2nd rib.

Grades I to IV refer to *mobilisation*, i.e. passive-movement treatment under control of the patient (see p. 121) and Grade V refers to *manipulation*, i.e. a single passive movement which is not under the control of the patient; it may be regional (V) or a localised (locV) manipulation.

Since different single joints and multi-joint articulations have widely varying characteristics, the grades of movement employed in treatment also need to be flexible, to meet these requirements.

A. For joints with a normally abrupt 'end-feel'

to the physiological range of movement (e.g. knee extension, elbow extension) the grades are depicted as follows: Fig. 11.4(a) Fig. 11.4(b)

For joint movements where the normal end-feel is rather more abrupt than soft (e.g. external rotation of tibia with the knee-joint flexed at 90°) the grades may also be represented in this way: Fig. 11.4(c)

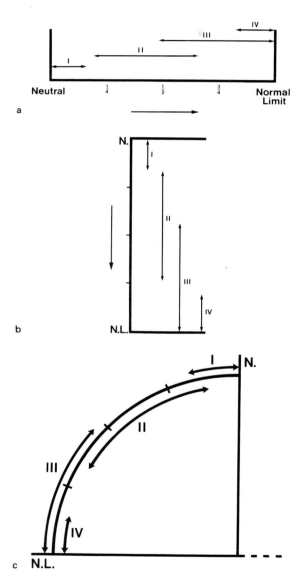

Fig. 11.4A, B and C The position and amplitude of the grades of mobilisation, represented (A) horizontally, (B) vertically and (C) on the rotation range, of the available excursion of movement in *normal* joints.

Each grade has:

(i) *position* on the *available* excursion of movement, and

(ii) *amplitude,* which is a proportion of it.

Grades I and IV are small amplitude movements at the beginning and end, respectively, of the *available* range, while II and III are larger amplitude movements at the middle and end, respectively, of available range.

Like 'grades' of anything and everything, the values overlap to a degree, and in practice minus or plus signs are used to indicate this modification (Fig. 11.5).

Movements of *abnormal* joints are usually, but not invariably, limited, and since the available excursion of movements is reduced, the grades of treatment are proportionately reduced (Fig. 11.6).

Thus, when the 'treatment grade' is expressed or recorded, it refers to grades on the *available* excursion and not the anatomical normal range, unless the range of movement is not limited, e.g. the abnormality is manifest by painful movement only. Searching tests will reveal that this is quite uncommon.

The initial grade of mobilisation depends upon the nature of the limiting factor (see p. 130) and it must not be assumed, of course, that mobilising

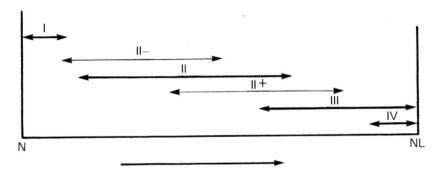

Fig. 11.5 Scheme to illustrate plus or minus values of Grade II, for example.

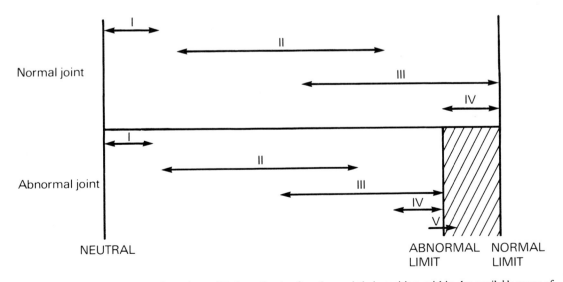

Fig. 11.6 Scheme to illustrate proportionately modified amplitude of grades, and their position, within the *available* range of movement of an *abnormal* joint. The particular treatment grade selected depends upon the degree of movement-limitation and the nature of the limiting factor.

movements occur along either the straight arrows or curved lines used in these schemes (Figs. 11.3, 11.4).

B. For joints with a normally soft end-feel, or with resistance rising through some degrees of movement to a maximum (e.g. cervical rotation, knee flexion, hip flexion) and in abnormal joints where the resistance may be capsular and/or muscle tightness, or muscle spasm, the grades need to be conceived a little differently.

There is also the paradox that a normally hypermobile, a normally loose, joint may temporarily be limited in movement, also painful and the prime source of the patient's complaint.

This can successfully be treated by mobilisation techniques, graded appropriately and accurately recorded.

To accommodate the proportionate use of grades for these 'soft end-feel' clinical requirements and for clarity of recording, the positions of Grades III and IV, on the horizontal line representing movement from neutral to anatomical limit are modified, i.e. Figure 11.7. Thus it is evident that Grade II is employed within the 'resistance-free' amplitude of movement, and Grades III and IV can be employed with minus and plus values, according to the existing

and changing requirements of the abnormal joint.

As one generally handles highly irritable joints and/or nerve roots, with much respect, and less irritable joints with less respect, technique grading is guided in the first instance by *pain:*

(i) If pain is constant even at rest and rises quickly on movement into range, or it appears early in the range and rises to a level sufficient to stop the movement well before the normal limit, the techniques should be of small amplitude, gentle and confined to the beginning of available range, i.e. grades I, I+ or II-.

(ii) If there is no pain at rest, and it only begins after more than half range has been traversed, then the mobilising technique can move into the pain a bit, and even up to the limit, with care.

(iii) A 'block' by spasm, more than pain, can be treated by a grade IV technique up to the point of spasm so long as it occurs beyond half range. If it occurs before that, one should use a lower grade — the earlier the spasm, the lower the grade.

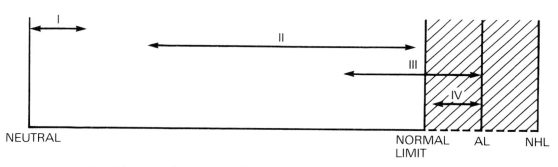

AL = Abnormal limitation or block to normally available movement in this hypermobile joint

NHL = Normal limit of hypermobile range

Fig. 11.7 Scheme to illustrate the conception of grades in clinical use for joints (or movements) with a normally soft end-feel. It is emphasised that Grade II is employed in the 'resistance-free' part of the available range, and to be noted that Grades III and IV are employed more gently (III- and IV-) or more firmly (III+ and IV+). The precise *nature* of the limitation governs initial grade selection.

(iv) A block by inert-tissue tension, or compression, with negligible pain or spasm, should be treated with a grade IV technique, and a grade V technique may be indicated.

During treatment, movement into pain depends not entirely on the pain as such, but also on its characteristics, its quality or its nature: with much pain and irritability, low grades are employed; with dull aches, one can often manipulate immediately, that is, use a single, short-amplitude, high-velocity thrust technique, a grade V, provided all other factors are favourable and there are no contra-indications.

The ability to grade techniques accurately depends upon a working knowledge, from clinical experience and trained perception, of the voluntary and accessory range of all vertebral segments. Yet when palpating we must always remember the patient's age and the natural varieties of individual spines, i.e. hard and springy; soft and springy; soft and yielding; inelastic, tight and tough.

In brief:

(i) Examination and assessment must elicit the range-pain-resistance relationship existing.
(ii) The depth of mobilising must be right for the range-pain-resistance relationship.
(iii) Subsequent assessment must be precise enough to guide technique and grading in accordance with the changing requirements of the abnormal joints.

Having decided whether one is treating *pain* primarily, or *resistance* primarily, the broad principles for choosing the patient's position, the technique and the grade are as follows:

Pain. Mobilise the range of accessory movements with the joint in a painless position, or use physiological movements in a painless part of the range.

Resistance. Both accessory and physiological ranges are mobilised at or across the limit of available movement.

Use of grades in treatment

It is not possible to describe the very many varieties of presentation of abnormal joints, with permutations of the 'Range-pain-resistance' relationship, but an outline guide to initial grade selection is useful provided subsequent selection is guided by careful assessment of results; the two factors of: (i) treatment position of the joint, and (ii) technique selection being given.

By combinations of five simple steps ((i) to (v) below) the 'Range-pain-resistance' relationship for any one movement can be clearly expressed.

Validity of programmes of research, into the nature and magnitude of movement-limiting factors in degenerative joint disease, would depend upon precise data and meticulous recording, but in clinical work the need is for a quick and clear graphic record of the assessment by which the treatment plan is formulated. Advantages of this method are speed and simplicity because the need for abscissae and ordinates, calibrated for joint range and for magnitude of limiting factors respectively, is avoided. The important clinical findings to record are: (i) the *point of movement-limitation,* as a proportion of normal range; (ii) the nature of the primary range-limiting factor; (iii) the nature and magnitude of secondary factors.

These can be clearly expressed and be read at a glance, and although easier to apply to careful manual tests of peripheral joint movement, the method has been found of much value in 'Examination-and-assessment' training programmes during which candidates, after some tuition and practice, are able to express their findings, after vertebral-segment tests, with a degree of inter-observer error which is gratifyingly small.

This is probably the best use of 'joint pictures', i.e. as a means of developing perception of the *characteristics of* joint abnormality as they differ from patient to patient.

Joint pictures may be used for each of two or more passive movement tests of single vertebrae or for two or more active tests of a vertebral region, but reach their most sophisticated development when employed for the single accessory vertebral movement which is being given priority as an assessment parameter during treatment.

Examples of findings follow, with a *method of graphic description* in which:

(i)   the horizontal line represents normal range and movement is from left to right
(ii) pain is depicted above it
(iii) spasm is depicted below it
(iv) movement-limitation is represented by a vertical line from the dominant factor responsible
(v)   resistance (other than spasm) is represented by a number of vertical lines which always cross the range line.

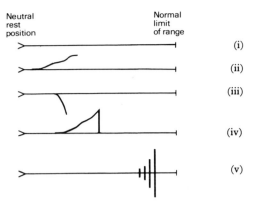

Assessment	Joint picture	Initial grade
1. Joint irritability is manifest with pain at rest and/or provoked early in the testing movement		I
2. Spasm elicited by the testing movement limits it quite early in the range, with pain less dominant		I or I+
3. Elicited spasm and pain inseparably limit the movement early in the range		I
4. Spasm limits the movement much earlier with a quick probe than with a slow probe, indicating latent irritability	Slow Quick	II
5. In the absence of resistance, slowly rising pain limits the movement after ½ range		II

Assessment	Joint picture	Initial grade

6. Pain and 'resistance' (as either spasm, other tissue tension or tissue compression) are *together* limiting the movement. The grade employed depends upon: (a) which is the dominant factor, (b) when the limit occurs

   (i) Pain and/or spasm encountered early in the range have been described in (2) and (3).

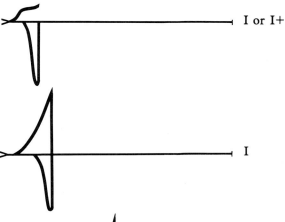

I or I+

I

   (ii) Limitation by pain and virtually spasm-free resistance in roughly equal proportions

      a. before ½ range

      b. after ½ range

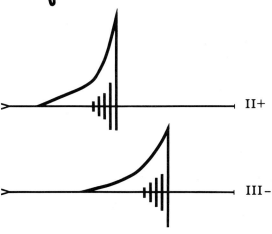

II+

III –

   (iii) Spasm limits the movement beyond ½ range with little pain

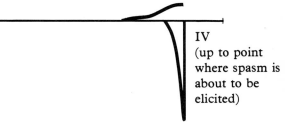

IV
(up to point where spasm is about to be elicited)

   (iv) Limitation by the resistance, without spasm, of tissue tension, or compression, is encountered at or beyond ½ range; pain rises to its maximum then but is much less dominant than resistance and by itself would not limit the movement

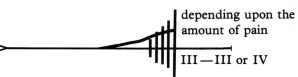

depending upon the amount of pain

III — III or IV

Assessment	Joint picture	Initial grade
7. In the virtual absence of pain or spasm, resistance limits the movement (a) either before, or (b) after ½ range	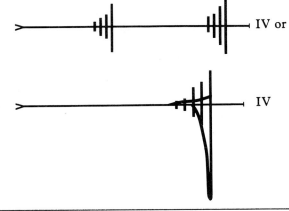	IV or
8. Resistance, including spasm, is encountered well beyond ½ range, with minimal pain		IV

Notes

1. The notion that grades denote progression of treatment in time is incorrect, since the nature of the movement-limiting factor governs initial choice of treatment grade and it has been shown that, from the first, this may be grade IV.

2. Neither do the grades symbolise an ascending scale of aggression in treatment. 'Grade IV' indicates a particular amplitude, and position, on the available excursion of movement, and not *necessarily* the greatest vigour in mobilising.

3. One should make up one's mind whether one is treating primarily *pain, or resistance,* because this is fundamentally related to the grade of mobilisation which is chosen. Most of the more serious manipulation accidents, a few of them catastrophes, which have been reported in the literature have followed overvigorous or rough treatment, more often to the upper cervical spine. But there is a dilemma here—certainly nothing untoward, but also nothing of any therapeutic value, is going to result from aimless, undisciplined, oscillatory waggling applied to the upper cervical area or any other body part.

Technique should be precise, specific and controlled, yet mobilisation is by no means always gentle—as it has frequently and erroneously been defined—and in the appropriate circumstances is quite vigorous. If mobilisations grade I to grade IV, and traction, do not produce sufficient improvement, it is time to consider the indications and contraindications for manipulative thrust techniques.

4. An intervertebral segment may present as (1) above while another segment in the same vertebral

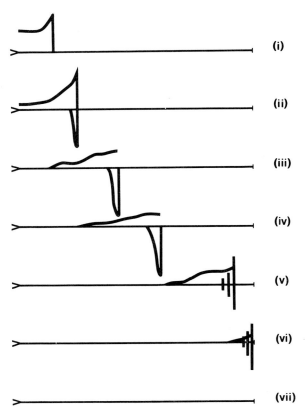

Fig. 11.8 Recording method example.

region will present as in (6 ii a). Treatment of the former should take priority.

5. When employing grade III or IV, possible treatment soreness should be alleviated by using lower grades on alternate days.

6. Indications for grade V techniques are on page 230.

7. *Recording method*
As an exercise for beginners it is useful to symbolise, as treatment proceeds, the changing relationship of pain, resistance and point of limitation of one movement; an example is given on page 132.

Not all joint problems require more than one treatment; for example if patients present with joint problems in stages (v) and (vi) a single localised grade V technique may be all that is indicated.

Abnormal 'end-feels' on passive testing

A general table of findings of segmental abnormality on passive testing is set out below, with general indications. They do not represent diagnoses and they cannot be considered in isolation from assessment of the clinical features as a whole; their presence *per se* does not necessarily amount to an indication for treatment.

The table refers *only* to the differing nature of what can be perceived by palpation, *per se*, and does not include the important factor of pain, and other clinical features.

(For more precise relationships between findings and grade of mobilising see 'Range-pain-resistance relationship', p. 130).

Type	Comment	General indication
1. Resistance (a)	Elicited spasm	Mobilise (grade I–IV)—degree of irritability governs initial grade
2. Resistance (b)	Negligible spasm; negligible voluntary guarding response. Tissue-tension limits movement before end of range, with elastic resilience detected when stressed. Other movements of the segment feel similar	Mobilise (grade I–IV) May manipulate (localised grade V) later
3. Resistance (c)	'Block'—no elastic resilience when stressed. 'Block' feels firm to attempts at moving it. Only one movement may be involved	Manipulate (localised grade V) if no preclusions (see p. 230)
4. Resistance (d)	Fairly 'hard end-feel' nature of limitation at end of movement, which is reduced. No possibility of much further movement, but may be slight elastic resilience. Other ranges likewise limited. (Chondro-osteophyte contact?)	Persistent mobilisation—and traction, provided adjacent segments are not hypermobile
5. Resistance (e)	'Springy-rubbery rebound' type of resistance to questing movement—feel is similar to that when trying to extend knee joint in fixed-flexion after IDK	Mobilise in positions which gap the joint surfaces—traction alone may be helpful. Only those manipulations (localised grade V) which gap the joint should be considered
6. Resistance (f)	Very little, if any, movement can be detected. Fused vertebrae, or degenerative ankylosis?	Refer to radiographic appearance
7. Hypermobility (a)	Normal physiological 'feel' (i.e. detectable elastic resistance at end of range) but range is greater than normal. May or may not be painful	If not causing symptoms, or provoking those reported, leave alone. If painful, mobilise within normal range for pain only
8. Hypermobility (b)	'Boggy', 'squashy' unphysiological feel; amplitude of movement is greater than expected, and 'end-feel' may not be encountered. May or may not be painful, but usually is. When elicited spasm is provoked, it is widely generalised	Likely to be serious pathology. Stop testing movements and do not treat. Check history again, and leave alone until indications for treatment have been reconfirmed

N.B. The development and sophistication of radiological methods, e.g. radiculography, stereo-radiography, epidurography and image-intensification techniques together with the highly detailed parameters adopted by radiologists[74] for clarifying the nature of mechanical changes depicted on plain film, might appear to be overtaking and overshadowing the usefulness of palpation as an examination method. The two are not really in conflict, because while these significant advances add valuable facilities for the better understanding of vertebral abnormalities, our perennial concern as therapists *in the clinical situation* will remain the articular signs and their relation to symptoms.

There is no effective substitute for passive movement and palpation as methods of seeking, segment by segment, to provoke or reproduce symptoms reported by the patients, by which we assess the need for mobilisation techniques of a particular nature, direction and grade, and further assess their efficacy as treatment proceeds.

Because we enjoy better means, and can apply more detailed criteria, when looking at abnormal joints, general medical and surgical indications are better appreciated; but where manual techniques *are* indicated, the treatment needs of the abnormal joints, and our methods and criteria for assessing these, remain the same.

The essence of good examination and assessment of joint problems lies in extracting, from all the material presented by the patient, a clear mental picture of the interaction between the various factors we can measure, or estimate, i.e.

(i)   The patient's story gives *some* information regarding the probable degree of joint irritability (i.e. undue reactiveness), the amount of pain at rest, and the functional restrictions

(ii) The active test of movement gives *more* information regarding the functional range, and its possible limitation, as described above

(iii) The passive test of functional and accessory ranges gives the *most* information (and often confirmation) regarding:

   a. amount of pain, and spasm and other resistance during applied movement
   b. their point of onset on the range of movement

c. the relationship between these factors
d. their rate of increase of effect, in bringing the movement to a halt
e. the primary nature of the limit to further movement.

Only this depth of attention, observation and perception during palpation will allow us to assess the 'Range-pain-resistance' relationship which gives us our treatment indications for each joint problem we handle. The nature of the range-limiting factor invariably decides the grade employed in treatment, and frequently also the positioning of the patient's joint, and the particular technique.

So far as movement applied to vertebral joints is concerned, it is probably naive to believe that there is any such thing as a truly specific procedure — all we can strive for is to localise our effects as much as possible by careful technique. It is not possible to move a practically rigid structure (e.g. a vertebra) without also moving all structures attached to it; connective tissues and muscles span more than one segment, and it is optimistic to expect that mere positioning, however carefully contrived, is all that is necessary to 'localise' a technique. Innocent structures have many times been injured by unthinking adherence to this notion. In the final analysis, all mobilisations and manipulations are 'soft-tissue techniques', and for the most part it is in the soft-tissues that the lesions we treat, and the effects we produce, are to be found.

MOBILISATION

The following *representative* examples of techniques, with observations about their use, are grouped according to the author's personal view (p. 120). A few examples of techniques for the limb girdle joints are included, since the treatment of vertebral joint conditions frequently requires some mobilisation of proximal peripheral joints.

For complete descriptions and illustrations of the great variety of manipulative methods (in the general sense), appropriate texts should be consulted.[58, 168, 135, 136, 137, 32, 125]

While some of Maitland's techniques (among others) are briefly described (p. 138), readers are referred to his textbooks. For applied movement which is *not* under control of the patient see page 143.

Where the techniques, or adaptations of them, described by Maitland[128] are illustrated, the grade of movement is given.

Some of the symbols used by the author are in general use; some are not.

Regional mobilisation

This description correctly applies to a wide variety of techniques, when defined as repetitive, rhythmic passive movement applied to vertebral *regions*, or at least to more than two segments, by reason of the area treated, the grasp and the nature of the movement.

Rhythmic manual or mechanical traction (p. 154) is perforce also regional mobilisation in this sense, although by careful positioning of the patient every effort may be made to produce the majority of the mobilisation or traction effect at a particular segment or locality of the spine.

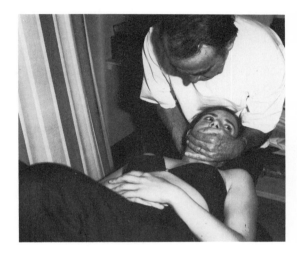

Fig. 11.9A 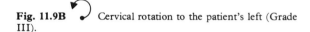 Cervical rotation to the left, within a grade I amplitude, for a C2–C3 joint problem. For lower cervical segments, the neck would be more flexed. Localisation, in the sense that a particular segment may be placed in its most favourable disposition for movement, is achieved by maintaining the neck in a neutral position for craniovertebral movement, with increasing flexion for successively lower segments. A further method of restricting the effect is to transfer the palmar surface of the index finger of the 'occipital' hand so that it unilaterally bears against the transverse process of C4, for example; the head and all segments to C4 are then rotated as a unit, with a localised effect on the C4–C5 segment.

Fig. 11.9B Cervical rotation to the patient's left (Grade III).

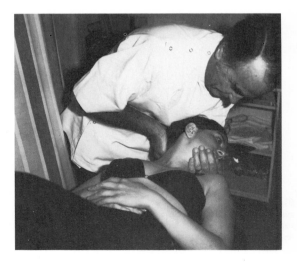

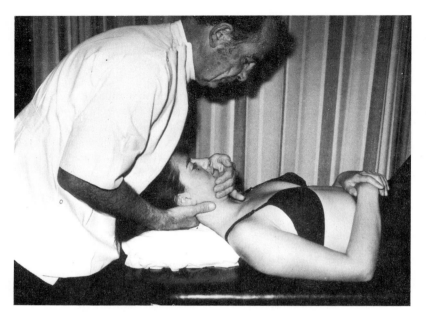

Fig. 11.10 ◄—•—► Oscillatory longitudinal movement.

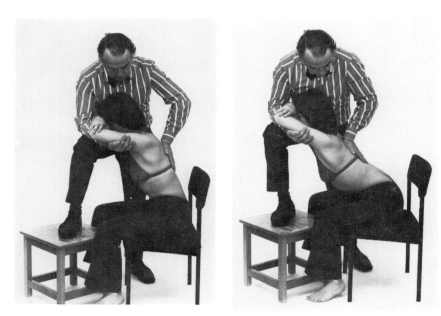

A   B

Fig. 11.11A and B. (A) Regional mobilisation technique for improving thoracic extension range. The patient sits, straddling the corner of a stool between knees. With one foot on the stool and his forearm of that side resting on his thigh, the therapist supports the patient's folded arms, on which she rests her forehead, and grasps the patient's far upper arm. The other hand rests on the mid-thoracic region. (B) By abducting his supported leg and slightly inclining his own body laterally in the same direction, a rhythmic extension movement is imparted to the patient's thoracic spine, in a to-and-fro manner.

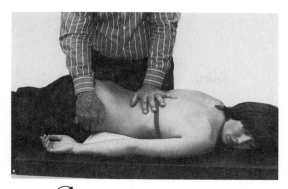

Fig. 11.12 ↻ A moderate range of lumbar rotation, which is more useful for encouraging relaxation (preparatory for other techniques) than for much else, can rhythmically be performed with the patient lying prone.

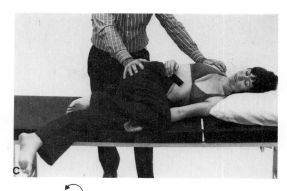

Fig. 11.13C ↻ A grade III lumbar rotation.

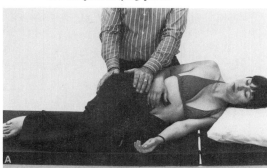

Fig. 11.13A ↻ Rhythmic lumbar rotation, to the patient's left side.

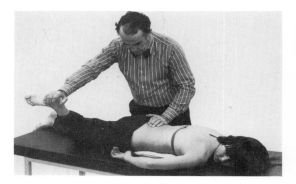

Fig. 11.14 Regional mobilisation. Gentle gapping/gliding technique for left sacro-iliac joint with left ilium stabilised. While the technique looks 'specific', a regional effect is hard to prevent. Precisely the same grasps can be used to passively stretch the *right* piriformis, and/or to improve its extensibility by hold-relax or isometric techniques.

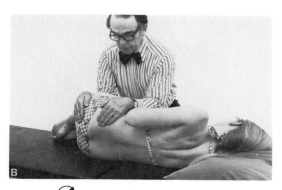

Fig. 11.13B ↻ Lumbar rotation (in grade II) by a slightly built therapist for a heavy patient.

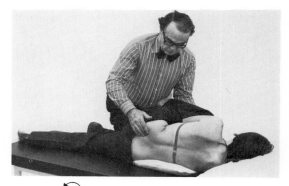

Fig. 11.15 ↻ A modest and undramatic sacro-iliac mobilising technique, when the painful side is that of a relatively depressed posterior superior iliac spine, and the lumbar spine is not involved. It is not necessary for sacro-iliac relationships to be 'changed' for pain to be relieved, and the precise nature of the lesion may remain undetermined.

Localised mobilisation techniques

Localised mobilisation techniques are those in which every effort is made to restrict the effect of movement to a single segment. This is easier in some anatomical locations than in others.

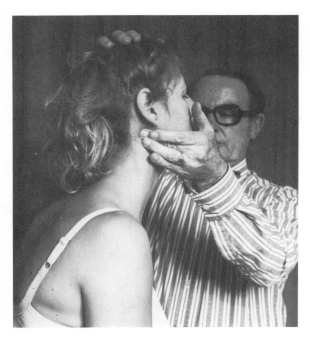

Fig. 11.16 To show the surface anatomy point for the tip of right lateral mass of atlas.

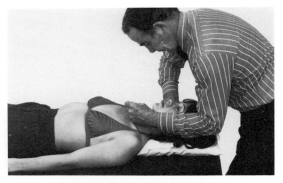

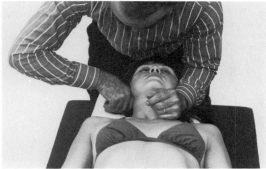

Fig. 11.18A and B ◄─●─ Transverse vertebral pressures, to the patient's left, of the atlas. Alternative technique. Because of a coexistent shoulder or upper rib-joint condition, the patient may not be able to lie on one side; the technique is adapted so that with the patient supine, the operator's arm replaces the firm pillow against the painful side, and the lateral aspect of the operator's second metacarpal head replaces the thumbtip contact with the lateral mass of atlas on the painless side. It is important to keep the forearm aligned with the gentle movements being imparted via the contact with the lateral tip of atlas.

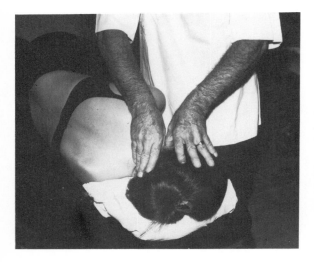

Fig. 11.17 ─●─► Transverse vertebral movement of the atlas towards the painful side.

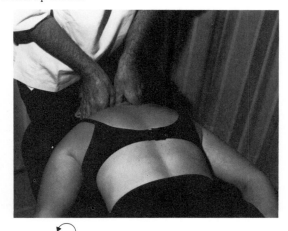

Fig. 11.19 ↓ Mobilisation of left rotation at the atlantoaxial (C1–C2) segment, near the extreme of rotation range.

Fig. 11.20 Side-lying techniques are valuable in the early stages of treating irritable cervical problems, and localisation can be very precise. The thumb positions illustrated are self-explanatory.

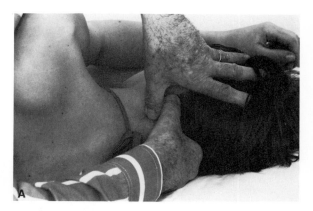

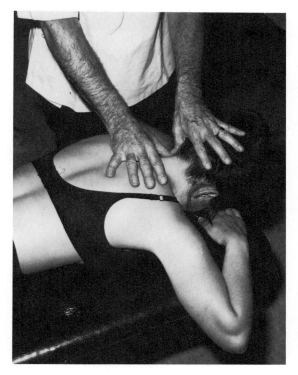

Fig. 11.21A ⟶•⟶ Transverse vertebral pressures to the spinous process of C2.

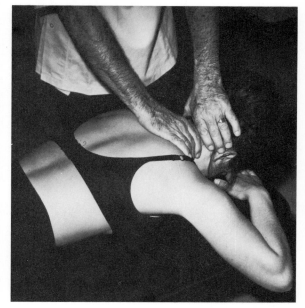

Fig. 11.21B ⟶•⟶ Transverse vertebral pressure to the transverse process of C2.

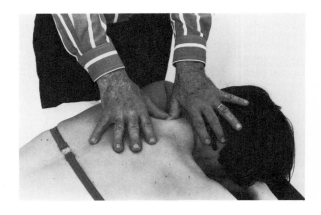

Fig. 11.22 ⟶•⟶ Transverse vertebral pressure to the spinous process of C6.

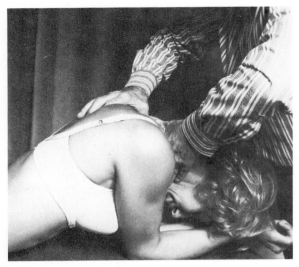

Fig. 11.23 ◄—● (C6) —●► (C7) Firm simultaneous transverse vertebral pressures, to the left on C6 and the right on C7 spinous processes, with the patient in the elbow-lean prone-lying position. This is a very localised 'push-pull' technique.

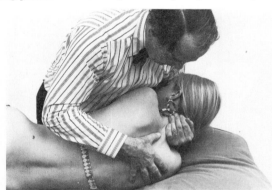

Fig. 11.24 Side-gliding of neck and C7 to the patient's left, on a stabilised T1. Compare with grasp in Figure 7.42 (p. 91).

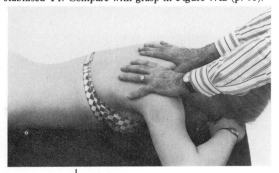

Fig. 11.25 ●—→ (1st Rib) Mobilisation of the right first rib by repetitive pressures, applied anteriorly to the upper trapezius and against the upper rib surface, and directed to the opposite hip.

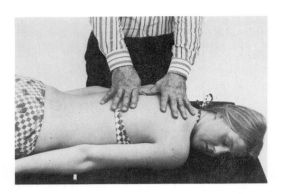

Fig. 11.26 —●► Transverse vertebral pressures to T5.

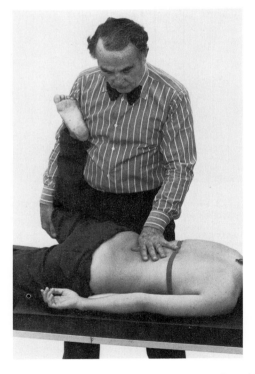

Fig. 11.27 —●► Transverse vertebral pressure to L4, with left leg abduction, which introduces a degree of gapping effect on the right side. The precise nature of the movement depends upon the configuration of the individual's lumbar facet-joints.

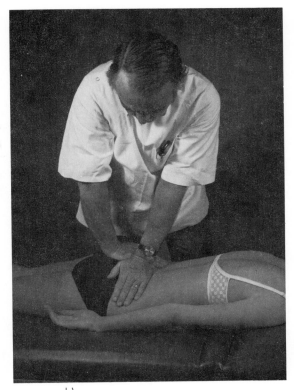

Fig. 11.28 (PSIS) Downward, outward and caudal mobilisation of the patient's right ilium, while the sacrum is stabilised with the opposite hand. From the painless side, the therapist leans over the patient.

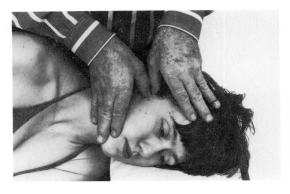

Fig. 11.29 Medial transverse movement of the right temporomandibular joint, by thumb-tip pressures on the lateral aspect of the mandibular condyle.

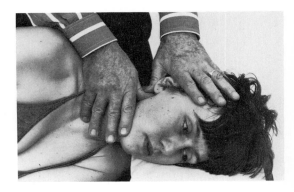

Fig. 11.30 Postero-anterior movement of the right mandibular condyle, by thumb-tip pressures against its posterior aspect.

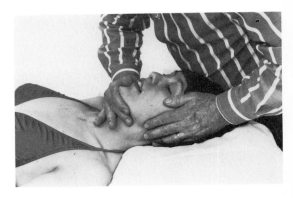

Fig. 11.31 Left lateral deviation of the mandible, pivoting on the left temporomandibular joint, if the movement is applied mainly at the chin. If applied more with the heel of the right hand, there is a degree of left mandibular shift. The grasp may also be used for a hold-relax technique to stretch the right deviator muscles, or to strengthen the right deviator muscles, after habitual left deviation because of a bruised left temporomandibular joint.

The temporomandibular and limb girdle joints

Painful upper cervical conditions are frequently associated with temporomandibular joint pain and appear to cause it; likewise, mal-occlusion of that joint is often associated with sub-occipital muscle tightness, tender cranio-vertebral joints, migrainous headaches (see p. 54) and neck problems. Vertebral pain syndromes are very frequently accompanied by associated painful conditions of the limb girdle joints. Their treatment by manual techniques is a comprehensive subject in its own right, and the few examples which follow may serve as an indication of the importance of gentle distraction techniques, and of improving the range of accessory movements which underlie normal active movements.

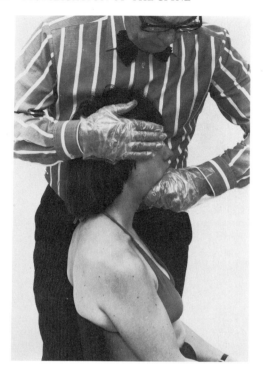

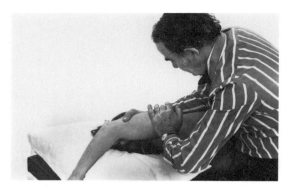

Fig. 11.34 Gaining the last few degrees of elevation at the glenohumeral joint, by small accessory movement anteriorly of the humeral head, with the scapula stabilised. The patient lies on the painless side with hips and knees flexed to 90°; the therapist stands behind the patient and elevates the arm, to the point of restriction, by grasping its medial aspect just above the elbow. This brings the flexor aspect of his near-side arm against the lateral border of the scapula, which becomes the method of stabilising it. By applying his other palm to the humeral head, just distal to the shoulder joint, and keeping his other forearm aligned at right angles to the patient's arm, the small-amplitude postero-anterior mobilising movements can be localised to the joint.

Fig. 11.32 Distraction of temporomandibular joint surfaces, with the patient's head stabilised against the therapist's abdomen. The technique is of value when the joint is locked in a partially-open position. The therapist's thumb-pad engages the biting surfaces of the lower molars, against which repetitive oscillatory depression is applied. If this is unsuccessful, the condyle is rocked forward and backwards, or from side to side, while distraction is maintained, holding the degree of opening close to the point of its limitation.

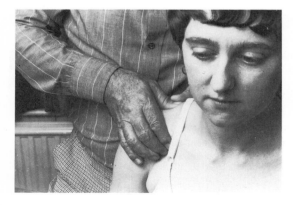

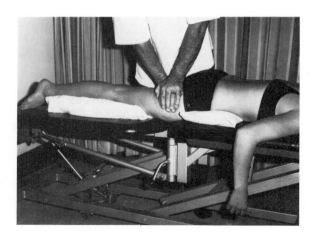

Fig. 11.33 Caudal oscillatory pressures to the superior surface of lateral end of clavicle.

Fig. 11.35 Gaining extension range at the hip-joint. The patient lying prone with flat hard pillows under ilium and upper femur allows a small but important degree of movement (probably stretch of anterior structures, with a trace of anterior gliding motion of femoral head) to be applied by postero-anterior pressures at the upper end of femur. The technique is unsuitable for other than slight or moderate restriction of extension.

Regional manipulation

It is sometimes necessary to employ grade V manipulative thrust techniques, near the limit of available range, when improvement in signs and symptoms achieved by progressive and adequate mobilisation (grades I–IV) has reached stalemate, and assessment of the condition indicates that further improvement is possible.

While the aim of manipulative procedures is more often that of influencing a particular vertebral segment, the term 'regional manipulation' is here taken to include the single, quick distraction techniques with a regional effect, after careful positioning of the patient, as well as the rotational manipulations for the cervical, thoracic and lumbar regions (Fig. 11.36) when manual contact with a bony apophysis of a vertebra for the purpose of localisation does not form part of the method.

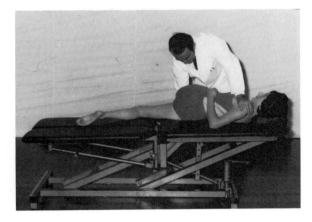

Fig. 11.36 This technique, of regional lumbar and thoracic rotation, is a prime example of 'environmental manipulation'. This is not to say that it does not succeed at times, which can be said of many other techniques, too, of course.

Localised manipulation

After careful and precise positioning of the patient, these techniques are single, high-velocity movements of short amplitude, and are not under the control of the patient, since the movement is completed before the patient can stop it. They are distinguished by the speed of movement, and are categorised as grade V techniques when vertebral *regions* are manipulated, and Localised grade V techniques when every effort is made to localise the

movement to a particular *segment*. There is probably no such thing as a completely segmentally localised vertebral manipulation; true isolation of effect to a single segment is virtually impossible.

Many descriptions and illustrations of localised or specific techniques plainly show that the positioning for, or execution of, them applies stress to many vertebral segments. This regional stress should not be ignored, and sometimes may well be a factor underlying the indifferent results of manipulative methods which, during the hot pursuit of localisation, overlook the regional stress imposed by positioning.

Care and delicacy of technique will minimise stress to uninvolved segments. The basis for preparatory so-called locking of vertebral regions prior to localised manipulation, by methods of positioning which employ combined movements, rests upon the differing nature of vertebral movement from region to region.

Generalised description of spinal movement and of limiting factors need not occupy us here. A detailed knowledge of the morphology of facet-joints is indispensable when devising manipulative techniques with the intention of 'localising' the effect, since the paired facet-joint planes are an important factor influencing the direction, the nature and sometimes the extent of movement in a vertebral district. There are, however, other factors which should not be overlooked, e.g.

1. The spine as a whole is not only an 'empilement' of individual vertebral bones of particular shapes, but also a flexible rod exhibiting three distinct curves in one plane. Its tendency to rotation, when bent in the plane at right angles to these sagittal curves, is no more than can be demonstrated by performing the same experiment with a green and flexible twig; thus an explanation of the physical behaviour of this living flexible rod does not depend entirely on the presence or arrangement of vertebral apophyses or facet-joints, except that by reason of their presence its natural physical characteristics are somewhat modified.

2. The effects of anomalies of bone structure and of facet-plane orientation, and of anomalies in the presence of adventitious fibrous bands with unilateral tethering effects which are present in many patients should not be forgotten.

When using specific or localised techniques, the

declared *aim* is that of moving one vertebral joint only, but since a single typical cervical vertebra, for example, takes part in the formation of 10 joints: 4 facet-joints, 2 intervertebral body joints, 4 neuro-central (or uncovertebral) joints, besides giving attachments to very many soft tissue structures which span more than one segment, the view that it is possible to move one joint only becomes untenable.

Similar considerations will apply to all other vertebral articulations. This is not to say that, by careful technique and a well-developed sense of tissue-tension, the skilled therapist cannot arrange the patient's position so that the manipulative effect is mainly exerted at a particular segment in a particular way, but only that notions of affecting 'a single joint' should not go unexamined.

Techniques of positioning for localised manipulative thrust techniques (grade locV)

The aim is to stabilise adjacent vertebral joints in such a way that the single, quick, short-amplitude thrust is maximally exerted at a single segment in a particular direction; it may be to neatly distract the two planes of a facet-joint, i.e. movement at right angles to these planes, or to translate or glide one upon the other in the existing plane.

Manipulative thrust techniques are not necessarily restricted to gapping synovial joints at right angles to their articular surfaces, or in the plane of those surfaces. The intended geometry of the combined manipulative movement may have a degree of variability between these extremes, and includes rotation, of course.

Thus the line of the thrust may be at an acute angle to the plane of the joint surface, the direction employed depending upon the purpose of the manipulation in that particular circumstance.

A further aim is protective, in that careful techniques of controlled fixation of neighbouring articulations where possible will prevent them from being subjected to needless movement; this is also the consideration underlying economy of vigour when applying the manipulative thrust. These are thus the aims.

Let us now examine these considerations, as applied to the cervical spine. In Figure 11.37(A) a scheme of the left lateral aspect of the cervical facet-joint planes shows that the planes would roughly converge somewhere in front of the eye. During side-bending to the patient's left, i.e. towards the viewer, the weight of the superimposed head will soon, but not immediately, cause each inferior articular facet to move *downwards,* and then *posteriorly,* upon the upward-and-backward-facing superior articular facet of the subjacent vertebra. On the opposite right side, each inferior articular facet-plane tends to move *upward* and *forward* on the one below. Thus rotation towards the direction of side-bending is imposed by the facet orientation (see Figs. 11.37(B) (C) (D)).

If, while holding the neck side-flexed to the left, we impose an opposite (right) rotation, the left facet-planes are markedly approximated, and those on the right strongly distracted. In osteopathic terminology, the left row of typical facets are regarded as being 'facet-apposition-locked', and the right-side row as being 'ligamentous-tension-locked'.

Thus, in the position described above, the 'facet-lock' occurs on the side rotated away from, and the 'ligamentous lock' on the side rotated towards, when the rotation imposed is *opposite* to the physiological tendency of that particular vertebral district.

These positioning techniques which tend to stabilise the vertebral segments of a region by locking do not *ensure* that a small-amplitude thrust will mainly move only the vertebrae to which it is applied, but with careful technique will make it more of a certainty than not.

'Here, however, is a difficulty. Spinal joints do not move separately, they are linked together. Long before the first joint reaches the limit of its movement, the next one has started to move. It is easy to go too far and at least partially lock the joint that one is trying to move. One of the things that one learns by experience is how far to go. In order to decide how far to go one must monitor with one's fingers. Monitoring can be either or both of two changes. First the movement of the joint. Secondly the tissue tension around the joint. Accuracy in this kind of palpation is much improved by practice. . . . The commonest mistake by beginners is to go too far and make their task more difficult by locking the problem joint!'[13]

Bearing in mind what has been said about the regional characteristics of vertebral movement, it will be plain that positioning techniques will vary

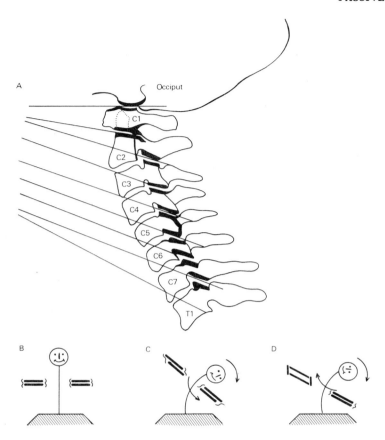

Fig. 11.37 (A) The cervical facet-joint planes are oriented so as to roughly converge at a point somewhere in the region of the eye. (B) Neutral position. (C) Physiological tendency is rotation to the same side on side-bending. (D) Opposite (right) rotation imposed. Facet apposition on (L) and facet gapping on (R).

On the (L) side, a 'facet-apposition-lock' or 'compression-lock' has been achieved by rotating the head and neck in an *opposite* direction to the physiological tendency.

On the (R) side, a 'ligamentous-tension-lock' has been achieved; the facet-planes are maximally distracted and the capsule of the joint is tautened.

from region to region, and that the techniques will need careful study and much patient practice before confident precision and economy of vigour gradually replace the hopeful shove.

It should be evident that a sound knowledge of the planes and angulation of the facet-joints, of the characteristics of spinal movement, of the importance of anomalies and individual variations together with a well-developed sense of tissue-tension, are important factors in positioning the patient immediately prior to the manipulative thrust. The German *Fingerspitzengefühl* (literally, the sense of perception by fingertip) expresses the importance of this sensitivity.

There is a further consideration, i.e. while the movement combinations of a typical *cervical* vertebra appear to be fairly well elucidated on the basis of facet-plane orientation, it is not so easy to adequately explain vertebral movement in the same way at all other regions.[70]

The osteopathic term 'locking' is unfortunate, since it conveys a finality of effect. Whether a true lock is ever achieved, excepting perhaps at the thoracolumbar mortice joint[34, 70, 126, 167] on full extension, is debatable. The facet-joint capsules are thin and loose, and even when full capsular tension is applied a rotatory slip or glide is still easily imposed, because the interposed discs (at least in the cervical spine) have the special quality of lateral distortion, which is the physiological basis of sagittal movement in the neck (see p. 9).

For analogy, the fact that the handles of a concertina have been distracted to their fullest limit does not mean that movement of the handles, at right angles to the line of distraction, is not easily applied. Nevertheless the arrangement of facets, and their effect on movement, are important, e.g. although the annular attachments of the strong lumbar disc would, on their own account, preclude a free range of lumbar rotation, the arrangement of the lumbar facets soon prevents this, anyway, by their being firmly approximated unilaterally like the flanges on a railway train wheel engaging the track. Other factors, e.g. bilateral ligamentous tension, are also brought into play to assist localisation of effect.[70]

N.B. It cannot be too strongly emphasised that manipulative thrust techniques, for the vertebral column but also for the peripheral joints, should not be used without instruction which includes a sufficiently long period of adequately supervised practical and clinical work. Manipulative thrust techniques cannot be learned from a text. There is no safe substitute for practical instruction by an experienced teacher, and close supervision in the early stages of clinical work. It is possible, of course, to learn from a textbook how to fly a light aeroplane, but only very rarely indeed would the process be without incident.

There are many ways of manipulating vertebral segments; the following selection (Figs. 11.38, 11.39, 11.40, 11.41, 11.42) is *representative of methods* employed to achieve a more localised effect.

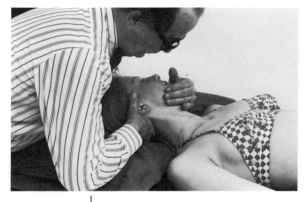

Fig. 11.38 (C1) Localised Grade V (loc V) manipulative thrust to right postero-lateral aspect of atlas.

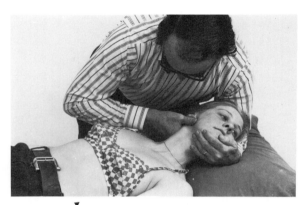

Fig. 11.39 (C3–C4) (loc V) A unilateral facet-joint gapping technique, in this case for the left C3–C4 segment.

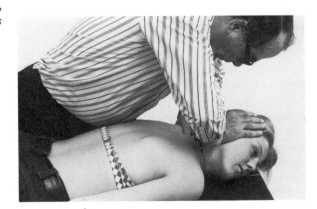

Fig. 11.40 (C7) (loc V) A localised manipulation thrust technique to gap the C6–C7 facet-joint on the patient's right side. Note that the therapist's forearms are aligned along the direction of application of both the right positioning hand and the left thrusting hand.

Patients with a leg-length discrepancy and thus an established mild scoliosis, secondary to a permanent lateral pelvic tilt, show that compensation has occurred because (i) a perpendicular dropped from the external occipital protuberance would pass through the gluteal cleft, and (ii) rotation of the vertebral bodies has occurred in some.

While this primary postural asymmetry may give rise to secondary joint problems of particular kinds, *we are concerned here only with those patients whose pelvis is level or virtually so but whose spine is secondarily deviated, or listed, to one or other side as a consequence of the primary joint problem;* a perpendicular dropped as above would now lie across the gluteal mass on the side to which the patient is deviated or listed (Fig. 11.43). Thus a

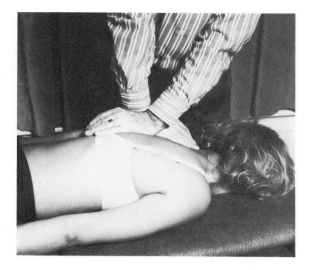

Fig. 11.41 The 'crossed-pisiform' technique for (i) freeing a fixed rotation restriction between T5 and T6, or (ii) freeing an extension restriction between the same segments. In (i) the pisiform bones of the therapist are applied one to T5 and the other to T6, on opposite sides, and depending upon the direction of rotation restriction, and in (ii) both are applied to the lower vertebra (T6) of the restricted pair. The technique is not suitable for the elderly, the osteoporotic or those with rheumatoid arthritis.

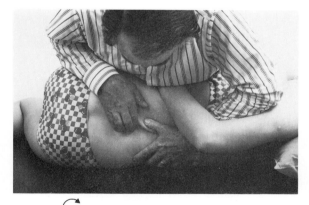

Fig. 11.42 (L3–L4) (loc V) Rotational manipulation to gap the L3–L4 facet-joint on the patient's left side.

5. CORRECTION OF LATERAL DEVIATION OF THE SPINE

While this postural variant, following presumed derangement, is quite as common in the cervical region as in the lumbar, the method to be described refers to the lumbar region[125].

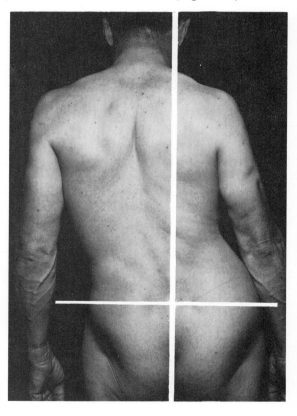

Fig. 11.43 Deviation, or listing, of the lumbar spine to the left side. Below the horizontal line, which joins both posterior superior iliac spines, the buttock contours are symmetrical and indicate a level pelvis. This deformity was secondary to joint derangement, but listing need not always be so. (Reproduced from: Bianco AJ 1968 Low back pain and sciatica: diagnosis and treatment. Journal of Bone and Joint Surgery 50A: 170, by kind permission of the author and the Editor.)

patient whose trunk appeared as 'wind-swept' to the left side would carry the head vertically over the left buttock, or at times over the left greater trochanter.

The lateral listing is sometimes compounded by a degree of postural flexion, too, or may show a component of pelvic rotation when active flexion is attempted, but the essential feature is the lateral list of the spine on a level pelvis.

The coexistence of lateral list and pain does not necessarily indicate that the list is solely secondary to the pain; what it does mean is that both factors are secondary to joint derangement. The list and the pain can vary independently. Pain may be completely relieved while the list remains, and presumably this reflects the continuing presence of a mechanical disturbance, or at least some tissue-abnormality which has a mechanical effect on vertebral carriage. Similarly, the list can be eradicated and the pain remain.

Straight-leg-raising is often normal and there are no neurological symptoms or signs. The segment involved may be L5–S1, or L4–L5, with the possibility that on occasions both segments may be contributing to the lateral spinal deviation. An alternating list and the more gross deviations are said to be more likely when derangement involves the L4–L5 segment, since the iliolumbar ligament stabilises the fifth lumbar segment.

McKenzie[125] observed that in two-thirds of 500 such patients the responsible segment was considered to be L5–S1 and in the remainder, L4–L5. Intrapelvic asymmetry in young people, consequent upon sacroiliac joint problems, may need to be included among the factors to be assessed, since it is not rare for lumbar discogenic problems and sacroiliac joint abnormalities to coexist.

Technique

With the elbow, of the side deviated towards, flexed and resting against his/her loin, the patient stands a little astride, and so far as is possible rests easily with body-weight equally on the feet. The therapist stands, with feet apart, on the flexed-elbow side, and applies either his chest (Fig. 11.44) or yoke area (Fig. 11.45) to the patient's upper or lower arm, respectively, and then reaches forward to interlace his fingers over the lateral pelvic region of the patient's opposite side.

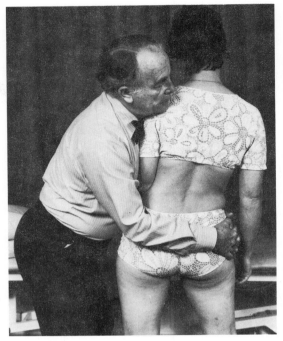

Fig. 11.44 Persuasive corrective pressure to the patient's upper trunk, for lateral deviation of the trunk secondary to joint derangement—when this is assumed to be the cause of the aberrant posture.

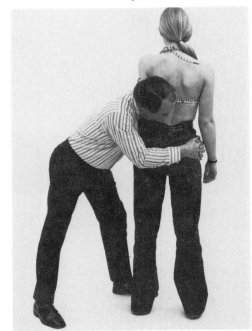

Fig. 11.45 Persuasive corrective pressure to the patient's lower trunk. How the pressures are applied for each individual is a matter of trial and error.

A persuasive and sustained corrective pressure is thus applied to the patient's trunk; now pressing, now relaxing for a little, then applying pressure again, with the aim of inducing a lateral gliding correction of the lateral list.

While pressure is being applied, the patient's part in the manoeuvre, which may take many minutes at each of several attempts during a single treatment session, is to remain as relaxed as possible, breathe quietly and report on the probable changing distribution and degree of pain. It is unwise to be aggressive or forceful at the initial attempt to over-correct the deviation, since many patients will experience impending syncope and some may faint.

The ideal combination is a co-operative patient and a therapist who is patient and considerate. Whether the pressure is applied higher or lower against the trunk depends on trial and error. Pain 'centralising' to the L5 region from unilateral buttock and upper thigh is a good augury, while pain spreading more peripherally suggests it is time to stop, at least for that session and until indications for trying again at another attendance, or reformulating treatment, become clearer. Successful over-correction of the lateral deviation should be followed immediately by a sustained and easy-resting lumbar extension posture (Fig. 11.46).

The manoeuvre, with its associated self-help regime as a home exercise programme, is fully described by its innovator McKenzie[125] whose work should be consulted.

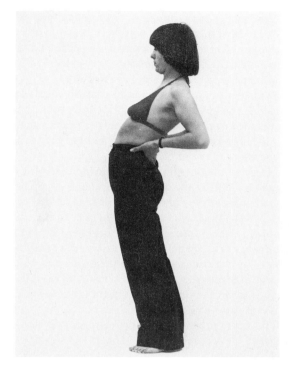

Fig. 11.46 Home exercise in the treatment of localised acute back pain with some loss of normal lumbar lordosis. The exercise is initially not suitable for those patients whose nerual arches have been painfully approximated by trauma or stress. Allowing the pelvis to sag forward means much less muscle work for the patient (and thus less pain) than bending the trunk backward. The subtle difference is important. The exercise is also unsuitable until the lateral postural deviant has been corrected, (Figs. 11.44, 11.45).

6. STRETCHING (A) (See also Stretching (B) p. 122)

Apart from the primary aim of *relaxation* when using soft-tissue techniques such as stroking during massage, the purpose of nearly all 'soft-tissue techniques' is to improve not only the vascularity and mobility of soft tissue, but especially its *extensibility*.

There is new evidence[45] to support the view that suppleness and flexibility of muscle and connective tissues are of prior importance. Long and continued occupational and postural stress, asymmetrically imposed upon the soft tissues, tends to cause fibroblasts to multiply more rapidly and produce more collagen. Besides occupying more space within the connective tissue elements of the muscle, the extra fibres encroach on the space normally occupied by nerves and vessels. Because of this trespass, the tissue loses elasticity, and may become painful when the muscle is required to do work in co-ordination with others. In the long term, collagen would begin to replace the active fibres of the muscle, and since collagen is fairly resistant to enzyme breakdown, these changes tend to be irreversible.

The single nerve-muscle-joint complex is not a simple mechanical entity, but one of many arthrokinetic systems which are functionally and reflexly interdependent with all others.

Abnormal *joint* function, increasingly better examined and increasingly better understood, is only one expression of motor systems impairment; the whole field of benign functional pathology of the motor system is as yet largely unexplored.

Janda[90] observes that muscles play an important part in the pathogenesis of various back pain syndromes, and Lewit[110] has drawn attention to the significance of iliopsoas spasm in the genesis of pelvic asymmetry in children.

Manifest changes in muscle are not random or incidental but follow certain typical and significant patterns. Selective tightness of some muscle groups, and lengthening with weakness of their antagonist groups, occur frequently in degenerative joint conditions of all spinal regions. A pattern emerges in which those muscles with largely a *postural* function appear to respond to pathological states by tightness, and those with mainly a *phasic* function respond by weakness and lengthening.

The differences may be broadly summarised as follows:

a. *Postural* muscle is phylogenetically older, can work for longer without fatigue, is largely concerned in the maintenance of static posture, is activated more easily and has a tendency to become shorter and tight.

b. *Phasic* muscle is phylogenetically younger, is fatigued more quickly, is primarily concerned in rapid movement and has an earlier tendency to become weak.

Those muscles which have a predominantly *postural* function, and tend to react to pain by increasing tightness are:

sternomastoid
pectoralis major (clavicular and sternal parts)
trapezius (superior part)
levator scapulae
the flexor groups of the upper extremity
quadratus lumborum
erector spinae, perhaps mainly: the longissimus dorsi and the rotatores
iliopsoas
tensor fasciae latae
rectus femoris
piriformis
pectineus

adductor longus, brevis and magnus
biceps femoris
semitendinosus
semimembranosus
gastrocnemius
soleus
tibialis posterior.

Those muscles with predominantly a *phasic* function, which tend to react to pain by weakening and lengthening are:

scaleni and the prevertebral cervical muscles
extensor groups of the upper extremity
pectoralis major, the abdominal part
trapezius, the inferior and middle part
rhomboids
serratus anterior
rectus abdominus
internal and external abdominal obliques
gluteal muscles (minimus, medius, maximus)
the vasti muscles (medialis, lateralis, intermedius)
tibialis anterior
the peroneal muscles

It is common experience that muscle imbalance tends to occur in typical patterns, e.g. as a rule, the upper trapezius, pectoralis major, lumbar sacrospinalis and hamstrings react to pain by increasing tightness, while others such as rhomboids, deltoid, abdominal muscles, glutei and anterior tibial muscles tend to show weakening and lengthening. *Yet the apparent chronological sequence of events may not be so.*

While muscle and other soft tissue changes (*vide infra*) frequently accompany joint problems, and can be seen as sequelae, e.g. muscle spasm in joint irritability (p. 133), *it is clinically evident that joint problems commonly occur as a sequel of chronic localised postural imbalance.*

The genesis of painful, degenerative joint conditions may frequently lie in more regional, and major, chronic imbalance of functional movement patterns, which place sustained and abnormal stress on joints.

Janda[92] observes that much present-day work and recreation occupations tend to favour postural muscles in getting stronger, shorter or tighter, as the phasic muscular system becomes weaker and more inhibited. More established tightness, and lengthening of antagonists, leads to chronic disturbances in functional movement patterns. By extended use, the imprint of abnormal joint function must be accompanied by abnormal imprints of neurone patterning.

The concept of connective-tissue tightness is not new. Mennell[136] has said,

It is very remarkable how widespread may be the symptoms caused by unduly taut fascial planes. Though it is true that the fascial bands play a principal part in the mobility of the human body, they are often conducive to binding between two joint surfaces. For obvious reasons it is of the utmost importance to restore the lost mobility in the joints, before attempting to stretch the fascial planes. On the other hand, if the mobility of these planes is not restored, recurrence of the binding in the joints is almost inevitable.

These concepts are a far cry from the 'if something is 'out', put it back' school of manipulation, yet they are a necessary part of any real attempt to fully understand the aetiology and nature of vertebral pain syndromes, their infinite variety of causation and presentation and our seemingly inexplicable therapeutic failures.

Weakened *phasic* muscle must be strengthened, and tight *postural* musculature and its connective-tissue elements must have their extensibility improved.

While the *soft tissue techniques* of Stretching (A) are intended to affect specific muscles or groups of muscles, they are essentially regional techniques by reason of their field of effect.

a. As a first step, chronically shortened tissues should be stretched (i) passively and steadily; (ii) after maximal contraction, and by this stretching the inhibitory effect on weakened antagonistic muscle will be lessened.

b. Other factors (age, chronicity, etc.) given, if a satisfactory balance between the opposed muscles and other soft tissue is not achieved after three to five treatments of the shortened postural muscles, a specific training programme for the phasic muscle group must begin.

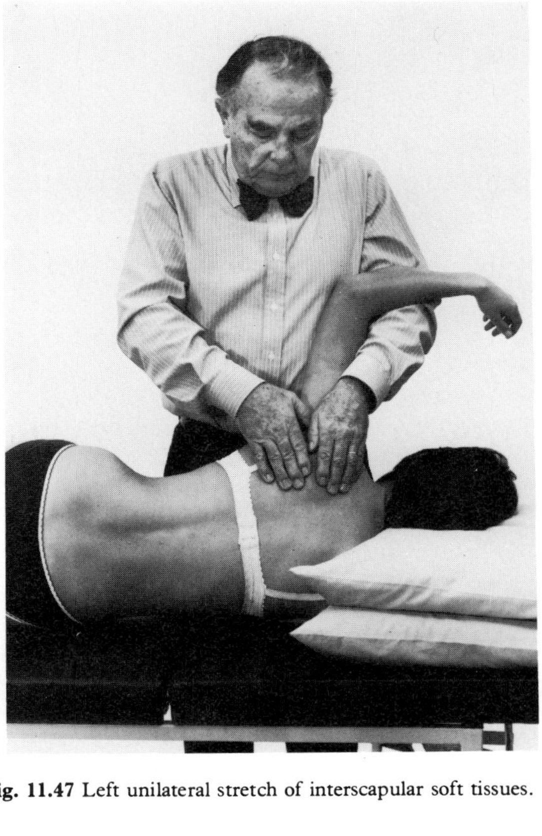

Fig. 11.47 Left unilateral stretch of interscapular soft tissues.

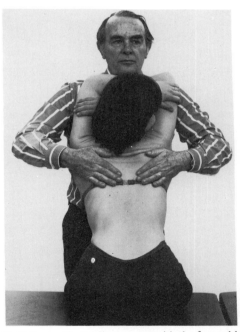

Fig. 11.48 By a walk-standing posture with the forward leg between the patient's knees, the therapist supports the patient's folded arms on his chest. The patient relaxes her forehead on her forearms. With his palms on her mid-thoracic region, the therapist repetitively stretches the pectoral soft tissues by rhythmically leaning backwards. A slight degree of localisation is achieved by placing of the therapist's hands.

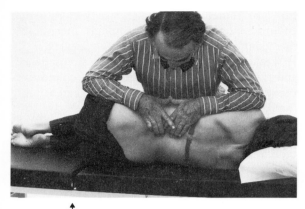

Fig. 11.49 ↑ Soft-tissue mobilisation of the paravertebral mass of the sacrospinalis muscle.

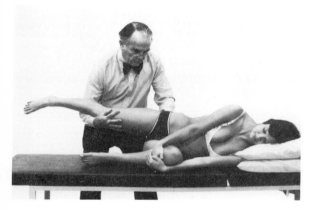

Fig. 11.50 A stretching technique for the right ilio-psoas and associated soft tissues. Stabilisation, by the patient, of the left hip and knee in flexion also stabilises the lumbar spine and prevents extension of it.

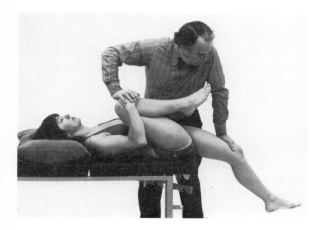

Fig. 11.51 An examination, as well as a treatment, technique for a tight left ilio-psoas muscle group.

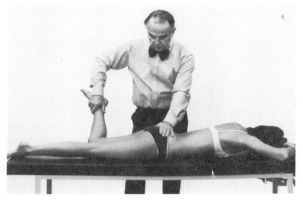

Fig. 11.52 If the hip flexion-adduction test (Fig. 7.30) reveals haunch pain without much limitation, or a lack of any real *resistance* to further probing, the cause may be a 'tight' piriformis muscle on the same side. This technique may be used to stretch the muscle, with its associated connective tissues, or to improve its extensibility by hold-relax or isometric techniques.

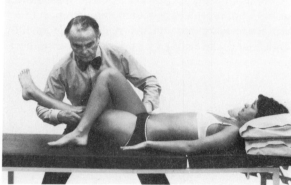

Fig. 11.53 Technique for stretching a tight left ilio-tibial band. The grasps are self-explanatory.

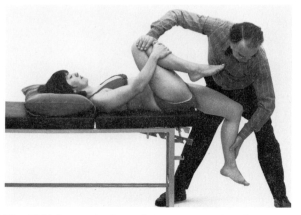

Fig. 11.54 An examination and treatment technique for a tight left quadriceps femoris muscle group.

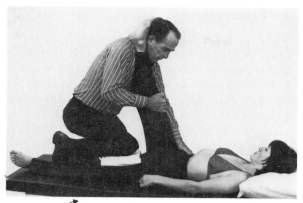

Fig. 11.55 Unilateral mobilisation of restricted range of straight-leg-raising when root or joint irritability is absent and *restriction*, rather than *pain*, is being treated.

7. MANUAL TRACTION AND MECHANICAL HARNESS TRACTION

Traction is only another way of using movement to treat benign painful abnormalities of movement. As in other methods, its use must be controlled, carefully assessed, and precisely recorded.

Like other treatments beginning to acquire some antiquity, consideration of the purpose and value of neck traction should include an appraisal of why it came into vogue in the first place.

Traction is classically used in various ways in orthopaedic practice, but its use in association with manipulative treatment of spinal joint problems in the recent past has been restricted to attempting to restore presumably shifted disc material to its 'proper' place, most often by way of a sustained pull repeated daily. However, Bourdillon[13] states: 'There appears no evidence to suggest that actual disc protrusion can be reduced by this means'.

So long as the nature of common pathological changes underlying neck pain and brachial neuralgia, and backache and sciatica, is basically envisaged as 'a slipped disc' and the sole basis for using traction is the notion of mechanically 'putting it back', or 'shifting it off the nerve root', the therapist is denied a much wider range of application of this useful treatment method.

Alternatively, if traction is conceived as a flexible and freely adaptable method of manual or mechanical mobilisation, including grade V dis-

tractive manipulation techniques, its field of usefulness is considerably broadened. *With regard to traction for neurological symptoms and signs:* 'Cervical spondylosis can only be regarded as a pre-disposing factor for the development of nerve root symptoms... It is quite amazing to what extent a nerve root can become squeezed and deformed by a slowly growing osteophytic protrusion, without any clinical evidence of irritation or dysfunction. Reactive fibrosis may also involve the root-sheaths and periarticular tissues, obliterating root pouches — yet the root remains functionally intact... Such changes, however, always make the root extremely vulnerable to all kinds of stress and pain'[59]. Duncan[43] and Sunderland[171] have also emphasised this factor.

When a nerve root is stretched or otherwise injured by trauma, in a mature patient, and begins to hurt, perhaps after months or years of being steadily squashed and distorted by slow, painless degenerative trespass, are we giving traction to try to reverse the serial tissue changes which have given rise to the current syndrome of root pain and root signs (i.e. 'put the disc back'), or would we do better to devote our time to gently trying to reduce the current inflammatory response?

Some effects of traction

Undoubtedly, traction is capable of producing both a measurable separation of vertebral bodies, and centripetal forces exerted by the traction applied to surrounding soft tissues.

Yet traction has other and equally important effects, some of which are likely to be most valuable when it is employed to produce rhythmic longitudinal movement rather than a frank distractive effect. Among them may be:

a. The simple mobilisation of joints with reversible stiffness.

b. Modification of the abnormal patterns of afferent impulse traffic from joint mechano-receptors, particularly at the cranio-vertebral junction.

c. Relief of pain by inhibitory effects upon afferent neurone traffic subserving pain.

d. The reduction of muscle spasm.

e. The stretching of muscle and connective tissues.

f. The improvement of tissue-fluid exchange in muscle and connective tissue.

g. The likely improvement of arterial, venous and

lymphatic flow.

h. The physiological benefit to the patient of rhythmic movement, and of the lessening of compressive effects.

Clinical experience often reveals that a relatively small poundage, sufficient to equal the natural apposition tendencies maintaining the integrity of resting joints, is enough to relieve pain and limitation of movement.

Joint apposition forces are small[7,8] being due to:

a. The slight elastic tension of muscle, tendons and aponeuroses; the joint capsule, and ligaments; periarticular connective tissues; deep and superficial fascia and skin.

b. The slight negative pressure within joints, some 5–10 mm Hg (0.67–1.33 kPa) below that of atmosphere.

The presence of elastic fibres has also been demonstrated in intervertebral discs.[62]

To summarise this point, it is often useful to regard traction both as a moderate (sustained, progressive or rhythmic) amplification of the effect of negating gravitational compression by simply lying down; and as another form of passive mobilising technique. To do this, it is not necessary to employ cumbersome apparatus which may resemble the weight and construction of a battleship, or use a harness resembling the trappings of a brewer's dray.

It has to be admitted that the mechanism of pain production in common joint problems is not yet completely understood, nor enough known in every case about why the procedures relieve the symptoms and signs. Neither is it possible to explain the puzzling fact that 5 to 15 minutes of daily traction can have potent therapeutic effects on a joint which is otherwise subject to some 12 or more hours daily of gravitational compression amounting to many times more than the poundage employed in treatment. In the face of this embarrassing ignorance, it is surely sensible to place the most reliance on what is much more clearly known, i.e. the relationship between common and uncommon sets of signs and symptoms, and the varying grades and types of treatment procedures.

Because there are both manual and mechanical harness techniques for every vertebral district, they may be considered in that order.

A. Manual traction

While these techniques could correctly be grouped under 'Regional Mobilisation' (p. 135) they are a special category in that, for the most part, movement is symmetrically applied along the axis of the vertebral column, with variations of position and grasp for the different spinal districts.

Despite the regional rather than segmental effects of these techniques, careful positioning of therapist and patient can often ensure that particular segments are placed in the mid-range of their available excursion of movement, for the purpose of evenly applying a gentle, moderate and sometimes firmer distractive effect to all aspects of it. The techniques can be tiring if not performed correctly, with a good stance, yet are surprisingly easy when mastered.

For obvious reasons, manual traction is more often rhythmic than sustained, and it is especially useful in its own right for those who may fear being treated in any kind of harness, those who cannot lie down because of hiatus hernia or dyspnoea and those who may relax more completely when feeling the reassuring contact of the therapist's hands.

This is a more important factor than the sometimes pejorative comments about 'the laying on of hands' may suggest. It is good assessment practice to perceive those patients who respond markedly better to manual rather than mechanical methods.

Although more difficult to 'grade' than specific mobilisation techniques, it is worth striving to do so. The techniques should never be used in a generalised way, without specific intentions and after-assessment, and require as much precision and care for detail as any other spinal mobilisation procedure.

They may also be used in preparation for other, more specific manual procedures when it is plain that 'the ground must be prepared' by gaining the patient's confidence and inducing relaxation. There are many variations of technique, including that detailed by Stoddard[168] where cervical traction is applied manually to the supine patient via a harness, spreader and spring balance, in series (Figs. 11.56, 11.57, 11.58, 11.59, 11.60).

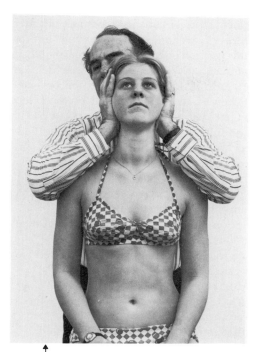

Fig. 11.56 ↑ Rhythmic manual traction to the cranio-vertebral region. Note that the head is in a somewhat military posture.

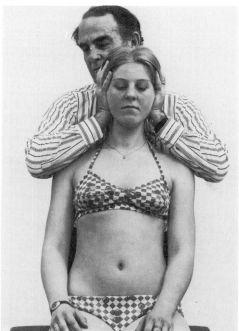

Fig. 11.57 ↑ Rhythmic manual traction with the mid-cervical region in neutral flexion-extension posture. Compare patient's position in Fig. 11.56.

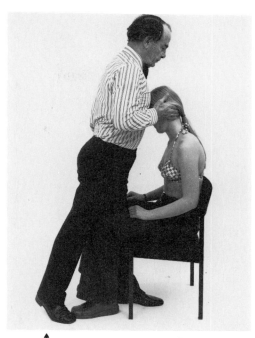

Fig. 11.58 ⊥ (Mid-upper-cervical) Rhythmic traction can be applied with the patient sitting and resting her forehead against the therapist's lower chest. With a walk-standing posture and his weight on the forward leg, the therapist gently places his palmar finger surfaces on the sub-occipital area, and applies the traction effect by small backwards movements of his own trunk, keeping the patient's head in contact with his chest. It is important to make only small excursions of movement.

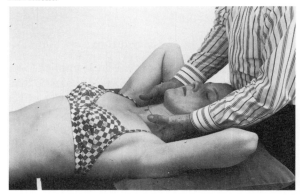

Fig. 11.59 ↦ (Cervico-thoracic region) With the patient in the supine neck-rest lying position, the therapist stands behind and reaches over the patient's forearm to apply the palmar surface of his fingers over the upper two ribs on either side. By a combination of ordinary skin traction and of gently lifting the patient towards his own sternum, a very comfortable distraction effect is imparted to the cervico-thoracic district. It is important not to pull with the fingers, but to 'lift' the patient. Ordinary gravity ensures that the resultant is distraction.

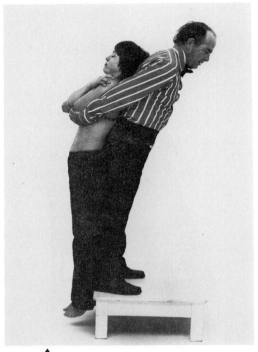

Fig. 11.60 ⊥ This distraction technique for the lumbar spine is sometimes of value in treating acute low back pain. Since it requires a physically able therapist and a cooperative, not too obese patient, its use is somewhat limited. It is not a good technique to be used repetitively, and two good attempts are sufficient to indicate its effectiveness (or failure) in relieving an acute episode.

B. Mechanical harness traction

Although harness traction is routinely applied in the longitudinal axis of the spine, techniques include arranging a degree of bias to the distractive effect, which is thus emphasised on one aspect of the joint.[166]

The introduction of bias has been especially developed in the techniques of auto-traction for the lumbar spine (see p. 211).[12,48,116]

Cervical traction

Signs and symptoms due to involvement of articular and periarticular tissues at the neck and upper/middle thoracic spine respond well to passive movement techniques, of which cervical harness traction (sustained or rhythmic) is only one.

Cervical traction should not be regarded solely as a

treatment in itself; patients sometimes benefit from a mixture of techniques. Some will improve on harness traction only, though manual mobilising can be more specifically localised to vertebral segments affected, and is often quicker in appropriate cases.

Flexion of the neck, without traction, separates the vertebrae posteriorly—it also increases the tension in the dura, meningeal ligaments and nerve roots;[19] this tension is increased if there is already a degree of *congenital* or developmental stenosis, and further increased if there is *acquired* stenosis due to: disc pathology; osseous bars and bosses; ligamentum flavum buckling; facet-joint changes.[17]

Flexion also aggravates the tension of meningeal adhesions.

The following findings can be derived from the literature[28,29,30,176,177].

a. Most experimenters, with poundages above 20 lb (9 kg), some of them very high, separated the vertebrae by about 1–1.5 mm per space, measured at posterior vertebral levels.

b. By far the greatest separation occurs posteriorly, and is greatest with increasing flexion (Fig. 11.61).

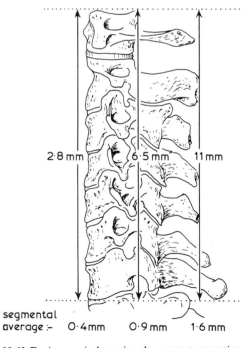

segmental
average :-   0.4 mm   0.9 mm   1.6 mm

Fig. 11.61 During cervical traction the greatest separation occurs posteriorly.

c. The normal cervical lordosis is eradicated at pulls of about 20–25 lb (9–11 kg).

d. A traction force of 30 lb (13.5 kg) for only seven seconds will separate the vertebrae posteriorly, the amount increasing with flexion.

e. At a constant angle, a traction force of 50 lb (22.5 kg) produces greater separation than 30 lb (13.5 kg), but the *amount* of separation is not significantly different at 7, 30 or 60 seconds.

f. When separation of vertebral bodies *is* desired, high tractive forces for short periods will achieve it.

g. Upper cervical segments do not separate as easily as lower cervical segments.

h. Rhythmic traction produces twice as much separation as sustained traction.

i. When traction forces are removed, restoration to normal dimensions is four to five times quicker in posterior structures. Restoration in anterior structures is much slower (Fig. 11.62).

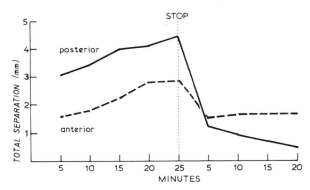

Fig. 11.62 Amount of cervical spinal separation (mm) during and after 25 min rhythmic traction with 24° rope angle, 30 lb (12 kg) poundage, 7 sec pull 5 sec release. Upon release of tractive force restoration to normal dimensions is four to five times quicker in posterior structures.

j. As would be expected, less separation occurs in 50-year-old patients than in normal 20-year olds.

k. In one comprehensive trial, patients with frontal headaches and vertigo-like symptoms did not do well on traction given in slight or greater flexion.

Da Lacerda[36] employed EMG findings to ascertain the effects of increasing angles of pull (10°–25°–30°) on the myoelectrical activity of the upper fibres of the trapezius, in seven young adult females with no history of cervical trauma. The angles were those between pull direction and longitudinal body axis; presumably the neck/trunk angle. No mention is made of that important factor in trapezius tension, the head/neck angle. At a standard 30 lb (13.5 kg) tension, electrical activity in the trapezius increased as flexion increased; the author suggests that this factor could aggravate soft tissue injuries.

Deets et al[35] showed that more separation, between segments C4 to C7, occurs when the patient is supine rather than sitting, and ascribed this to increased comfort and better relaxation.

Notwithstanding that the aims of cervical traction do not necessarily include 'vertebral separation', the properly-supported and comfortable *half-lying* position, which many patients prefer to lying supine, produces full relaxation and promotes confidence in a significant proportion of patients, especially in those who are just not able to lie down comfortably. In a study of the biomechanical influence of traction (of 150 N, about 15 kg) on the cervical spine,[63] widening not exceeding 1 mm was seen in only a minority of discs. It was not correlated to radiographic evidence of degenerative disc disease nor to the clinical features.

Since heads and necks are dissimilar in shape and size, a supply of different harnesses is useful. A desirable harness is adjustable in all three dimensions — occiput to spreader, chin to spreader, and chin to occiput — this allows comfortable adjustment of the head/neck relationship without necessarily affecting the degree of neck flexion which may be required by the treatment. Single pulleys and weights are often used but a double pulley with a small spring balance (or better still, a tensiometer or statimeter) in series allows a more graduated application and removal of traction.

Localisation of effect: The main traction effect should be directed to the vertebral segment involved and the patient so positioned that the segment is at midpoint of its available sagittal movement.

It follows that: (a) interpretation of the segmental significance (if any) of the distribution of signs and symptoms, (b) palpation for extra spinal tenderness, local guarding spasm, thickening around joints and diminished accessory movement, and (c) a passive test of physiological movement to find the mid-range of affected segment(s) are necessary parts of examination.

It also follows that: (a) the patient's position (e.g. sitting, lying, half-lying), (b) the angle of the neck with head, and neck with trunk, (c) the adjustment of harness straps to individual requirements have a bearing on the effects produced and are therefore important.

Generally, since the most movement is achieved when a joint is positioned at the midpoint of all its available ranges, the occiput —C1 and C1 —C2 joint should be treated in the neutral or slightly extended head/neck relationship, with increasing flexion of the neck for lower cervical and upper thoracic levels, but the best position for each patient is entirely governed by the requirement to produce the movement (traction effect) at the vertebral level intended, and by the response to the initial treatment. Hence, assessment of effects produced is also important.

The duration of treatment and amount of force applied to the vertebral column in all of these techniques need not be as great as is commonly employed; good results are often achieved with minimum poundage. Occasionally up to an hour's traction with heavy poundage (30–40) (13.5—18 kg) is required; in these cases a few minutes' rest half-way is wise.

A more or less standard force/duration 'recipe' for all patients does not amount to planned treatment, neither does a steady progression of one or both factors as a routine procedure.

No passive movement technique should be continued beyond that necessary to relieve signs and symptoms.

Assessment

Accurate assessment is possible only when the dispositions of patient and apparatus, and precisely known magnitudes of tension, are repeatable — only then do effects become a significant basis for modifying the numerous variables in treatment. A moment's consideration indicates the formidable number of variables which need to be controlled. For example, with the patient in half-lying, the *resultant* of the longitudinal forces applied to a given segment of the neck (Fig. 11.63) is a function of:

a. The disposition and weight of neck and head.
b. The presence, degree and distribution of contracture of cervical soft tissues, of osteophytosis and segmental ankylosis.
c. The weight of harness and spreader, and cord

between harness and pulley.
d. Friction between occiput and pillow.
e. The angle between body and direction of pull.
f. Discrepancy between the nominal poundage and the degree of force dissipated, by the change of direction of pull and by friction.

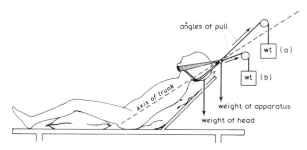

Fig. 11.63 Some factors to be assessed during neck traction in the half-lying position. When pulling along the axis of the patient's trunk, or as (b) the mandibular strap will apply most of the tension owing to the weight of the head, the distance between the occiput and symphysis menti and the consequent 'beer handle' effect. Set-up (a) is more likely to apply tension along the neutral axis of the neck.

We should bring under control as many variables as possible.

While we cannot actually weigh the head of each patient, the ratios derived from several section weight/body weight cadaver studies have produced reliable anthropometric data suggesting that the head weighs some 7.0–8.1 per cent of an individual's body weight; thus a rule of thumb might be 7.5 per cent of body weight.[108]

Spring balances in series, each on either side of the pulley, will testify that some 2–3 lb (1 kg) less than a nominal weight of some 10–15 lb (4.5–7 kg) is actually being applied to the spreader and harness. These discrepancies are greater at higher magnitudes, and are critical when giving sustained pulls of low duration and poundage for severe cervical root pain.

For this reason, it is necessary to devise means whereby *the tension actually being applied to the patient* can be precisely known, and where apparatus is successively being used by many in the bustle of clinical work, a neat but sturdy spring balance attached to the spreader, and thus in series with the pulley cord, is indispensable (Fig. 11.64).

In the near future, it is likely that more sophisticated devices will be incorporated. Tensiometers or statimeters (which measure tension without undergoing any change in length) are

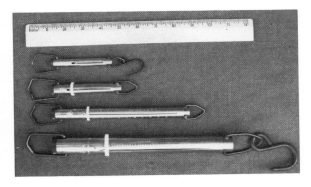

Fig. 11.64 A selection of tubular brass spring balances, which are necessary for incorporation in series with the traction cord, to measure the tension *actually being applied to the patient*.

already available but very expensive. Digital electronic force gauges may soon take the place of spring balances, and an alternative possibility is the strategic placement of several thin film beam load cells at different points on the traction apparatus, enabling precise measurements to be made across the whole range of procedures. The load cells would provide electrical output signals for a single remote digital display fitted with a selector switch.

Bearing in mind the condition and diagnosis, i.e. the whole nature or family of pathological changes which might have occurred, its unique presentation in any one patient, the effect it is hoped to produce, and co-existing conditions which may complicate techniques, there are about a dozen factors to be considered:

a. The type of apparatus and suspension points available.
b. The physique and weight of the patient.
c. The position of the patient.
d. The head/neck angle lie (i.e. the relative lengths of occipital and mandibular straps).
e. The neck/trunk angle (i.e. the rope angle, decided by position of the fixation point).
f. The poundage or force applied.
g. The weight of apparatus, between neck and attachment point.
h. The duration of the traction.
i. Whether sustained, progressive or rhythmically varied, and the periodicity of pull and release phases.
j. The frequency of traction sessions.
k. The presence of difficulties, such as an over-

tender sub-occipital area, a painful arthrotic temporo-mandibular joint, badly-fitting dentures, and so on.

What are we doing it for?

Pain production in common joint problems is not yet completely understood, neither is enough known in every case about *why* procedures relieve the symptoms and signs. The idea that cervical muscle spasm and pain are interdependent could bear inspection[70].

The association is not as straightforward as is commonly believed.

Again, the immense amount of information now available about the inter-vertebral disc and the great variety of biomechanical and physical changes which can occur in it and its closely related structures, should warn us not to conceive of it simply as a sort of badly-packed suitcase. The clinical field covered by that nebulous phrase 'cervical spondylosis' is a very comprehensive one[16]. It is concerned far more with the four essential factors of vascularity, inflammatory response to stress, aberrant neurophysiology, and soft-tissue tethering effects, than with notions expressed by the catch-all label 'disc lesion'.

Technique

Sustained traction with patients lying or half-lying. (Traction in neutral can be done with the patient sitting under the apparatus. A tilting dentist-type chair is then useful for altering the neck/trunk angle, for traction in flexion). (Figs. 11.65, 11.66). It is probably better to avoid trying to give 'neutral' traction with the patient lying, and pulling with the rope parallel to the horizontal plinth, because there is always a tendency for the mandibular strap to apply the lion's share of the tension; also, the amount of friction between head and pillow precludes the best estimate of the amount of pull actually being applied to the upper cervical structures.

To produce a pull the resultant of which is virtually in the longitudinal axis of the upper neck, it should be arranged that the rope angle is some 10°–15° above the horizontal, counteracting the effect of gravity on the head; this arrangement ensures a pull in the neutral position (Fig. 11.63). Yet there is still the factor of friction to be considered, and for this reason neutral cervical traction is probably best applied in sitting (Fig. 11.65) with a double-pulley and spring balance set-up, because the tension then being recorded is that being applied to the patient (less the weight of the harness and spreader, which are between spring balance and the patient) and it may be necessary in the early stages to pull with low tension, i.e. just sufficient to allow the beginning of movement to be perceived by a palpating finger.

(i) *Initial treatment:* Explain procedure to patient.

Lay patient down, with head supported on pillow(s) while harness is applied. It is often more comfortable for patients to have knees flexed. If using adjustable harness, secure straps so that pull is comfortably and evenly applied to occiput and mandible, and the head/neck relationship in sagittal plane is consistent with the need to produce the main effect at specific intervertebral levels.

Fix spreader and pulleys, etc., and arrange attachment of upper traction hook and the height of pillow(s) so that the intended angle of *neck flexion on trunk* is produced (this may need to be adjusted after assessment). The line of the rope is usually at a slight angle to the longitudinal axis of the neck. For this reason, traction in flexion is best done in lying or half-lying, and traction in neutral in sitting, although traction in slight flexion while sitting can be done.

By gently applying and releasing moderate traction force (8–10 lb) (3.5—4.5 kg) in a rhythmic way, and by palpation between spinous processes, ensure that the movement produced is occurring mainly at the vertebral level intended. Adjust angles of pull until this is achieved, and note the minimum poundage required to do so. Increased the latter if intervertebral movement cannot be detected.

Then give a short two to five minutes pull at this poundage.

Remove traction and reassess salient signs and symptoms.

N.B. Behaviour of symptoms *during* traction is of no special significance (relief of signs or symptoms during traction by no means indicates that they will remain relieved *between* tractions, which is the aim of the treatment) and it is not an infallible guide to modifications of technique, except, if very severe pain is dramatically relieved during the first gentle traction treatment, carefully take the harness down at once and reapply with reduced poundage and

duration on next attendance. These patients may suffer a prolonged and severe exacerbation afterwards if care is not taken.

It is the assessment immediately preceding the treatments which should dictate modifications (if necessary) of angle and pull, force applied, and duration of traction, but, *for the first treatment,* apply the minimum amount of traction necessary to improve the signs and symptoms when assessed immediately following (Figs. 11.65, 11.66, 11.67, 11.68, 11.69, 11.70).

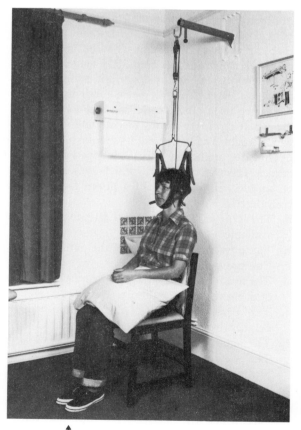

Fig. 11.65 ⌐ Cervical traction in the neutral craniovertebral posture, for upper cervical joint problems. Note the spring balance in series.

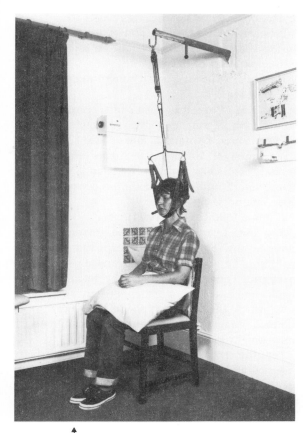

Fig. 11.66 ↕ Cervical traction in the slightly flexed position, for mid-upper cervical joint problems. Note the spring balance in series.

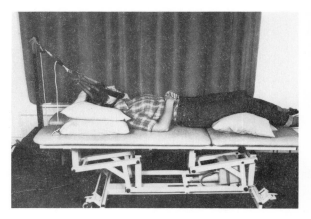

Fig. 11.68 ⊢→ Cervical traction in supine lying, with a further degree of neck flexion. Compare pillow arrangement.

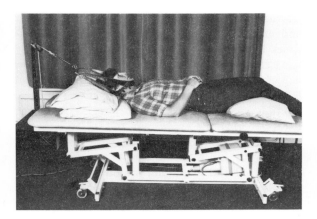

Fig. 11.67 ⊢→ Cervical traction in supine lying, with slight flexion. Note spring balance in series, and arrangement of pillows.

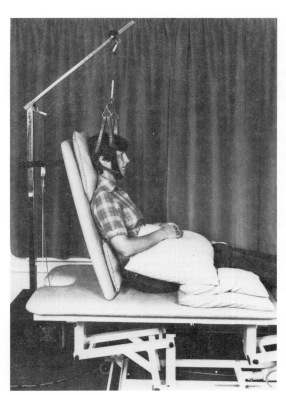

Fig. 11.69 ⊢↗ Cervical traction in half-lying (or long sitting) with a slight degree of flexion, for the mid-upper cervical segments.

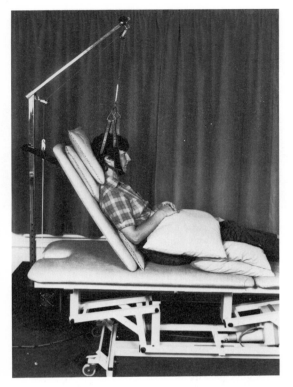

Fig. 11.70 ↰ Cervical traction in half-lying for the lower cervical segments. Note spring balance in series, and the position of back-rest, compared to that in Fig. 11.69, also type and arrangement of pillows.

Guides for action are:

a. If adequate subjective improvement (i.e. symptoms) and adequate objective improvement (i.e. signs) are evident, repeat treatment at subsequent attendances with same position/poundage/duration, as long as adequate improvement continues.

b. If worse, do no more at first session, but modify apparatus for head/neck angle, and fixation point for rope angle, at the subsequent attendance.

If no change, add 3–5 lb (1.5–2 kg) and repeat traction with same duration; if still no change, repeat increased poundage with duration increased by five minutes.

(ii) *Subsequently* (if patient is having traction treatment only): Assess changes in signs and symptoms before each treatment, and if the patient continues to improve adequately there is no need to alter angle, poundage or duration. Cervical traction is not necessarily like a 'progressive weight resistance' exercise regime.

Patients having traction and manual mobilising during the same sessions should be assessed after each application of technique.

N.B. Try to achieve results with minimum duration and poundage.

As a rule of thumb, patients of average physique should have treatment progressed, when indicated, by increments of 3 minutes and/or 3 lb (1.5 kg), with a maximum of 20 for both; higher amounts are necessary for some patients. Traction is unlikely to help if significant improvement has not occurred in three attempts.

A guide follows (Fig. 11.71).

Rhythmic traction (or variable traction). Technique is not very different, except that the many varieties of modern electronically-controlled apparatus require the inertia of the patient's weight for operation and many patients try to 'go with the rope' when the pull is applied. They need to be reminded to remain still and relaxed, and allow their body weight to act.

Set the poundage, duration and periodicity required and proceed then as for sustained traction except that: with severe symptoms — relatively long periods of 'hold' and 'rest' should be employed (i.e. less movement); as symptoms become less severe — shorter 'hold' and 'rest' periods are more effective (i.e. more movement).

Thoracic traction

The not infrequent clinical finding, that cervical traction is capable of provoking pain from a latent and undeclared middle/lower thoracic, and sometimes lumbar, problem is a useful reminder of the mechanical interdependence of the vertebral column, and of how far into the thoracic area cervical traction is felt. In general, the principles governing thoracic traction are the same as for other regions, with the exception that the application of tension is not as direct. Cervical and lumbar harnesses can be designed to utilise convenient bony configurations, e.g. occiput and mandible, contours of upper loin area, lower loin and iliac crests, but because there are no conveniently shaped body areas which allow an upper attachment for traction to be applied specifically to the thoracic spine, the treatment requires adaptation of:

Symptoms	Signs	Procedure Duration	Weight	Notes
Improved	Improved	→	→	Be slow to increase if joint is irritable; otherwise be quick to increase duration, and then weight, if adequate improvement is not maintained
No change	No change	↑	→ or ↑	*—Care if irritable*
Improved	No change	↑	→	
Improved / Worse	Worse / Improved	→	→	
Worse	No change	→	↓ ½	
Worse	Worse	↓ ½	↓ ½	

Fig. 11.71 A guide to modification of duration and/or tension, when necessary, after the initial treatment by traction.

a. the cervical traction method, for the upper three-quarters of the thoracic spine (T1—T9), and

b. the lumbar traction method, for the lower quarter of the region (T9–T12).

Segments T1–T9. When applying experimental cervical traction with a horizontal pull to a supine subject of average physique, a pull of around 60 lb (27 kg) is required before the traction is sufficient to overcome body weight and friction, and begins to move the patient bodily along the plinth towards the attachment point. (The pull required will vary somewhat with the patient's physique and clothing, and the nature of the plinth surface.) For this reason, when giving thoracic traction via a cervical harness, the weight of an inert and relaxed patient is often sufficient to provide counter-traction with pulls below 50 lb (22.5 kg); poundage of this order and sometimes above may be required when attempting to influence thoracic joint problems below the T6 segment. With higher poundages counter-traction by the lumbar traction pelvic harness may be necessary. Down to the T6 level, lighter poundages are quite effective, and for the T1 to T3 segments, pulls in the middle and upper ranges of cervical traction poundages are usually sufficient (Fig. 11.72).

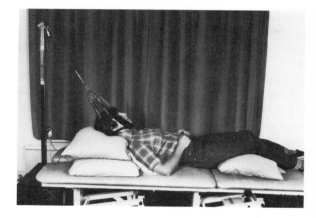

Fig. 11.72 ⊢⟶ Traction for upper/mid-thoracic segments, by arrangement of pull via the cervical spine, with rope angle at some 45°. As is evident, this does not mean that the longitudinal axis of the neck is also at 45°. Note extra pillow under scapulae. The angle of pull may need to be increased by additional attachment of the angled mast.

It goes without saying that any degree of cervical pain, and irritability, will preclude this method of harness traction for the thoracic spine problem, and manual mobilisation (including manual thoracic traction) must be the treatment of choice.

Breig[17] has described in clear detail the potential dangers of giving cervical traction, especially traction in flexion, in cases of cervical myelopathy.

When the free mobility of spinal cord and meninges is already restricted, or nervous tissue is distorted, by the space-occupying and/or tethering effects of degenerative or traumatic changes in the neck, a further increment of physical stress by traction may be critical.

Similarly, the arrangement of a pull, via the cervical harness, to affect the upper two-thirds of the thoracic spine should never be employed in the presence of frank cervical spondylotic change, cervical irritability or when neurological symptoms and signs, in one or both lower limbs, are considered due to thoracic changes.

Technique. By a passive test of thoracic flexion and extension in sitting, assess when the segment to be treated is in the mid-position between extremes of these sagittal movements and try to reproduce the general thoracic posture which accords with this requirement when the patient lies down.

Existing postural curvature differs widely between patients, of course. Raising the end of the plinth and placing two or three pillows under the patient's head and upper thorax may be necessary.

The cervical harness is applied and the fixation point arranged so that the next/trunk angle is around 45°; this may need modification following a pretreatment manual test of whether the traction is affecting the segment intended. This is palpated by the therapist as test pulls of the selected treatment poundage are rhythmically applied with the therapist's other hand. A double-pulley system reduces manual effort.

Before proceeding, assess joint irritability, intensity of pain and nature of the pain; providing no exacerbation has occurred following the test pull, and the traction is clearly reaching the affected segment, apply the traction for four mintues, then reduce the tension slowly and considerably. The signs and symptoms are then assessed as for cervical traction with the exception that when poundages around 50–60 (22.5–27 kg) are being employed for the middle/lower thoracic segments, and there is no change after the initial session, repeat the four-minute pull but with the same poundage. If there is still no change, do no more at that session—the guide for subsequent sessions is as for the cervical spine (Fig. 11.71)–bearing in mind that proportional increases in poundages, as for cervical traction, are not always desirable when the middle/lower thoracic

segments are being treated.

Dissipated force factors

The effect of friction between patient and plinth, and thus the amount of applied pull which is dissipated because of it, is not easy to assess—many factors (termed 'dissipated force factors' by B. D. Judovich)[95] contribute to the proportion of applied poundage required to overcome resistance, e.g. (i) the weight of the patient; (ii) the surface area of contact; (iii) the nature and shape of the contacting surfaces. Added to this, the weight of the patient's head and neck, acting downward at an angle of approximately 135° to the line of the rope, when the latter is at 45° or so, contributes to the fraction of the poundage which is neutralised so far as clinical usefulness is concerned.

For example, during horizontal lumbar traction on a fixed plinth surface, a force equal to some 25 per cent of the patient's body weight must be subtracted from the poundage selected, the remainder representing the force actually being applied to the lumbar joint structures; and while dissipated forces of this order would not apply to the T1–T9 thoracic traction method described, it remains a factor to be eliminated, or reduced as much as possible.

The poundage dissipated is very much lessened by a non-friction, rolling half-section of the plinth, but not quite so completely as in horizontal lumbar traction because of the large angle between the lines of pull and the direction of the rolling section movement, at least when the patient is propped up by two or three pillows and the fixation point is somewhere overhead.

When a rolling plinth-section is not available, simple methods which help to reduce the proportion of dissipated force are: (i) placing a small nylon sheet, doubled, between patient's upper trunk and pillow; (ii) carefully lifting the patient's trunk, after poundage has been applied, and then lowering it back on the pillow. The lower the segment being treated the more important are these considerations. Forces applied can be measured in various ways, e.g. by a statimeter or a tensiometer in series with the rope, by a single spring balance reading up to 56lb (25.5 kg), or by a bank of two light spring balances, reading up to 25 lb (11.2 kg) each, and arranged in parallel by common attachment points at either end of the bank. With this method, which is somewhat cumbersome, each balance shows a half of the tension applied.

Segments T9–T12. This may be done in two ways: (i) with the patient supine on a flat table as in supine lumbar traction (described below), or (ii) with the patient in a degree of half-lying on a raised back-rest, employing the cervical traction mast and strong cervical spreader for attachment of the thoracic strap (Figs. 11.73, 11.74).

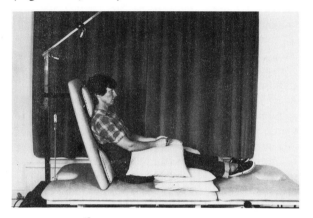

Fig. 11.73 ⊢↗   Thoracic traction in half-lying for lower segments, with thoracic harness and strong cervical spreader. Note the fairly upright position of the patient, spring balance in series partly obscured by neck pillow and the lumbar support pillow.

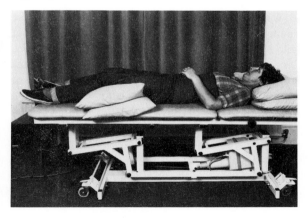

Fig. 11.74 ⊢→   Thoracic traction in supine lying for the low thoracic region, with the segment to be treated placed opposite the junction of the gliding and fixed sections of the table. Spring balance in series between patient's calves.

In both cases, the thoracic harness must be attached cranially and not caudally to the segment to be treated, and the axillae suitably protected. For women patients, padding to protect the bosom should take account of individual needs.

In technique (i), the degree of flexion of hips would be the important factor deciding the mid-position of the segment to be treated, which should, of course, be placed directly over the division of the table. The lumbar traction plinth and harnesses are employed with the thoracic belt applied higher than when treating lumbar segments. Small folded towels may be needed in the axillae to prevent discomfort. The pelvic harness is applied as usual.

Vertebral mobility in the sagittal plane is *least* at the T9–T10 segment, amounting to 2°–4° only, and the mid-position of this range is more difficult to assess. So long as the supine lying posture is comfortable, and the patient is relaxed, the mid-position is achieved in many patients. Nevertheless, it is always worth ensuring that this is so because, depending upon the patient's posture type, pillows considerably placed beneath the knees 'for comfort' may well put the low thoracic segments into an undesirable amount of flexion. The amplitudes of movement are small, and therefore critical.

The aim of localising the pull to the segment concerned is more likely to be achieved by placing the segment immediately over the division between fixed and rolling sections of a friction-free plinth.

Technique. The initial test treatment, and immediately following assessment, are conducted virtually as for lumbar traction, bearing in mind that treatment on a non-sliding section plinth requires incorporation of the dissipated force factors into assessment of the tensions needed. There is also the factor of the fraction of pull which is effectively neutralised by the springy thorax, and the slightly extensible vertebral segments lying in series between the low thoracic spine and the sacrum.

In technique (ii), flexion of the knees (and thus further flexion at the hips) also puts a low thoracic segment into a flexed position—this can be ascertained by palpating the segment and raising/flexing the knees with the other hand. It is frequently necessary to place a flat pillow between the support and the patient's low back.

Lumbar traction

Some reports[115,117,132] in the recent literature indicate that clinicians are investigating lumbar traction in new ways, and attempting to provide added information on its application and usefulness. Yet in a majority of papers the writers appear to remain preoccupied with the factors of:

(i) Increasing the height of the intervertebral space
(ii) Altering the profile of the annulus fibrosus
(iii) Reducing the intradiscal pressure and thus creating a suction effect
(iv) Exerting centripetal pressure by increasing the tension of circumferential soft tissues.[87, 97, 122, 133, 134, 156]

Probably because there have been clear demonstrations that conditions favouring these effects are readily produced by traction, questions of its efficacy continue to be largely discussed only in relation to disc trespass, sciatica and neurological deficit,[106, 107, 180] yet it has been estimated that motor weakness occurs in less than 15 per cent of hospital cases of sciatica.[185] For example, brief reports of four trials, all of which admitted patients with sciatic pain, many of whom also had neurological signs, are of interest. Some reported good results, others indifferent results:

(i) Thirty-seven patients with sciatica, neurological deficit and positive myelographic signs were treated by rhythmic traction of one-third body weight on a friction-free table. A control group of 35 with similar clinical findings were treated by simulated traction with trivial poundages for the same period. There was no significant difference in treatment results, in these 72 patients with clear evidence of root involvement.[180]

(ii) Forty patients, most of them with neurological signs, were treated by 55–70 lb (25–32 kg) rhythmic traction on a friction-free table for 20 minutes daily, producing 'excellent' results in 6 cases, 'good' in 15 and 'poor' in 19.[87]

(iii) A double-blind controlled trial of sustained traction excluded patients with recently acquired neurological deficit, although one criteria for admittance was the presence of sciatica, defined as severe and well-delineated pain in the limb. The 'control' group (14 patients) received simulated traction with trivial poundage. Improvement in the treated group (13 patients) did not achieve statistical significance, albeit the groups were small.[134]

(iv) Sixty-two patients with low back pain, and sciatic pain of more than a month's duration, were assigned to one of three groups comprising: (a) heat, massage and exercises, (b) hot packs and rest only, and (c) 20 minutes rhythmic traction in the Fowler position with pulls of one-third body weight plus 30–40 lb (13.5–18 kg), combined with abdominal and hip extensor muscle strengthening. Briefly, the patients in group (c) showed a significantly greater improvement than groups (b) and (a).[115]

Some other conclusions derived from research findings are:

(i) With high poundages, the L4–L5 space is increased by 1.5 mm and the L3–L4 space by 2 mm, i.e. narrowed disc spaces are returned to something like their normal width, but the spaces return to their pretraction level after release of tension and on standing up.[39]

(ii) *Vide* other reports, high poundages are apparently not necessary; in general, pulls of half, or a little more, of a normal subject's body weight will increase the lumbar vertebral space by about 1.5 mm, if this be the aim of treatment, and reduce the intradiscal pressure by about 25 per cent.[145]

When some of these reports prompt unfavourable opinions in medical journals of international standing, wholly questioning the value of traction and suggesting that it should be abandoned as a routine treatment,[106, 107] there is justification for reiterating the value of traction used in other ways and for other reasons.

When selecting manual and mechanical passive movement techniques in the treatment of lumbar and lumbo-sacral joint problems, there may well be an advantage in setting aside the classical and almost automatic tendency to associate (a) sciatica with or without neurological signs, and (b) sustained traction.

Perhaps a greater flexibility of approach, based primarily on the signs and symptoms *per se* and the degree of joint and root irritability, rather than on classical concepts of mechanical changes as the necessary causes of these clinical states, may lead to wider appreciation of the infinite variety of their presentation, and the formulation of a wider and more appropriate field of indications for using traction.

Lumbar traction should certainly not be regarded as a treatment apart from other mobilising techniques. It is a passive technique which can be interspersed or changed with others as indicated.

Perhaps we are optimistic to expect that prolapsed disc material can be restored to its former position by traction. Many patients who benefit from this treatment may not have sustained this particular type of joint derangement, and if we believe that some have, it is not necessarily the sole cause of all the symptoms. Consequently, it is not easy to know precisely why traction is beneficial, especially when applied with low or moderate poundage.

The object of treatment is to relieve signs and symptoms *between* treatments and relief of pain *during* traction does not always indicate that this object will be achieved, although the initial trial of traction can be employed to note its subsequent effect.

Technique—sustained traction. Initial procedure is broadly the same as for cervical traction (q.v.) and it is assumed that a modern friction-free table is being employed.

Know the patient's salient signs and symptoms before applying traction, and assess them after the initial trial; subsequently, assess before each treatment session.

Shoes, belts, corsets and restrictive clothing should be removed. Shirt or petticoat may be kept on but should be loosened upwards before straps applied.

On a flat treatment table, low lumbar lesions are better treated supine with hips and knees flexed, and mid/upper lumbar with less flexion, though the optimum position for each patient must be found by assessment.

Arrange thoracic and pelvic bands on the table before the patient lies down and test the salient sign chosen as the assessment marker (often straight-leg-raising). Estimate the angle at which limitation, if any, occurs, noting its characteristics, e.g. if painful, where the pain is being provoked, and record it on the patient's card.

Notes:
    a. Explain what the treatment involves and what reactions may be expected.
    b. Instruct the patient not to have a heavy meal before treatment.
    c. Warn the patient to try to avoid sneezing or coughing while on full traction.
    d. Patients should expect a possibly

irregular improvement, with some stiffness immediately following each treatment.

Movement on and off the treatment table. Patients who are unable to modify their functional movements to lessen pain should lie down and get up from the plinth with the lumbar spine held in the neutral position.

Lying down.
    (i) Sit on plinth with back straight and a right angle at hips, knees and ankles
    (ii) Keep knees and ankles together all the time and lower the trunk sideways to a side-lying position with the back held still. As the trunk is lowered the legs are raised sideways, the body moving as one piece
    (iii) Roll on to back
    (iv) Stretch out legs.

Getting up. This is an exact reverse of this procedure. Do *not* allow the patient to get up by initially raising the head and shoulders forward. Legs must flex first, then roll on the side, then sit up.

Stretcher patients should roll, or slide with knees bent, on to the treatment table from trolley placed alongside.

(i) Padding: Some harnesses need to be padded; most are better without padding.

(ii) Thoracic band: Patient puts arms through the thoracic harness and the straps are secured. The band should be placed immediately below the greatest diameter of the thorax (i.e. its upper edge at the xiphoid level) so that it cannot slip upwards, and securely fastened. Respiration is bound to be somewhat restricted; try to achieve a good pull with the minimum discomfort to the patient.

(iii) Pelvic band: The band is secured resting on the iliac crests (or sacrum, if prone)—some patients prefer it resting on the greater trochanters, and if it can be comfortably secured in this position there is no objection to this; it makes no difference to the ultimate effect but compression of gluteal vessels may produce transient paraesthesiae. Secure the thoracic straps to the head of the apparatus, taking up all slack by hand. Steadily pull the straps of the pelvic harness, and take up all slack by hand before securing them to apparatus. The patient should wriggle a little to settle harness comfortably, and do this again during the application of the traction. The pelvic band should be settled round the patient's pelvis at right angles to the horizontal and tilted anteriorly, or posteriorly, if assessment of early treatment shows the subsequent need for this.

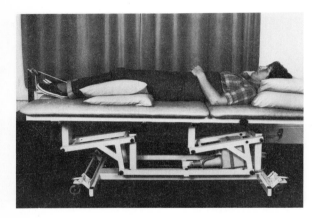

Fig. 11.75 ⊢──→ Lumbar traction in supine lying for a mid-lumbar segment.

First application. It is good practice to initially apply the set poundage or tension *before* releasing the sliding section of the table. This allows slack to be taken up and the harness to settle snugly on the patient's torso. As applicable, set and start the traction machine, or manually wind out slowly and progressively to about an indicated 40 lb (18 kg), and check straps; friction effects will reduce the applied tension to about 20–30 lb. Switch off the machine, or manually reduce the pull, and check the patient's comfort and position of harness. Then release the sliding section of the table and re-apply the tension, setting the treatment timer also. The patient's reaction to a short and gentle initial pull of ten minutes or less provides valuable information for future procedures, and his confidence is gained if he is introduced to an unusual experience gradually. He is told to report the slightest discomfort.

N.B. If severe pain is dramatically relieved with the first gentle pull, lessen it carefully at once,

otherwise a very severe pain reaction may occur.

On tables which are not friction-free, around 25 per cent of the force of the traction is 'mopped-up' by the springy thorax and soft tissue generally, and by friction between patient and plinth (which is lessened considerably with a sliding friction-free platform). The spring balance will show a decrease in pull, but the decrease during treatment will be negligible if slack is taken up efficiently beforehand. If the straps are slipping they must be reapplied more effectively after slowly winding the patient in.

End of treatment. Wind in slowly and smoothly until all straps are slack. Carefully assist the patient to lift buttocks a little, so that sliding platform can be gently closed up and locked. Release straps carefully and slowly—a sudden release of a tight thoracic band can be severely painful. Warn patient not to inhale deeply immediately as this can also be painful. After treatment, the patient should lie for a minute or two to collect himself. Assist him up by the method described. Instruct the patient to get off the table after a short rest by rolling onto side with knees and hips bent, and lowering legs as trunk is brought to the vertical.

Notes: a. Since the traction is virtually 'friction-free', poundage indicated on the dial is probably that being applied to the joint.

b. Some patients may need to be helped down.

c. Patients may also be treated in the prone position, with standard or reversed application of harness.

Assess results immediately afterwards, as described for cervical traction, (p. 162) employing duration increments of five minutes and poundage increments of 10–15 lb (4.5–7 kg).

Subsequent treatments. Pull in an indicated range of 40–100 lb (18–45 kg) (very occasionally up to 150 lb (67.5 kg), depending upon the physique of the patient) and for up to 20 minutes daily, although 15 minutes often suffices, using the 'guide' (Fig. 11.71) given for cervical traction but with the increments mentioned above. The main assessment is carried out the day after treatment, i.e. prior to the next one.

A basic treatment has been described but there are many variations. Patients may be treated prone or supine, one or both bands may be used upside-down. (Figs. 11.75, 11.76, 11.77, 11.78).

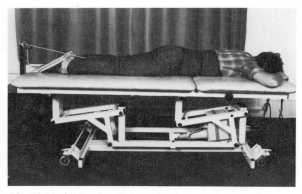

Fig. 11.76 ⊢→ Lumbar traction in prone lying, and a degree of lumbar extension, for the L4–L5 segment. The magnitude of distraction effect, with the same indicated poundage, would be less than in Figure 11.77, of course.

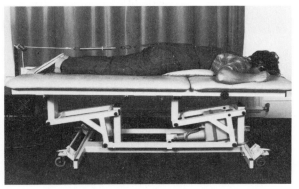

Fig. 11.77 ⊢→ Lumbar traction in prone lying, with a degree of lumbar flexion by reason of the reversed harness and flat pillow under abdomen.

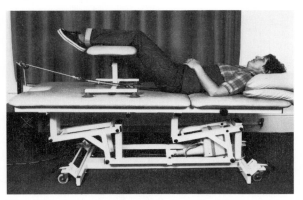

Fig. 11.78 ⊢→ Lumbar traction in supine lying, with hip and knee flexion, for the L5–S1 segment. Whether a patient be treated in this degree of hip flexion would depend upon the purpose of the traction. If the purpose is to stretch the dorsal lumbosacral soft tissues, hip flexion is considerable.
N.B. The posture depicted is an example only — the position for each patient is a matter for assessment, and there is no 'standard' position.

Spinal traction is effective but often undramatic; it involves the patient in some discomfort, and so the length of treatment should be kept as short as possible by giving an adequate session at each attendance.

It is usual to start with most patients supine on a firm surface and thereafter to modify the technique individually according to findings — we cannot know exactly how the lesion is affecting the joint and we can only find the most effective procedure by trial and error with each patient. The consistent factors are (a) a steady pull repeated daily at first, and (b) assessment of suitable poundage by behaviour of signs and symptoms, and the patient's physique.

Intermittent or repetitive rhythmic lumbar traction with sliding plinth sections.

The principles governing the use of rhythmic rather than sustained traction are the same as those for the cervical spine (p. 162). Rhythmic traction is to be preferred, although the gentlest sustained pull is obligatory for manifest nerve root and/or joint irritability.

Patients having sustained traction for severe root pain should be carefully checked for the appearance of neurological signs at each visit, because a lessening of pain may actually be the change which often accompanies increasing root compression and this may indicate the need for a short trial of increased poundage and duration; watchful assessment of effects is important at this stage. As the pain becomes less severe and less variable, rhythmic traction can be substituted with advantage.

N.B. The physical behaviour of the clothed lower half of the torso, lying on a sliding-section platform and being subject to intermittent longitudinally applied tension, is not the same as that of a simple helical spring; it is likely that a degree of residual or resting elongation remains, even when the pulling cord is slack during the rest phase of rhythmic pulling cycles.

It is important to bear in mind that once an initial distraction to the set maximum has been applied, a sliding-section platform will rarely go back to rest in the previous fully closed-up starting position after the pull phase has been completed, unless a system of springs or some such is provided to draw it back.

A moment's experiment will demonstrate this, and so long as there is no provision for both the sliding-section platform and the patient's lower half to be incorporated into a single mass which is distracted *as a whole,* notions of what happens to body tissues between pull phases may be fallacious.

This is a factor which must be included in any consideration of the use of this or that traction method, and what is believed to be happening during its application.

Much the same considerations probably also apply to cervical traction in supine, but less so in the half-lying position and probably not at all to traction from a suspension point directly overhead, when the patient is seated.

Similarly, the physical behaviour of a torso, under rhythmic or sustained traction, is not the same when prone as when supine; the differences can be reduced if the harness is always arranged so as to be in contact with the sliding-section, but this may not always suit the aims of the treatment method and the differences will remain. An experiment will verify that the nether end sliding-section will be distracted more (for a given tension) when the patient is supine, and the harness straps under the patient, than when the patient is prone and the harness is arranged to pull on the dorsal aspect of the trunk. With the latter arrangement, excursion of the moveable part of the table is lessened and the benefits of a sliding-section table are considerably reduced.

Traction should be abandoned when (a) there is no improvement after three sessions, or (b) there is deterioration in terms of increased pain and/or further movement restriction during the first two days, despite variations in the application of pull.

Oudenhoven and Lossing[154,118] describe *gravitational lumbar traction* as a method of treating pain considered secondary to nerve root or sinuvertebral nerve inflammation (Figs. 11.79, 11.80).

By employing the thoracic harness only, and tilting the support in progressive increments, distraction is applied to the lower half of the torso, gravity beginning to produce a traction effect at about 35° of tilt. Hence frictional resistance is progressively negated.

Inpatient treatment sessions are 30–60 minutes, six to eight times daily, depending upon tolerance. The angle of traction is progressively and regularly increased, and when pain is relieved, treatment

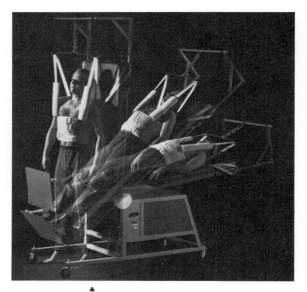

Fig. 11.79 ⊢→ ⊥ Gravitational lumbar traction, from the lying to suspended erect position (see text).

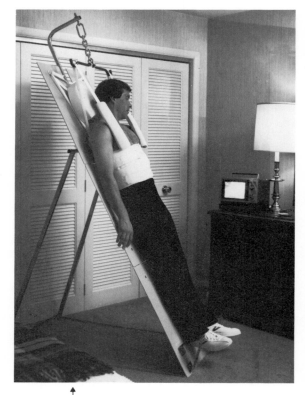

Fig. 11.80 ⊥ Apparatus for gravitational lumbar traction at home. The illustration is self-explanatory. (Figs. 11.79 and 11.80 reproduced by courtesy of Camp International Inc, Michigan).

sessions are continued at this angle of tilt for similar durations for a further three days, after which the patient is discharged to continue a home traction programme as indicated.

The treatment was considered unsuitable for referred pain from the lumbar musculature or apophyseal joints, and to this end the differential was established by the response to local anaesthesia of the posterior primary rami at L3, L4 and L5 bilaterally — the injections were under fluoroscopic control.

Those patients whose pain was relieved for the duration of the anaesthesia were considered unsuitable for gravitational traction.

The study was not intended to assess forms of conservative treatment other than gravitational traction, although the patients in this review had failed to benefit by other conservative measures.

The 121 patients were divided into:

Category I: those who had had no previous operation — 87 (72 per cent)

Category II: those who had undergone one or more surgical procedures — 34 (28 per cent)

In Category I, 69 (87 per cent) of the 81 patients without a true disc herniation were no longer occupationally disabled, and in Category II, 13 (45 per cent) of the 29 patients who had not had a spinal fusion continued to have good pain relief.

It was postulated that the treatment failures in Category II may have been due to postoperative fibrosis, and Oudenhoven suggests that the technique of gravitational lumbar traction warrants careful consideration in the management of chronic back and leg pain.

Autotraction (see p. 211)

Traction equipment

After gathering a consensus of opinion among therapists as to the best arrangement of apparatus, angles of pull, type of support and so on, the manufacture of treatment tables has usually to be something of a compromise. To a degree, traction method may have to be dependent upon the apparatus-maker's concept of what is required. It is uncommon for an individual clinician to have made a completely 'one-off' apparatus system which satisfactorily meets his/her every demand and preferred clinical method. Commonly, variation of patients' posture, and options of treatment method, are a little restricted by plinth design and the type of accessories provided as standard by the maker. Given this, and the notion that more chrome, more electronics and seemingly more treatment-position options necessarily mean better clinical effectiveness, the therapist should not be too beguiled by glossy brochures and a multitude of chromium plate, knobs, switches, dials and ingenious mechanical contrivances, nor allow gleaming and costly machines, in themselves, to become more important than their only purpose, i.e. the delivery of precisely reproducible tensions for repeatable durations, with similar control settings, on patients who are correctly supported, relaxed and comfortable.

If this is not possible across the full range of clinical requirements, and variations of patients' physique, the apparatus should be modified before the clinical method.

Clinical indications are primary and apparatus as such is secondary. It must remain the tool, and should not be allowed to become the arbiter — as sadly, it sometimes does.

12

Clinical method

Like all good and ultimately productive habits, precise recording is onerous. Yet the need is inescapable, and the benefits make it infinitely worthwhile. Precise assessment of the effects of treatment is not possible without precise recording.

Paradoxically, we learn more from our therapeutic failures than from our easy successes, and we will make this timeless agent of real learning work much more effectively for us when full and precise recording allows a retrospective analysis.

USE OF SYMBOLS. Notation method for passive movement techniques

It is not possible to symbolise every technique suggested, since they incorporate much from many teachers. A single straight, angulated or curved black arrow, with dots, on the white page can symbolise only a finite number of techniques, of which there are thousands, of course.

Even then a degree of familiarity with this or that system would be a pre-requisite to understanding them.

Thus any system of recording symbols must remain something of a makeshift (even when a single advocated system is being described) until something like the comprehensive notation of a musical score, or the *Benesh system* of symbolising movement, is formulated for the infinite variety of manual and mechanical therapeutic movements. The major difficulty, in symbolising methods of passive or active movement, is that of trying to represent three-dimensional movement on a two-dimensional surface.

The following are examples of symbols used by the author and some are a modification of those developed by Maitland.

Pending an internationally agreed system (a formidable undertaking), they constitute no more than a contribution for perhaps further modification or development by others. The inclusion of a lateral or medial bias to left or right, or a cranial or caudal bias, should be noted, i.e.: postero-anterior unilateral pressures on the left side, with a slight medial bias, would not be written thus ⊢• but thus ⊢• ; a lateral bias would be written ⊢• .

A cephalic or caudal bias could be written, ' •⊢ ceph', or ' •⊣ caud', and combinations of caudal and lateral bias can be expressed by ' •＼ caud', for example.

Symbols which are carried to the reader's right of the centre spot indicate the *patient's* right side, whether standing, sitting, side-lying, prone or supine.

Where a symbol indicates a unilateral technique to the patient's right, the symbol is reversed when it represents a *left* unilateral technique.

Vertebral mobilization and stretching techniques

Unilateral transverse soft tissue stretch of paravertebral structures (region to be specified)

Successive unilateral transverse soft tissue stretch of paravertebral structures, to each side (region to be specified)

Unilateral longitudinal soft tissue stretch (region to be specified)

Bilateral longitudinal soft tissue stretch (region to be specified). (One side at a time, or together)

Postero-anterior central vertebral pressures

Postero-anterior unilateral vertebral pressure (on patient's left)

Postero-anterior unilateral vertebral pressure (on the patient's left) with simultaneous lateral flexion to the right

Postero-anterior unilateral rib pressure (on patient's left)

Postero-anterior unilateral pressure over rib and vertebra together

Bilateral postero-anterior rib pressures (specify whether specific or regional)

Unilateral antero-posterior rib pressure on the supine patient's right

Bilateral antero-posterior rib pressure (supine)

Unilateral antero-posterior cervical transverse vertebral pressure on the supine patient's right

Bilateral antero-posterior cervical transverse vertebral pressure (supine)

Transverse vertebral pressure (specified whether spinous or transverse process) towards patient's right

Transverse vertebral pressure, to the prone patient's left side, with an anterior bias

Transverse vertebral pressures, in opposite directions, successively or simultaneously on two adjacent spinous processes, which should be named.
N.B. When applied to the left and

then to the right at a single segment, the segment should be named

Transverse vertebral pressure to the left, with the subjacent spinous process (or sacrum) stabilised

Oscillatory longitudinal movement (patient lying supine)—cervical spine, cervicothoracic region or one lower limb (specify)

Oscillatory longitudinal movement grasping both legs (neutral)

Oscillatory longitudinal movement, one lower limb in flexion

Oscillatory longitudinal movement, two lower limbs in flexion

Oscillatory longitudinal movement in sitting or standing

Manual or mechanical harness traction in sitting or standing (record whether rhythmic or sustained)

Manual or mechanical harness traction in half-lying

Manual or mechanical harness traction in supine or prone lying

Rotation, of head, thorax or pelvis, to patient's right (add 'Sust.' if sustained)

Cervical, thoracic or lumbar lateral flexion, to patient's right

Combined regional cervical side-flexion and rotation to the right

Posterio-anterior unilateral vertebral pressure, on the left during rotation to the left (C1–C2)

Straight-leg-raising stretch (left leg)

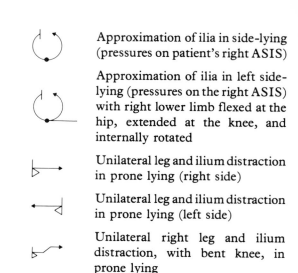

Straight-leg-raising stretch (right leg)

Passive lumbar flexion without crossed legs

Passive lumbar flexion with crossed legs

Sacrospinalis stretch exercise in standing (see p. 215)

Lumbar rotation to patient's left, with legs crossed

Gravitational adduction, over edge of support, of uppermost hip in side-lying, with the under hip and knee flexed and stabilised

(right)

(left)

Correction of deviation or listing by pressure to patient's left

Correction of deviation or listing by pressure to patient's right

Approximation of ilia in side-lying (pressures on patient's right ASIS)

Approximation of ilia in left side-lying (pressures on the right ASIS) with right lower limb flexed at the hip, extended at the knee, and internally rotated

Unilateral leg and ilium distraction in prone lying (right side)

Unilateral leg and ilium distraction in prone lying (left side)

Unilateral right leg and ilium distraction, with bent knee, in prone lying

Examples of notation for *sacroiliac joint* mobilisation techniques are given below. Where appropriate, indicate the side treated.[70]

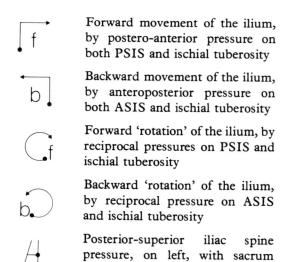

f — Forward movement of the ilium, by postero-anterior pressure on both PSIS and ischial tuberosity

b — Backward movement of the ilium, by anteroposterior pressure on both ASIS and ischial tuberosity

f — Forward 'rotation' of the ilium, by reciprocal pressures on PSIS and ischial tuberosity

b — Backward 'rotation' of the ilium, by reciprocal pressure on ASIS and ischial tuberosity

Posterior-superior iliac spine pressure, on left, with sacrum stabilised

Sacral apex, or sacral base, pressures (specify)

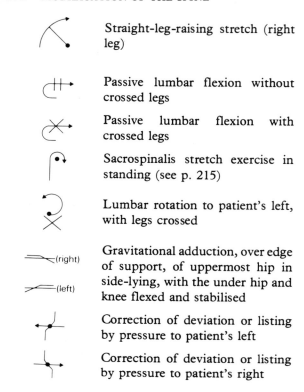

SELECTION OF TECHNIQUE

Much has been written about applied anatomy, congenital anomalies, pathological change with or without root involvement, clinical syndromes, examination method, assessment in examination and techniques of mobilisation, manipulation and traction.[70] It will have become apparent that our certain knowledge of the changes underlying common joint problems amounts to an island of knowing in an embarrasingly large sea of ignorance. Similarly, following examination and initial assessment, the times when a therapist is confidently able to forecast precisely *which* technique, or treatment approach, will get the patient better, are not as frequent as we would like.

The reminder to 'assume *nothing*' merely states the same truth in a different guise.

Tabulated suggestions of what to try first have a tendency to become permanent rules of thumb, albeit qualified; they should be nothing of the sort, since their intention is only that of providing the novice with an initial basis for guidance. As experience is gained, the now more confident therapist will have perceived why the suggested sequence was arranged in this particular way, and will have acquired the clinical basis to know more surely when to transgress the sequence.

For those who have received their initial training in a particular manipulative school, the matter is relatively simple, because their selection of treatment procedures has been inculcated from the first. Those with some experience of many schools may find tabulated schemes irksome, since it is highly likely that they have evolved their own favoured sequence, anyway.

The question uppermost in the tyro's mind is: 'When to do what to which, and how gently or forcefully to do it', i.e. the selection and use of technique. Therefore in the teaching of manipulation, the frequent question: 'I have done a good examination, and found such and such, now what do I do?' must be answered by:

1. Giving the 'Summary of Rules of Procedure' (p. 181).
2. Providing demonstration of the approach of various schools of manipulation to a given set of signs and symptoms, to show that there are many ways of starting and none of them are 'wrong', necessarily.
3. Teaching contraindications, which help to show when procedures may be unsafe.
4. Producing basic guides for selection of first and subsequent mobilisation and manipulation technique (see below), and stressing the importance of continuous assessment.
5. Assurance that all manipulators have this trouble and that it becomes less troublesome with experience, although all profit from the experience of those who have gone before.
6. Arranging opportunities for course members to be in pairs, ideally, and to work for many weeks on the clinical shopfloor with an experienced teacher.

The following seemingly modest selection of techniques has a very wide range of clinical application; increasing experience of their potential for resolving the signs and symptoms of degenerative joint disease (when their use is correctly applied to the 'range-pain-limitation' relationship, p. 129), is a salutory exercise, and will rightly cast doubt on the proposition that technique must always be based on facet-joint plane geometry. A thorough knowledge of the clinical application of these modest and undramatic procedures is the very best basis for more advanced work.

Selection of technique by distribution of pain

(i) Central pain, or bilateral symmetrical pain

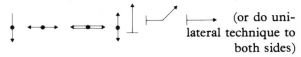

(or do unilateral technique to both sides)

(ii) Bilateral asymmetrical pain

Usually a good plan to treat as two separate unilateral pains unless they can be shown to be associated, or both pains arising from a segment or adjacent segments, when the pains can be treated as bilateral symmetry.

(iii) Unilateral pain (e.g. left side)

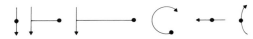

Initially, rotate *away* from the side of pain, and be cautious about rotating *towards* or into the pain, in the cervical region; this guide is modified with experience.

If the initial *lumbar* rotation away from the side of pain is not successful, the opposite rotation is then used without fear of untoward effects because of the direction of rotation itself, other factors given.

Selection of technique in order of efficacy for spinal regions

Traction is mobilising technique, and should be employed as such (p. 156). It is just as correct to change from a manual mobilising technique to harness traction, or vice versa, as it is to change from one manual technique to another. The factor that harness traction may need some three or four *sessions*, before assessment can reasonably be made, does not negate the proposition that it is correctly used in this way, i.e. as a mobilising technique.

Maitland[128] provides a detailed tabulation of effects of the individual mobilising procedures (Figs. 12.1, 12.2).

For more experienced therapists, who have mastered the techniques of careful regional and segmental examination, and understand the prime importance of accurately localised treatment procedures, a précis

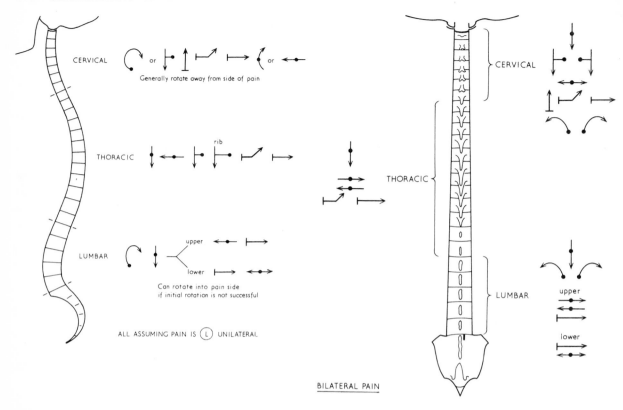

Fig. 12.1 Spinal techniques in order of efficacy (from left to right).

Fig. 12.2 Spinal techniques in order of efficacy (from above downwards).

of clinical method (with some reiteration) might be arranged as follows:

1. During the 'observation' part of the examination for *all* vertebral regions, check leg-lengths, and pelvic symmetry, in sitting as well as standing.

2. Always check the lower limbs neurologically when dealing with neck problems in mature patients.

3. Always check the sacroiliac joints in any case of thoracic or lumbar pain.

4. Note the regions of soft tissue tightness.

5. During palpation, be awake to segmental hypermobility, as well as stiffness and irritability.

6. While primarily seeking the segmental locality of a joint problem, bear in mind the important junctional regions (p. 113) and the covert effects of degenerative change there.

7. Treat specifically at all times, but within the context of regional changes which may also need treatment.

8. Never forget the functional and the neurophysiological interdependence of the vertebral column.

9. Proceed on the basis of:
   a. Specific or segmental joint mobilisation (or manipulation if indicated) by appropriate method
   b. Regional soft tissue techniques, to release tightness
   c. Regional mobilisation, when indicated
   d. Segmental exercises to maintain mobility
   e. Segmental and regional exercises to improve stability, if indicated
   f. Ergonomic advice and guidance
   g. Always aiming to instil the patient's *confidence* in the durability of their vertebral column. Nothing lasts forever, not even joint pain.

N.B. (i) The treatment factors are added in the sequence suggested, as clinical features declare the need, but the set routine may not be necessary, e.g. the gentle release of a recent vertebral joint derangement at C2–C3 may be all that is required.

(ii) Vertebral segmental exercises are given for the same reasons as exercises for individual peripheral joints.

10. Never lose sight of the whole, while pursuing one's self-education in the many approaches to the treatment of vertebral pain syndromes.

An additional suggested sequence, in broad terms, of localised and regional manual and mechanical techniques, for those with more experience, is given below. Each technique can and should be transposed according to clinical findings, with selections guided by assessment of effects.

Many experienced therapists are competent in the use of techniques derived from various manipulation schools and because this text is not solely devoted to teaching any particular manipulative method, not all of the suggested recording symbols are included in the sequences.

Some standard techniques will be recognised, but it should be borne in mind that in mobilisation of a first rib, for example, the patient may be in the supine or prone position; this variation applies to many procedures, by individual preference.

This tabulation can be no more than a personal recommendation, since a single technique often achieves different effects in different hands.

There are many other procedures for successfully treating the segments and regions concerned, and none should be considered in isolation from the need to restore extensibility and pliability of soft tissue where necessary; some soft tissue techniques have been included. (Figs. 12.3, 12.4).

Selection of Grade V manipulative techniques is not included, for two good reasons:

(i) they are less important and thus less used nowadays
(ii) learning to use mobilisation methods efficiently is far more important than 'learning to how manipulate'.

Yet this does not negate the real value of understanding the technical basis of Grade V procedures (p. 144), in terms of combined-movement positioning and so-called vertebral 'locking' techniques, because this skill is also employed in the less dramatic post-isometric relaxation techniques, although not in the same way. Sometimes, there is nothing for it but to manipulate — but first things first. As one's clinical mileage of patients treated steadily mounts, the knack of more successfully choosing the first technique comes more easily to hand, but acquiring it is a slow process.

Alike in the early and advanced stages in manipulative work, there is no substitute for clinical self-education by step-by-step analysis, expressed by the mnemonic SOAP:

S   Subjective examination
O   Objective examination
A   Assessment
P   Plan of treatment.

The *only* difference between the novice and the advanced worker, in terms of cerebral activity, is that the latter has experience to call upon and progressively works more quickly. At no time does the clinical routine of segmental analysis become redundant.

Assessment continues during treatment (p. 181) and the response to what is done initially, and subsequently, provides guidance for the next step in treatment. Thus it comes about that, by a logical and orderly method of examination, followed by treatment which is planned solely on the basis of the signs and symptoms in themselves, patients are frequently relieved of painful disablements without the therapist ever really knowing the precise nature of the changes underlying these conditions. At times it is possible to be reasonably sure, but more often than not there is insufficient basis for complete confidence that the diagnosis is correct, or has other than a supposed relationship to the changes causing the patient's attendance.

The need to reach a diagnosis is important, but this need is not met by facile, snap decisions which often appear to be made on a patently inadequate basis.

As manipulation, in the general sense, remains largely an empirical form of treatment, so diagnosis, in its precise and clinical sense, often retains some empiricism when applied to common musculo-skeletal conditions. For this reason, it is not wise to

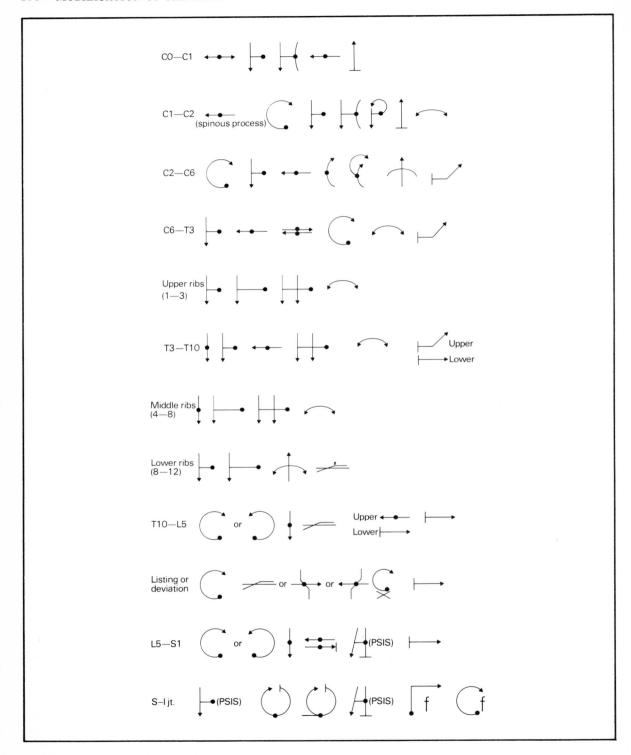

Fig. 12.3 Unilateral, i.e. (L) sided pain.

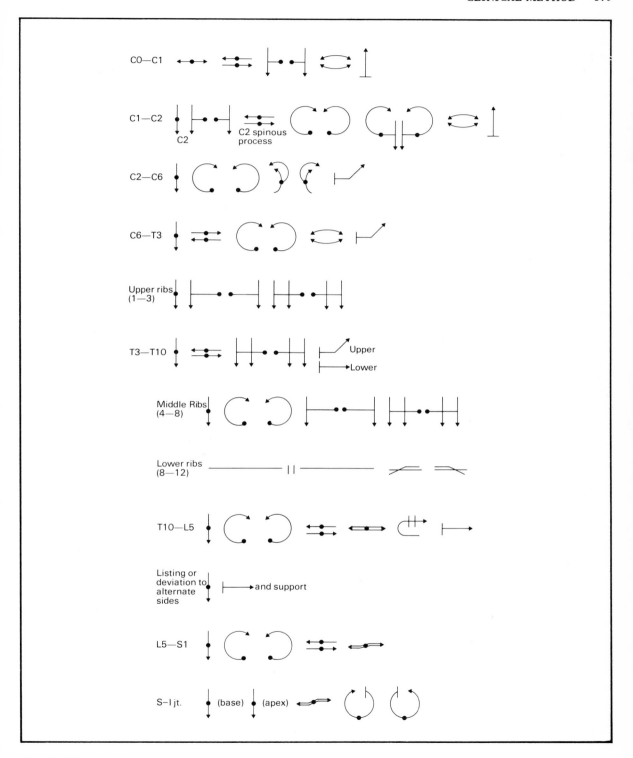

Fig. 12.4 Bilateral pain.

base the selection and use of passive movement techniques on diagnostic concepts only, although there are certain important clinical features which must be respected for what they infer. For example:

— backache in a patient with a history of neoplastic disease
— joint problems in a patient with advanced diabetes
— mid- and low-lumbar pain in the presence of radiologically-evident osteoporosis
— low backache in a patient with advanced Scheuermann's disease

Nevertheless, the principle is that of formulating treatment on the *unique* way in which signs and symptoms present in each patient, while coexistent disease or factors indicating caution are borne in mind. Further, since we do not know exactly what mobilisation or manipulation actually does to a joint and to its associated tissues, we can only use the treatment intelligently, i.e. select and modify it, on the basis of signs and symptoms and how these change as the treatment proceeds. The response of the joint, to the initial procedures selected, is the dominant guiding factor, e.g. in the case of testing the response to one of the pressure techniques or a trial of traction.

Thus *clinical method* is considered under the two headings:

1. Use of technique in general terms
2. Assessment during treatment.

1. USE OF TECHNIQUE IN GENERAL TERMS

Other factors given, the *aim* is to make the joint 'clear', i.e. able to sustain grade IV mobilisation without pain, but it is not always possible, nor advisable, to aim for full restoration of movement, and if symptoms have been relieved it is often better not to attempt to influence joint limitations which are clearly the result of adaptive shortening.

Since the object of treatment is to produce movement, and most movement will occur when a joint is positioned in the mid-position of all the other ranges of which it is capable, the lordotic areas of the spine (cervical and lumbar) should be positioned more in neutral or slight extension when treating the upper parts, i.e. C1–C2, L1–L2, and in increasing flexion as the lower areas are treated, i.e. C6–C7, L4–L5. *This applies especially* when using regional techniques to affect single segments, e.g. rotation.

Two good uses of a technique, in the appropriate grade, at one session, are enough to assess its value in a particular case at a particular time.

In cases likely to progress slowly, four or five *treatment sessions* are sometimes required, before the value of techniques can be assessed.

Unless progress is obviously going to be slow, the therapist should move through the techniques fairly quickly to find the value of each, but this should be well controlled throughout, with techniques adequately peformed and with reassessment of signs and symptoms guiding selection at all times. This is quite different from a haphazard and willy-nilly use of whichever technique happens to spring to mind — it is important always to keep the treatment firmly in hand, with a clear grasp of how the signs and symptoms are responding to applied procedures.

Slightly altering the angle when using pressure techniques, or the joint's position in rotation techniques, is often necessary to extract the most benefit. The technique itself need not always be changed.

A technique which produced no change, yet no deterioration either, should be repeated with a higher grade, i.e. more firmly. If the condition continues to remain unaffected, the technique must be changed.

If a procedure helps, it should be continued with. If not, it must be discarded for something that does. There is no gain in persisting with pointless techniques, simply because they may be the therapist's favourites.

Techniques which do not help in the initial stages of a treatment are often found to be successful in the later stages — the therapist should change his ground as the signs and symptoms change theirs, which they will do as the localisation of stress changes during treatment, but he should not discard a particular treatment method until it ceases to help.

When a patient has two or more areas of pain from separate lesions, or a large area of pain appears to have more than one lesion (e.g. a cervical segment and a high thoracic segment) contributing to its existence, it is better to clearly know the effects of treatment procedure on one of these, before a second technique is added in during the same session.

When treatment soreness is such as to make assessment difficult, treatment should be stopped for a day or two to allow the soreness to settle.

When improvement by manual mobilisation has reached a limit, traction should be added or substituted for a little while, after which manual techniques may be taken up again.

It is not always necessary to pursue signs and symptoms with treatment to the bitter end. Often, treatment can be stopped before they are completely cleared, although the patient *must* always be assessed at the end of a few days, when it is frequently found that the joint problem has continued clearing without further treatment.

Gross cervical and lumbar rotational manipulations (grade V) can be repeated two or more times in a single session with benefit (other factors being equal) if the improvement in signs indicates this.

Localised specific manipulations (grade loc V), when indicated, should be done as a rule only once to each side (but see p. 230), and should not be repeated until soreness has settled down in a few days, and then only if signs indicate that a repetition should be useful.

Summary of rules of procedure

(i) Bear in mind contraindications, and the conditions requiring extra care and gentleness. DO NO HARM.

(ii) Examine thoroughly, and carefully assess patient's signs and symptoms for indications of initial technique and likely progress.

(iii) Always try to localise the problem(s) and work in a specific way, i.e. localise the treatment, too.

(iv) Begin feeling your way forward by exploratory mobilisation, or traction, and keep the treatment under control by frequent reassessment and precise recording.

(v) Each step should be reasoned, and governed by the response to the previous steps in treatment.

(vi) Use manipulative procedures only if necessary; for the most part only when adequately applied mobilisation is not achieving the degree of improvement reasonably expected.

(vii) If a technique is being effective, do not

substitute another until it ceases to produce adequate improvement. Discard or modify techniques which are unproductive.

(viii) Remember to warn patients about treatment soreness and temporary after-effects; this relieves their unnecessary anxiety between treatments.

(ix) Do not overtreat; when signs and symptoms are cleared, STOP.

(x) NEVER push through the spasm when it is protecting the joint you are treating; treat joint irritability with respect.

2. ASSESSMENT DURING TREATMENT

In close accordance with the detailed findings during examination and treatment, each session has a beginning, a continuation and an end. The guides for starting, continuing and finishing are solely provided by assessment — there are no criteria other than those wittingly or unwittingly presented by *the patient*. Perceiving when to stop is as important as knowing how to start and recognising how to continue. The better the assessment, the fewer the treatment sessions. Practice makes perfect — there are no short cuts.

Taking as our enemy the changes causing the patient's distress, and regarding the clinical shopfloor as a front line, we are more likely to win battles if we see to our military intelligence, endeavour to objectively understand the nature of the enemy, resist intimidating propaganda about him, do a thorough reconnaissance of the terrain and of his present positions in relation to it, and make an appraisal of the possible moves open to him during the battle and of his present and future intentions. We are also likely to be more successful if we fully understand the nature and potential of our own weapons, economically use our firepower to the best effect and do not deploy our heavy artillery when good marksmanship with a rifle may suffice. Thus we do our best to avoid desecration of the countryside not presently occupied by the enemy.[70]

These observations transpose themselves into the importance of:

a. Developing a comprehensive examination procedure, which allows the joint to speak for itself, and then listening to what it is saying. We will not hear successfully with the deaf ears of preconception.

There are many examples of wide differences in the behaviour of body systems, and a diversity of clinical features which follow tissue damage or abnormal stresses.

While there must be reasons for this biological plasticity of behaviour in what appear to be similar changes and we may have elucidated some of the reasons, our certain knowledge remains limited; until it is more complete, attempts by instructors to impose an overall regularity and seemingly reasoned and logical order, where none can yet exist, are highly misleading for beginners.

No explanation at all is better than authoritarian nonsense.

b. Recognising the biomechanical, neural, vascular, and thus functional interdependence of vertebral structures. This interdependence is a constant factor underlying clinical presentation and further, a constant factor to be borne in mind when examining, assessing, choosing techniques and formulating plans of treatment.

So far as treatment of the joint itself is concerned, the effects of precisely localised and graded passive movements in treatment are better noted if the patient attends daily at first. Once the responses of

the joint condition during treatment are understood, attendance can be less frequent.

Not only does assessment give guidance during the continuation of treatment, it also provides the basis for knowing with assurance when treatment can safely be discontinued. Depending upon the nature of the joint condition, and its consequences, attendance will vary between one session and frequent sessions for two or three weeks.

It is important for the therapist to decide (p. 114), 'Can I expect a quick result or is progress going to be slow?' and also decide (p. 130), 'Am I primarily treating pain or resistance (in its various forms)?'

Assessment of the presenting and then the changing relationships during treatment of pain with movement is a fundamental skill which can be learned, as can the assessment of whether a joint is normal or not. Any joint which is not causing symptoms should be able to accept a certain amount of stretch at the limit of its ranges, without pain. Similarly, Mooney and Cairns[143] have observed that there is every reason to expect that a joint unable to proceed through its full anatomical range is abnormal. These considerations have to be exercised in the knowledge of the known, or likely, diagnosis.

In Figure 12.5B, where the flexion range is

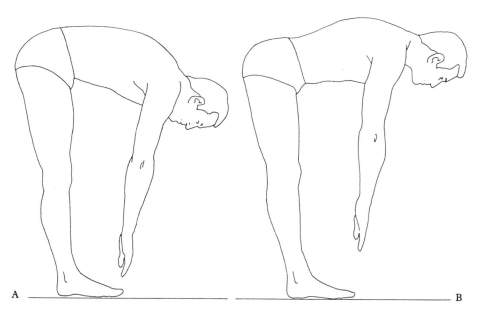

Fig. 12.5 Normal (A) and abnormal (B) lumbar flexion (see text).

reduced and the spinal contour is plainly abnormal, it is necessary to relate these clinical signs to possible causes, of which there are many, e.g.

— chronic postural abnormalities due to occupational stress, the stooping posture of a tall man or the effects of heavy, pendulous breasts
— ankylosing spondylitis
— osteochondrosis (Scheuermann's Disease)
— established contracture of lumbo-dorsal fascia
— a degree of postural spasm of lumbar extensor muscle groups
— old wedge fracture of a lower thoracic vertebra
— any combination of these.

These two signs *per se* are not pathognomonic of any one condition but are the common expression of many spinal conditions.

Assessments of the changes produced by treatment will be inaccurate unless *all* the factors of a movement abnormality are precisely known. Maitland[127] has well exemplified this:

The behaviour of pain with movement is very important, as is borne out in the following examples of equally restricted lumbar flexion, each with a different pain pattern. The differences are important because they guide the treatment and because, if they are not appreciated, the patient may be made worse by treatment without the physiotherapist realising. In all of the examples which follow, the patient has an ache in his lower back which extends down his leg into his calf. On forward flexion, he first feels a change in his pain when his fingertips reach his knees. With further movement he can reach halfway down his shin with the following differences in the behaviour of his pain:

(i) There is no alteration to the pain, 'half-shin' being the normal limit of his range.
(ii) His back pain increases in intensity until the increase in this pain prevents him from flexing further than halfway down his shin. His thigh and calf symptoms are not affected by the flexion.
(iii) As movement increases the pain spreads into his buttock but it is stiffness which prevents him from flexing further than halfway down his shin.
(iv) As movement increases so the pain spreads down his leg to his calf.

(v) As movement increases the pain in his back disappears but his calf becomes increasingly painful as the movement reaches the limit of his range.

When the pain behaves as indicated in (v) the patient must be treated with much more care than when it behaves in a manner similar to (i). The first indicates a nerve root pain which may be harmed by too zealous treatment. If we are treating a patient such as in (i) and do not take note of the behaviour of pain throughout movement and then his pain may change to that of (v) without our appreciating it.

Accurate assessment of the nature of abnormal 'endfeels' on passive testing (see p. 133) will also indicate when further mobilisation (grades I-IV) is pointless, and a grade V thrust technique is indicated. In some cases, this will be indicated from the first, in which case the joint is manipulated, provided there are no preclusions (see p. 230). Confidence in safely recognising the indications is based mainly upon methodical assessment of the nature of the range-limiting factor (see p. 130).

Assessments are made: (a) after each use of a technique, during one treatment session; (b) prior to the next treatment.

A selection of two important 'markers for assessment' enables a quick estimate of progress to be made without repeatedly going through the whole examination procedure. The changes in *one symptom*, e.g. the length of time a patient can sit, and *one sign*, e.g. the intensity and precise distribution of pain and/or paraesthesiae during a particular movement, are adopted as parameters; thus assessment of the value of each technique during the treatment session usually hinges on the sign, and the effects of the treatment between attendances upon the symptom, with other information spontaneously proffered by the patient.

Criteria will vary considerably between patients, e.g. an improvement of 2 in (5 cm) in the range of flexion may be significant in one patient, but in another may be judged inadequate improvement to justify continuing with a particular technique.

Choice of the best parameters for assessment is a matter of experience, but patients usually present the dominant symptoms first in their history and this helps selection for *subjective* assessments.

For *objective* assessments, selection is easy if only one movement is painful and/or limited, but it may be necessary to choose the movement which produced the greatest spread of pain, e.g. if both flexion and extension of the lumbar spine aggravate or produce calf pain, it is extension which should be chosen because limb pain on spinal extension movement is a more sensitive index than flexion. This usually also applies to the upper limb.

Although changes in a salient sign and a salient symptom are chosen as the immediate markers of treatment effects, assessment as a whole can be likened to an intensive care unit, in that many factors are continually monitored. Examples are, of course, ranges of movement (both active and accessory), intensity and distribution of pain and of para-esthesiae, neurological signs, degree of tenderness, range of straight-leg-raising and its effects, decrease or increase in asymmetry of movement, changes in the degree of postural deviation, changes in postural spasm and elicited spasm, and so on.

While the routine procedure has been outlined, it is important to make the right interpretation of what patients report. A laconic, 'Not so bad' from a patient who is known to be somewhat monosyllabic, should perhaps be given about the same assessment value as the effusive, 'It's been absolutely marvellous' from a patient who appears unable to make the simplest statement without fulsome embroidery.

If distal pain has become more proximal during the interim, even if the more proximal pain is increased in intensity, this generally indicates improvement. 'The longer the pain the slower the gain', and the progressive centralisation of pain is an important assessment marker which indicates progress. If a patient reports that pain has remained in the same distribution, has come on at the same time of day, and at the same intensity, but its *duration* is 75 per cent less, this is progress. Similarly, if the straight-leg-raising test provokes a grimace at 45°, when it did so at 35° the day before, this is progress, however dramatic the grimace.

Hence the therapist's grasp of the patient's symptoms, and their behaviour according to time, posture and movement, must be complete; patients must be helped to be as precise as they are able. A handful appear incapable of doing other than producing confusion (see apophthegm, Fig. 12.6),

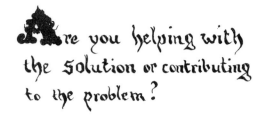

Fig. 12.6 Apophthegm.

and a bit of courteous firmness may be a good idea, i.e. 'You're either better, worse or no different—which is it?'

Improvements are not always due to treatment: in mature/elderly patients, whose resilience and powers of recovery are somewhat diminished, it is often more profitable to find ways of reducing joint stress rather than repeating specific treatment which does not hold its improvement. An elderly patient whose pain is always bad on Thursdays, when she carefully negotiates her shopping trolley over pavements by rotating the head to the right to look behind, can be relieved of her regular Thursday pains by learning to pull her shopping trolley with the opposite hand, especially if the regular exacerbation of her right C2–C3 chronic joint problem, by right cervical rotation when pulling the trolley, is undoing the improvement of specific treatment.

Mobilising techniques are grouped as:

a. Localised mobilisation by vertebral pressures
b. Rotation
c. Longitudinal movement and traction.

Examples of treatment guided by assessment follow:

1.Where a quick response to treatment is expected

If, in these cases two uses of the first choice in group (a) do not result in adequate improvement, it is better to proceed next to group (b) than to immediately try all other pressure techniques. If rotation does not produce satisfactory progress, a short traction treatment may be tried, but the next most profitable step is to work through pressure techniques again to find the most effective. The ultimately successful combination of procedures should be achieved solely with the guidance of assessment; wishful thinking and therapeutic favourites are no substitute for objective evaluation of results.

While the patient's report, of changes in symptoms immediately following a technique, are important, some discrimination must temper their face value. For example, if a pain is reported during treatment and it is other than worsening of the particular symptom taken as the marker for subjective assessment, this is not necessarily a negative thing, especially if the signs are unchanged or slightly improved. Transient pain and other symptoms during treatment sessions can be an artefact of treatment, and need not ring alarm bells, unless they infer: incipient or increasing root pressure; vertebrobasilar ischaemia; a deterioration in joint function. For example, during lumbar rotation techniques, the patient may report what appears to be a 'rib-stretch' pain in the uppermost hemithorax. Slight modification of the patient's position will relieve it, and it is of no consequence.

When treating distally referred pain from the lumbar spine, it may transpire that a low-grade rotation technique has moderately worsened the symptoms; the same technique applied in small amplitudes at the limit of available range will frequently produce improvement. The guides for action are (i) that the initial attempt did not worsen the signs, (ii) it was not vigorous enough to have affected the underlying changes, and (iii) it did not produce an exacerbation *during* its application.

2. When it is obvious that treatment will span weeks rather than days

Small improvements or deteriorations in how the patient is troubled are important, and thus the initial examination must be full and precise enough to allow these significant straws in the wind to be recognised. Improvement in symptoms may not keep step with improvement in signs, and vice versa. For example, a patient may report being able to sit for longer, or be able to bend the head over reading or sewing for longer, for some days before any significant change in articular signs occurs. Again, signs may steadily improve for some days before the patient ceases to report 'no change' in symptoms.

In both above cases, the improvements would justify continuing the treatment which produced these results.

If the passive-neck-flexion test (in supine lying) provokes the existing sciatic pain from low back to heel, and after the chosen procedure the test provokes low back pain only, this is improvement.

The patient who, after sitting for 30 minutes, cannot rise directly from the chair and walk away, but has to cautiously 'unwind' and stand awkwardly for some 10–30 seconds before moving, requires patient and persuasive mobilising techniques which can be monotonous to perform, but which are shown to have been the correct approach when the patient returns and reports being able to more quickly stand from sitting.

When limitation of lumbar flexion in standing is accompanied by buttock and posterior thigh pain being provoked at the point of limitation, and mobilisation of a stiff lumbar joint allows an immediate increase of flexion, yet with precisely the same amount of pain, it is very likely that while *movement limitation* was due to the stiff joint, *pain* must be due to some trespass upon the pain-sensitive structures within the neural canal. Hence treatment must be modified to aim at these, and the addition of lumbar traction for example, should be considered. *The point being emphasised here is that pain and movement limitation are not necessarily related.*

If an otherwise fit and strong patient is steadily but slowly improving on mobilisation techniques, and there is no after-treatment soreness or increased irritability, completion of treatment aims should be speeded up.

Articular signs on active tests need not be the only assessment parameter; a reduction of segmental tenderness on palpation, less provocation of pain on segmental accessory movement or provocation of the same pain requiring further excursion into accessory range, are all indications of improvement.

A report that 'my head feels too heavy, I feel I can hardly hold it up' does not necessarily imply cervical segmental instability. Many patients with neck problems appear to have a type of 'pain inhibition' or a mechanical disturbance of joint function which interferes with postural control of the head, and which very frequently clears up satisfactorily by localised mobilisation of the abnormal segments.

The frequent combination of neck and arm pain need not imply a single cause; many patients will have neck and arm symptoms from a C5–C6 joint problem, together with scapular and arm pain from the T3 segment. It is necessary to be precise about the changing distribution of pain as treatment progresses, and to be aware of combinations of effect.

In contrast, the patient may stoutly say that his or her symptoms are improving while steady deterioration in joint function is objectively plain; the treatment techniques manifestly need modifying in this case.

Examples of signs and symptoms indicating deterioration, and the need for modification or cessation of treatment, are:

The patient's report that a particular symptom is more easily and more quickly provoked.

Periodic symptoms occurring more frequently, with more intensity and for longer duration.

An increase of distal pain, or a proximal pain beginning to spread distally.

Symptoms invoking a suspicion of increasing vertebrobasilar ischaemia (q.v.).

Symptoms changing from an ache to a sharper and more delineated pain, in the same or more distal distribution.

Increasing limitation of movement.

Spinal deformity, or deviation during a movement becoming apparent.

Symptoms of incipient root involvement, e.g. the advent of paraesthesiae, or sensibility loss.

The emergence, or increase, of neurological signs.

The advent of sphincter disturbance, indicating increasing trespass upon the pudendal nerve.

Neurological involvement. Where the possibility, or probability, of nerve root involvement is suspected, by reason of the patient's description of the *type and distribution* of pain (p. 31), it is wise to carefully monitor the clinical features from session to session, and to include neurological tests, for root tension and of reflexes, as the assessment markers.

When considering *neurological symptoms*, for example, if on cervical side-flexion to the painful side, there is a 12-second latent period for provocation of paraesthesiae in the fingers, and at the next treatment session the latent period is now 3 seconds, this indicates increasing root irritability and the need to modify treatment. Conversely, if the 12-second period has increased to 20 seconds, this gives an assurance that, for the time being at least, the treatment is succeeding.

So far as *neurological signs* are concerned, it is important to distinguish their import in relation to the condition; for example, the patient with spinal stenosis who has been sitting in a waiting room for 30 minutes before being assessed prior to treatment, may present without neurological deficit, yet if the same patient be asked to walk around the block or stand for 30 minutes immediately prior to examination, a transient neurological deficit may well be present.

If spinal articular signs are in part diminishing, i.e. greater range of some movements before being limited by pain, but the straight-leg-raising test indicates possible pressure on the nerve root because this passive movement is more reduced and painful, the patient's condition has obviously deteriorated.

An increase, or the advent of, a neurological deficit, and more particularly a report of sphincter disturbance indicate, respectively, the need for a modification of treatment and an *urgent surgical opinion*.

3. Assessment on symptoms only

Treatment may be necessary for intermittent symptoms which occur during some particular activity during evening hours. There may be very little in the way of joint signs to provide for an objective assessment *during* patient's attendance, and in order that procedures and their effects may be clearly related on assessment prior to treatment at the next attendance, it is necessary to keep the variety of techniques employed at one session to a minimum, otherwise ascribing good or bad effects to any one of them becomes difficult, and the necessary guides for action are not clear. It is useful to remember that in general, changes in barometric pressure and weather will affect symptoms more than signs.

Relief, or improvement, directly related to treatment procedures will show that treatment was correct, though does not necessarily show that the diagnosis was also correct, since we cannot always know.

If both were incorrect, it is better not to have made the patient worse, or the condition more serious; for this reason alone, a fundamental principle is economy in the use of vigour.

In our increasingly technological milieu, the value of subjective and objective clinical assessment should not be discounted or diminished. The predictive value of several highly sensitive and specific serological tests, including the latex fixation test for rheumatoid factor, were subject to investigation.* There were appreciable differences in sensitivity and reproducibility, and some widely used measurements appeared to have little if any real value. Where patients had kept a detailed daily record of morning stiffness and other symptoms, these reports proved to be as useful a measurement as any, and appeared to greatly reduce the variability of assessments by more technical methods. In short, the best measurement of all appeared to be that of asking the patient: 'How are you?'

N.B. The foregoing remarks on clinical method apply in general terms to the use of any technique, of course, whether passive, active-assisted or active-resisted, and to treatment by free active exercises. They are included in this part of the text only because they do refer mainly to passive movement techniques.

In summary. Passive movement treatment is flexibly adapted according to presenting signs and symptoms; as these change, so should treatment. The guides for action depend upon assessment. This requires concentrated attention at all times; it may be demanding, but it is infinitely more exciting and rewarding than the pedestrian performance of generalised textbook procedures.

*Leading article 1977 Reliability of tests for rheumatism. *British Journal of Clinical Practice* 31:173.

13

Manually assisted or manually resisted movements

1. SELF-CORRECTION OF LATERAL DEVIATION OF THE LUMBAR SPINE

This is merely a progression, in terms of self-help, of the passive correction of deviation described on page 147. Having manually achieved over-correction and instructed the patient how to move the lumbar spine into a sustained lordotic posture, it is necessary to teach self-correction, and manual guidance helps the patient to perceive what is required.[125] The therapist stands in front of the patient, placing one palm on the lateral pelvis of the side deviated away from, and one hand on the opposite shoulder, i.e. of the side deviated towards. The patient is encouraged to learn, by the proprioceptive assistance of the therapist's hand pressures, the corrective technique of actively deviating his own trunk, to the opposite side, on a self-stabilised pelvis. He should practise this in front of a mirror, without the guiding pressures of the therapist's hands, before leaving, and must continue the corrective drill at home as prescribed.

2. POST-ISOMETRIC RELAXATION TECHNIQUES

These terms indicate the patient's active participation, by muscular contraction and/or inspiration or expiration, during manual treatment techniques,[13, 48, 60, 64, 101, 112, 113, 114, 140] and rest on the prime importance of *soft tissues*, particularly muscles, as opposed to the skeletal elements of joint structures, in producing various moderately abnormal states of joint pain and movement-limitation. The technique may be used to mobilise restricted joints, stretch tight muscle and fascia, strengthen weak muscles and improve local circulation. Since much writing and clinical preoccupation has tended for the last two or three decades to be centred almost entirely around *the joint* as such,[62, 119, 179] it should not be surprising that attention has begun to turn once more to the importance of *muscular* abnormalities in the genesis of vertebral pain syndromes.

Bourdillon[13] suggests that the muscle dysfunction — shortening — appears to be a self-perpetuating over-action of the gamma motor neurone system. If this shortening persists the muscle cannot return to its normal resting length. When resting length is shortened the muscle is still able to contract further but relaxes only to its shortened position. It appears that the pain is produced in some way by its inability to relax to full resting length. 'If this hypothesis is correct, it follows that the limitation of joint movements is a result of the muscle tightness and not the cause of it.'

Plainly, this must be less so when frank morphological changes, such as chondro-osteophytosis and markedly thickened and contracted peri-articular soft tissues, are producing limitation of movement on mehanical grounds other than simple tethering — yet the techniques are useful for these degenerative states, too.

Together with tethering by muscle tightness or shortening, so familiar in the psoas, muscular imbalance includes lengthening and weakening of antagonists, of course.[91]

In many cases, the problem cannot be that of simple shortening only, although it is probably a matter of degree.

While Goodridge[64] suggests that 'treatment in which the patient actively uses his muscles, on request, from a precisely controlled position in a specific direction, against a distinctly executed counterforce' is a form of osteopathic manipulative treatment; the basic principles of these techniques have been an integral part of physiotherapy for three decades[101] although practical applications and indications differ a little. So far as the spine is concerned, these techniques appear to be really only proprioceptive neuromuscular facilitation methods (PNF) with the vertebral joints manoeuvred into combined-movement postures, the slight muscle contractions being elicited after precise positioning. Yet there are essential differences, one of which is that PNF techniques, particularly for the limbs but also for the trunk, tend to emphasise the importance of a *rotation* component in normal functional activities.

In post-isometric techniques, the important consideration is the particular type of three-dimensional combined movement posture which will best localise the effect to a particular vertebral segment or rib joint. While this very frequently includes rotation, this type of movement is not given importance in quite the same way as in treatment by PNF.

Further, while these procedures may resemble the hold-relax techniques of PNF, there is a great difference in the degree of resistance; the active contraction asked of the patient in post-isometric treatments is very slight. Localisation of force is more important than the intensity of force. The combined movement postures frequently take all of the three main degrees of freedom of a vertebral district to their combined existing limit, and are carefully devised to isolate effects—so far as is possible—to particular movement-limitations of specific segments. This requires a high order of perception by palpation, also considerable skill in localisation, together with active co-operation by the patient; *yet they are not a wrestling match with the patient.* Because the techniques are more gentle, they can be used in treating those for whom high velocity manipulation thrusts (Grade V techniques) would be unsafe. In specialist descriptive texts[64, 140] unfamiliar terms may be encountered, but these need not cause difficulty. The term 'roto-scoliosis', for example, is merely shorthand recognition that scoliosis is frequently but not invariably accompanied by rotation, and the term 'motion-barrier' will be plain anyway.

Clinical workers use terms like 'up-slip' of the 'hemipelvis', and 'latexion' and 'rotexion'; the latter

are less employed now.

Post-isometric purists group spinal lesions into Type 1 and Type II, the former occurring in the spine with normal a–p curves, when the facet-joints are bearing little or no weight. On other than sagittal movements, side-bending occurs *before* rotation, which is towards the convexity of the curve; thus side-bending and rotation occur to *opposite* sides, and this type of combined motion enjoys the word 'latexion'.

Type II lesions occur where a scoliotic curve crosses the mid-line; in this type, some facet-joints are partially weight-bearing and thus influence functional movement. There is asymmetry of movement between the painful facets at segmental level, and sometimes at more than one segment. Since the chronology of events is not always clarified in descriptions of lesions, a distinction must be made between an existing postural scoliosis (for whatever reason) which has caused secondary joint problems at particular segments, and a unilateral facet-joint lesion which has induced a secondary scoliosis (either postural or during sagittal movements) in a previously straight spine (see Fig. 13.1).

A Type II lesion is considered present if, on flexion and extension, a vertebra rotates and side-flexes to the *same* side. The distinction is that in these cases, rotation *precedes* side-bending, and it is presumed that capsular, ligamentous or intrinsic (segmental) muscle tension has restricted side-bending, and thus rotation must precede it, to relieve the constraints imposed by the tethering effect and allow movement to continue. This type of side-bending and rotation occurring to the same side has been called 'rotexion'.

Type II lesions can be further sub-divided into (i) those which present with asymmetry evident in the neutral 'normal' posture, the asymmetry becoming exaggerated on flexion, and (ii) those with no asymmetry evident in the neutral position, but with adventitious or distorted movement plainly occurring on flexion.

While segmental capsular and ligamentous 'lesions' have been postulated above, there is reason to believe that the resting tone of intersegmental muscle (particularly intertransversarii and multifidus) may be increased, i.e. a degree of intersegmental muscle spasm. This may not necessarily be accompanied by symptoms nor by

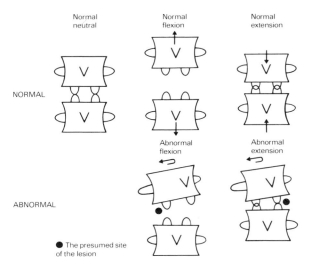

Fig. 13.1 Scheme of normal and abnormal sagittal movement. Viewed from behind, the paired facet-joint planes are normally districted during flexion and approximated during extension.

In the example of abnormal *flexion*, the left inferior articular process of the vertebra above is tethered, thereby inducing left side-flexion and thus also left rotation of the upper vertebra on the one below. The site of the lesion is marked ●.

In the example of abnormal *extension*, the right inferior articular process of the vertebra above cannot approximate, or glide backwards and downwards, as it should. Thus left side-flexion is again abnormally induced at that segment, and with it left rotation. The site of the lesion is marked ●

Both are examples of Type 11 lesions.

N.B. It must be noted that these are purely mechanical considerations, and that the vertebral column also exhibits, besides a mechanical interdependence, a neurophysiological and vascular interdependence. Many people with these 'lesions' are not necessarily in pain, nor functionally restricted.

functional restrictions, yet it seems reasonable to assume that it would be, sooner or later, if the abnormal localised tension were not spontaneously resolved, which they probably frequently are.

The tension in itself will produce a distorted 'guidance' of movement of a vertebra, with a shift of the normal instantaneous centre of rotation, and thus the probability of disturbed movement.

Hypothesising about the genesis of common vertebral lesions, based on a wealth of steadily mounting neurophysiological research,[103] is a fascinating and beguiling occupation, yet the lesions we see on the clinical shop-floor do not change, as may fashion in therapeutics; nevertheless, there can be new ways of seeing familiar lesions.

Well-tried, effective methods of manual treatment should not be abandoned simply because a new application of an old way of thinking is upon us. We need to understand, digest and utilise what is good about the new, but not completely discard all of the old, since there is nothing really new in this world.

What *is* especially welcome about these methods[13] is their substitution for the almost routine Grade V procedures of times past, and this is to be encouraged.

In accordance with others[42] Mitchell et al[140] have suggested that 'the most frequently used, *perhaps overused*, technique is the high-velocity low-amplitude thrust.' (My italics) There are various ways of classifying the 'new' techniques; one approach is to broadly divide them into:

a. Direct action techniques — in which the patient attempts to produce movement *towards*, into or across a motion barrier, and

b. Indirect action techniques — in which the patient attempts to produce motion *away* from the motion barrier, i.e. the movement–limitation is attacked indirectly.

We can then tabulate various applications of the method like this:

	Contraction	Muscle	Opposing force	Use
Direct	Isotonic-concentric	Shortens	*Less* than the patient's force —the movement is produced towards, into or beyond the motion barrier	Where joint mobility is impaired because of a temporary loss of muscle performance
	Isometric	Static length	Counterforce is *equivalent* to muscle force elicited —no movement occurs	Useful both in *'direct'* and *'indirect'* spinal joint mobilisation techniques, employing moderate and not maximal contractions
Indirect	Isotonic-eccentric	Lengthens	Counterforce is *greater* than the patient's lengthening contraction, thus movement occurs	Hard maximal contractions are used when the aim is to stretch shortened muscle and fascia, i.e. myofascial fibrosis.

Mitchell et al[140] add a further category, using a coined word—'isokinetic'—and also borrowing a word from the terminology of haemolysis—'isolytic' —which need not concern us.

Isometric techniques, which merit most attention, can be used in both 'direct' and 'indirect' joint mobilisation techniques, employing slight or moderate muscular contractions, since excessive force tends to tighten joints and defeats the object of mobilisation.

Lewit[113] employed the technique of post-isometric relaxation to treat restriction of movement in vertebral joints, employing minimal reistance three to five times, for at least 10 seconds, followed by relaxation and stretching as far as relaxation allowed.

He produced not only marked muscular inhibition but also a striking analgesic effect on the muscles and also at their tender points of insertion at the periosteum.

Treatment was unsuccessful if there was little or no muscle spasm, if a 'block' in the relevant vertebral segment persisted or if it was technically impossible to act on those muscle fibres which were in spasm.

Greenman[67] described the same tehniques for the thoracic cage (Figs. 13.5, 7.23) mentioning in passing that manipulators tend for the most part to give much attention to the posterior components of the ribs, and take insufficient notice of the lateral and anterior aspect of these long bony levers. He suggests that it is at the sides and front of the thorax that rib-joint dysfunction is most easily detected; and also observes that the intercostal muscles appear to have more of a stabilising function on the thoracic cage, their participation in respiratory movement being of less importance.

The steps of an isometric technique, to lengthen shortened muscle assumed to be restricting movement, are as follows:

(i) therapist carefully positions the patient and the body part, nudging against the motion barrier

(ii) then explains the patient's participation, i.e. the *direction* in which to actively move the head or trunk or limb, the *magnitude* of the active muscle contraction and the *duration* of it, and also how the therapist will resist it

(iii) the patient contracts

(iv) the therapist offers resistance equal to the patient's force (isometric contraction)

(v) the therapist maintains the resistance for 3–5 or more seconds

(vi) the patient and therapist, respectively, cease contractions and counterforce

(vii) after the patient has not only stopped the muscular effort but has also fully relaxed (sometimes a two-stage phase) the therapist moves the patient or body-part up to the new motion-barrier, when steps 1–6 are repeated two or three times. Movement of the abnormal joint is then re-assessed.

N.B. The amount of counter-force will vary with the size of the muscle-group concerned, yet is never excessive, and the procedure should be painless.

Bourdillon[13] suggests that the isometric techniques may succeed by re-setting the 'gain' of the gamma moto-neurone system, allowing lengthening of muscle fibres. Some examples follow:

a. C1–C2 restricted rotation (Fig. 13.2)

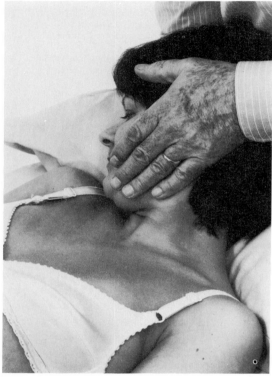

Fig. 13.2 Indirect post-isometric relaxation technique to improve right rotation range of the C1–C2 segment (see text).

Rotation is virtually isolated to the atlanto-axial joint when the neck is gently and fully flexed.

Standing at the head of the supine patient, the therapist flexes the neck fully, and without inducing side-flexion gently rotates the neck to the point of right rotation limitation.

(i)   The patient attempts to rotate the head back to the neutral position, against resistance of the therapist's hand. The indirect isometric contraction is held for some seconds, when the patient relaxes

(ii) when relaxation is complete, the therapist rotates the head further, to the new restriction point

(iii) the steps are repeated 3–5 times

(iv) right rotation range is re-assessed.

b. Upper half of thoracic spine, e.g. T5–6 (Fig. 13.3)

Assuming a Type 11 lesion of T5–T6, when there is restriction, on flexion, in that T5 is tilted to the left and rotated left by reason of a 'tethering' lesion of the

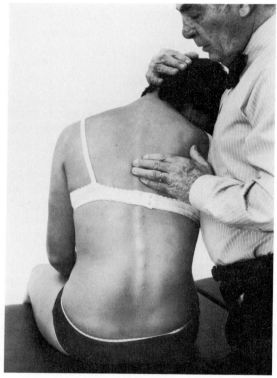

Fig. 13.3 Indirect post-isometric relaxation technique for a flexion restriction of the T5–T6 segment (see text).

left T5–T6 facet-joint, the procedure is as follows:

(i)   the patient sits across the end of the plinth and sags trunk backward against the therapist, who stands with body against her right scapula

(ii) the spine is flexed (sagged) until T5–6 is at the apex of flexion

(iii) the therapist curls right arm and forearm around the patient's head, placing fingers over the occiput; one finger of the other hand palpates the left T5–6 interspace

(iv) patient's head is side-bent and rotated away from the T5 left rotation, until movement begins to be felt at the palpating finger

(v) patient lightly attempts to neutralise head and neck position, for some seconds, and then relaxes

(vi) therapist takes head and neck further, by the sequence of first side-bending, then rotation, then flexion

(vii) the stages are repeated, to a total of 3–5, and T5–T6 joint range then re-assessed. The series is repeated if necessary.

c. Right side-bending restriction of two to three adjacent mid-thoracic segments, e.g. T5-6-7, when in neutral sagittal position (Fig. 13.4)

In this Type 1 lesion, these vertebrae will not fully side-bend right or rotate left.

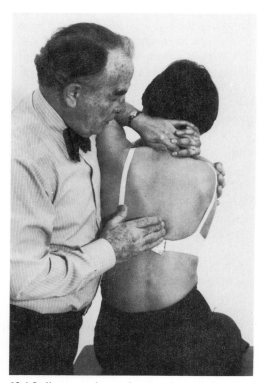

Fig. 13.4 Indirect post-isometric relaxation technique for right side-bending and left rotation restriction of mid-thoracic segments. The technique is 'indirect' in the sense that there is no attempt by the patient to move into the restricted ranges as such (see text).

The patient is seated across the end of the plinth, and clasps neck with interlaced fingers — alternatively, right hand behind neck while left hand grasps right elbow. Standing behind and to the left, with his chest against her left scapula, the therapist reaches his left hand under the patient's near arm to grasp her right shoulder, and places the palpating finger of right hand over the transverse process at the 'apex' of the restriction, e.g. T6. Maintaining *the neutral sagittal position*, the patient's trunk is passively side-bent to the right, and rotated a little to the left, until restriction is perceived by the palpating finger.

(i) The patient attempts, with some 10–12 lb force, to push sideways to the left against the therapist's left pectoral area, for three seconds or so

(i) the patient relaxes

(iii) the therapist side-bends the patient up to the new restriction, and then adds left rotation to the same point

(iv) the steps are repeated to a total of 3–5 times, and movement is then re-assessed, or spinal symmetry is assessed in prone lying.

d. The ribs

The basis of assessing so-called 'inhalation or exhalation restriction' of rib movement is made by noting which rib group stops moving earliest during testing the ranges of inspiration movement.[67]

During assessment, forward and upward motion of the upper 4–6 ribs is felt with the hands on anterior thorax, while the outward motion of ribs 6–10 is perceived with the therapist's hand placed antero-laterally on the rib cage. A refinement is then to identify the 'key' rib, i.e. that with the most restricted motion. Most lesions of rib dysfunction involve a little unilateral district of the thorax, and symmetry of *function* is more important than symmetry of structure.

(i) So far as the *first and second ribs* are concerned, they appear at times to be a little elevated by reason of scalene muscle tightness, or postural spasm, this particular 'exhalation restriction' apparently having little to do with joints since improvement of scalene muscle extensibility alone releases the rib restriction, also allowing freer and less painful neck movement. The examination technique (Fig. 7.23) is easily adapted as a post-isometric relaxation treatment technique, adopting the steps described on page 191.

(ii) Following active testing movements in sitting, and accessory-movement testing in prone-lying, a not uncommon finding is that of a little district of three ribs, e.g. 6th, 7th and 8th, with tender angles, pain on side-flexion and rotation to that side and discomfort on full inspiration. Since palpation antero-laterally may reveal a degree of seemingly restricted but painless rib movement on the *opposite* side, and complete bilateral symmetry of movement does not exist, the basis for 'inhalation and exhalation restrictions' may not be as secure as we would like.

Nevertheless, post-isometric techniques can help (Figs. 13.5(A) and (B)). After stabilising the angles of ribs, with finger-tips just lateral to them, a gentle caudal and lateral stretch is applied by taking the patient's arm of that side across and downward, for a few seconds (Fig. 13.5(A)).

In the second stage, the patient's arm is considerably taken into a degree of elevation, with elbow flexion (Fig. 13.5(B)) until the tension is perceived at the rib angles.

By the patient lightly attempting to move her arm away from her ear, against the therapist's resistance, the steps described on page 191 are repeated some three to five times, and the active movements of side-flexion and rotation are then re-assessed.

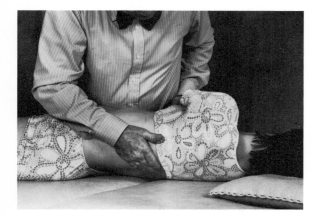

Fig. 13.5A Gentle caudo-lateral stretch to soft tissues associated with left rib-joints 6, 8 and 8 (see text).

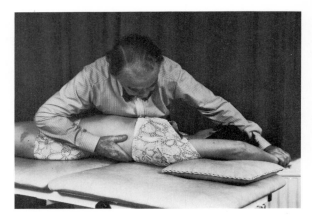

Fig. 13.5B Post-isometric relaxation techniques for 'fixation' of left 6th, 7th and 8th ribs (see text).

e. The low back

In treating a Type 11 restriction of full flexion, accompanying palpable left side-bending and left rotation of a low lumbar vertebra (see Fig. 13.1), the patient sits on a stool, with feet apart and flat on the floor. The left arm hangs between the patient's knees. The therapist stands on the patient's left side, straddling the patient's near knee and reaching across with his left hand to grasp the patient's right shoulder. The opposite hand palpates the vertebral interspace between spinous processes immediately below the most left rotated transverse process.

   (i) The patient is slumped until the segment being treated is most prominent posteriorly (Fig. 13.6(A))

  (ii) pressing his left pectoral area against the patient's left shoulder, and maintaining the flexed position, the patient is side-flexed away, i.e. to the right, reaching to the floor with right hand (Fig. 13.6(B))

 (iii) the therapist then rotates the patient away from himself, i.e. to the right, until tension is perceived at the segment being palpated

 (iv) the patient attempts to reach for the floor with the right hand, this movement being resisted by the therapist

  (v) she then relaxes, after which the therapist takes up a further increment of first side-bending, then rotation, then flexion

 (vi) steps (iv) and (v) are repeated to a total of 3–5 times

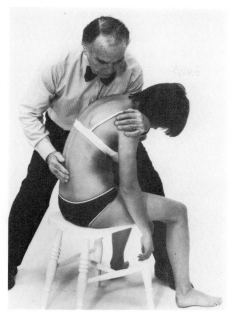

Fig. 13.6A Indirect post-isometric relaxation technique for restricted lumbar flexion due to 'block' or 'fixation' of a left lumbo-sacral facet-joint. The patients slumps until the segment is most prominent posteriorly (see text).

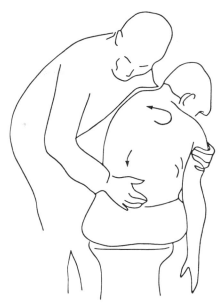

Fig. 13.6C Stage (vii), when the patient pushes against the therapist's left pectoral area with her left upper thoracic region, i.e. a combination of left-side flexion, left rotation and extension (see text).

(viii) the patient relaxes, when step (v) is repeated

  (ix) standing now a little behind the patient, while maintaining the rotation and with a hand on each shoulder, the patient is instructed to reach for the floor with the left hand (Fig. 13.6(D))

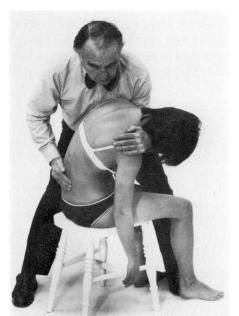

Fig. 13.6B The second stage of positioning the patient (see text).

(vii) the patient then pushes against the therapist's left pectoral area, which is resisted (Fig. 13.6(C)) for a few seconds

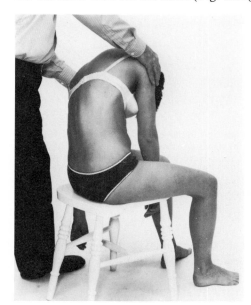

Fig. 13.6D Stage (ix), when the patient reaches for the floor with her left hand (see text).

(x) the patient then reaches to the floor with the right hand, too, until fully flexed

(xi) the patient is returned to the erect position, passively, against her slight resistance

(xii) flexion range is re-assessed

N.B. Not all stages are illustrated.

Goodridge[64] describes a variant (Fig. 13.7) in that, with the same positioning, the patient is instructed to move both shoulders in a left and upward gliding or translation movement, against the operator's chest, while the vertical relationship of the patient's shoulders does not change.

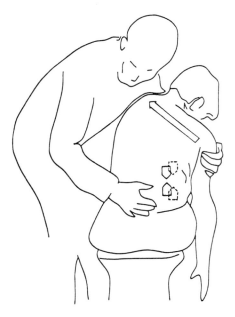

Fig. 13.7 A post-isometric relaxation technique in which the patient attempts to move both shoulders in a left and upward gliding or translation movement (see text). (Figs. 13.6(c) and 13.7 are reproduced from Goodridge J P 1981 Muscle energy technique: definition, explanation, methods of procedure. J Amer Osteop Assoc 81: 249, by courtesy of the Author and Publishers.)

On subsequent relaxation, right rotation is again imposed up to the new 'motion barrier', and the process repeated as described. He classes this as a 'concentric isotonic' technique, since there is right lateral flexion during the movement. The end-result is the same.

f. The tight ilio-psoas muscle

Tightness of these muscles is more common than weakness. The supine patient hangs the leg over the end of the plinth, flexing opposite hip and knee and gripping upper shin to maintain them so (Fig. 13.8).

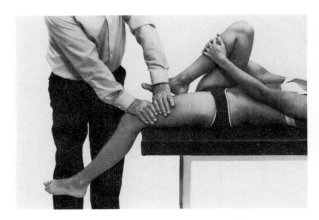

Fig. 13.8 Post-isometric relaxation technique for 'release' of a tight psoas-iliacus muscle group (see text).

The therapist stands on the medial side of the hanging leg, and flexes his far knee so that his shin can resist against the medio-plantar aspect of the patient's foot. Where the degree of tightness is slight the patient must have her buttocks at the edge of the plinth.

(i) the patient attempts to flex and externally rotate the hip — both movements are opposed, flexion by the therapist's hands and internal rotation by his shin

(ii) after a few seconds of isometric contraction, the patient relaxes, after which the therapist moves the hip further into extension

(iii) the steps are repeated to a total of 3–5 times.

g. The sacro-iliac joint

With the patient lying on the unaffected side, the therapist stands facing her at the pelvic level and flexes the upper knee and hip to engage her shin against his lower abdomen (Fig. 13.9).

My own preference is to stabilise the patient's under leg by placing my near leg on the plinth against it.

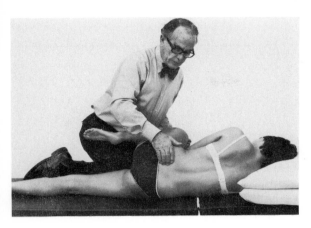

Fig. 13.9 Post-isometric relaxation technique for a presumed fixation of left sacroiliac joint, by reason of a palpably 'anterior innominate' restricting posterior movement of ilium on sacrum (see text, and Fig. 11.15).

The therapist's far hand supports the patient's knee; the near hand monitors movement in the upper sacro-iliac sulcus, as hip-flexion is passively imposed to the point where resistance is perceived there.

(i) the patient attempts to extend her hip against the therapist's resistance for a few seconds, then relaxes

(ii) the therapist increases hip flexion to the point of resistance again

(iii) the two steps are repeated to a total of 3–5, when the articular signs are re-assessed.

Manually-resisted isometric contractions to stabilise hypermobile vertebral segments

While these techniques are proper to this category, they are described in Chapter 14 Active movements, (i) Regional or localised active exercises, since they do naturally take their place in the section devoted to *stabilisation* of a segment rather than *mobility* of it.

14

Active movements

1. REGIONAL OR LOCALISED ACTIVE EXERCISES

Voluntary exercises, in many forms, are often necessary to complement passive movement techniques, and at times exercises may comprise the main form of treatment. Alternatively, many orthopaedists and therapists appear to hold that the patient has not had a 'proper' treatment unless the therapist has demonstrated and supervised exercises; treatments without exercises being traditionally regarded as incomplete. The suggestion that this or that particular patient does not *need* exercises, because they are not indicated, tends to evince pained astonishment in some.

Common assumptions underlying the general view that 'exercise is a good thing' could probably bear some examination. In a comprehensive analysis of the behaviour of low back pain,[10] it was clear that, 'Patients who regularly participated in physical exercise did not show any dissimilarity in the course of back pain compared to patients who only occasionally or never took exercise.'

In active people and juniors, for example, and also in many mature patients, exercise for the sake of exercise has little point when there are no indications for prescribing exercise with a clear purpose.

The current surge of interest in health, strength and athleticism (for want of a better word) behoves the clinical therapist to be clear as to what therapeutic exercise is about. The generalised, progressive improvement in joint mobility, muscle power, co-ordination and endurance, and enhancement of physical well-being in people who basically are fit and healthy, is a different prospect to the correction, by therapeutic exercise, of painful musculo-skeletal abnormalities suffered by those who may be mature and not especially athletically-minded.

While many competent therapists can equally well cater for both populations, the prescribing of exercises is sometimes too generalised, and appropriate aims of treatment not always clearly perceived.

Often enough we, and the patients, have to be content with less than the ideal, despite best efforts on both sides of the counter.

Often, a change of job is much more important than exercise. The load-carrier driver on building sites, who is bounced about on a pitching bucket seat, and the middle-aged telephonist who sits and reaches for heavy directories for hours each day, would reduce stress on low lumbar discs by changing to occupations with more standing, where feasible.

Alternatively, the administrator's chair-bound-backache problem tends to disappear with more physical activity, a better set of abdominal muscles and less weight, the last being rather an indicator of general physical fitness than having much to do with reducing stress on lumbar discs, as is often supposed.[49]

Patients can lose confidence in the capacity of their backs to stand up to the stresses of life.

Reassurance and a positive approach during treatment are in some cases more important than the treatment itself, because a fixed idea of spinal inadequacy is profoundly disabling, and not often justified.

There is considerable interest in new methods of treating chronic pain disability, by a goal-oriented programme aiming to reduce medication intake, to reduce avoidance of activities because of pain, to increase ambulation and selected exercise tolerance and to increase general social and work involvement.

Fordyce *et al.*[53] refers to 'operant conditioning' as the principles by which the rate, strength and frequency of occurrence of operants may be increased or decreased. Graded exercise programmes form an important part of behaviour-modification techniques, and actively involve the patient in the improvement process.

Mooney and Cairns[143] refer to the value of the therapist in the training and monitoring of progression through the strengthening exercises.

Group exercises can be a useful method of strengthening vertebral musculature, of improving physical endurance and general locomotor condition and of training in lifting and handling techniques. There is some variation in the organisation of group exercise programmes, since the approach to vertebral joint problems may differ considerably between departments of orthopaedics and rheumatology.

Unless some care is devoted to the clinical examination of each individual whose treatment is solely that of exercises in a particular group, there is a tendency for the person conducting the group treatment to learn very much more about giving exercises to groups than about the precise characteristics of joint problems in the patients being treated.

Individual exercises have many aims. For example:

a. The need to stabilise hypermobile joints by strengthening the environmental musculature, both regionally and segmentally.

b. Mobility exercises for joints liable to become stiff; these may also be regional and/or segmental exercises.

c. Postural retraining exercises, to diminish the effects of gravitational stress upon particular spinal regions or segments, e.g. where operation is not indicated or is delayed, as in spondylolisthesis or spinal stenosis; and preventive or prophylactic exercise, to restore reduced lumbar and upper thoracic extension range, and prevent recurrence of low back and upper/mid thoracic pains associated with flexed postures.

d. Progressive exercise programmes to generally improve muscular strength and physical endurance, and confidence in ability of the spine to stand up to stress.

e. Individual handling instruction, with practice of performance (see p. 210).

The aims are often combined.

a. (i) Strengthening the environmental musculature in treatment of a hypermobile low lumbar joint

While passive mobilisation techniques are used to reduce the *pain* arising from a segment which may be hypermobile, it is necessary that *stability* of the segment be improved.

If the spinal extensor muscles are considered to be weak, or to require extra strengthening, exercises to strengthen them should avoid inner range hyper-extension movements, and the starting position arranged so that the resisted movement occurs in middle range and the excursion ceases when normal postural length of the muscle is reached.

Exercises need to be selected with care, since those which stress the joint structures in extreme positions of flexion, extension or rotation are liable to exacerbate the condition. A potent cause of aggravation of low back pain, due to hypermobility, is that of active forced extension in the starting position of prone-lying. *It is a very familiar clinical experience to meet the patient who has been religiously performing 'back extension' exercises of this type, and has just as regularly been suffering recurrence of the pains for which these vigorous exercises were prescribed. They are mentioned only to be condemned as a potent source of continuing back trouble in a particular group of patients.*

During manipulative treatment, with or without anaesthesia, and any other treatment for that matter, including exercises, one of the most common errors is failure to recognise the hypermobile lumbar segment.

Recurrent aggravating backache[120] is one of the most common manifestations of degenerative changes associated with segmental hyperextension, and most of these patients are suffering from recurrent hyperextension strains of posterior joints, or chronic approximation of neural arch structures. *Again, the exercise of lying supine and slowly raising the straight legs together, 'to strengthen the abdominal and psoas muscles', is one of the ways in which the symptoms of hypermobile lumbar segments are recurrently aggravated.* In the initial few degrees of the movement, the posterior neural arch structures are painfully approximated by the powerful muscle action, as the lumbar spine is drawn into excessive lordosis by the muscles acting with reversed origin and insertion.[23] Similarly, some of the more exotic yoga hyperextension exercises may painfully approximate facet-joint structures, and in the author's recent experience these have more than once initiated an acute and very painful back problem in overenthusiastic patients.

'In the neutral position, moderate extension strains are not painful'[120] but a segment held in hyperextension has no safety-margin, so that painful capsular lesions result—and keep on resulting as a consequence of repetitive strains.

When progressively stronger isometric 'hold' positions are maintained against the resistance of gravity, with the joint in fairly neutral positions, muscle power may be improved without further joint strain. So far as disc pressure is concerned, isometrically performed exercises are less likely to provoke further pain and disability since it has been demonstrated that they load the lumbar spine less than isotonic exercises.[145] When isometric exercises comprise the only treatment, or they are used together with traction, the results are an improvement upon ordinary flexion and extension routines.[70]

Isometric exercises to improve the power of abdominal muscles are also of value in the treatment of low back pain (*vide infra*)[146] although postural re-education in the importance of reducing the lumbar lordosis by isotonic exercises can be very helpful for a proportion of patients and Cailliet[23] provides a few simple and good examples.

There are many types of isometric exercise, and gravitational resistance is not always a necessary component. The following exercises, of which there can be many variations, are suggested as a basis for progression:

Abdominal wall (upper)

Starting position: The patient lies supine (Fig. 14.1) with hips and knees flexed and the feet flat on the support, and hands on opposite shoulders
Exercise: The trunk is raised forward, while toes press on support and feet are plantar-flexed, to inhibit action of psoas.[92] The patient must breathe freely while holding the posture for a few seconds
Progressions: Hold posture for longer. Add weight (e.g. sandbag) to chest, as illustrated

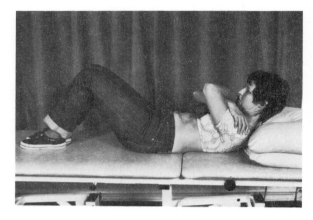

Fig. 14.1 Exercise for upper abdominal muscles. Note sandbags on model's sternum, for progressively increased resistance (see text).

Abdominal wall (lower)

Starting position: The patient grips sides of plinth, with legs in crook-lying (Fig. 14.2)
Exercise: Raise buttocks off plinth, bending hips until shins are parallel with plinth surface, and breathe freely
Progression: Sustain posture for longer

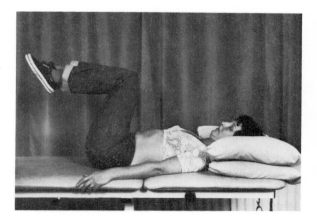

Fig. 14.2 Exercise for lower abdominal muscles. The patient should now grip the sides of the plinth (see text).

Abdominal wall (oblique)

Starting position: Crook lying with hands on shoulders (Fig. 14.3)

Exercise: Raise trunk forward, directing right elbow towards flexed left hip and knee. Hold posture while breathing freely. Repeat to opposite side

N.B. Clasping hands behind the neck is not recommended, since the over-enthusiastic patient can easily provoke latent cervical joint problems, or initiate new ones, by vigorously pulling the neck forward.

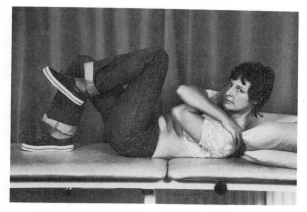

Fig. 14.3 Exercise for oblique abdominal muscles. Clasping the hands behind the neck is not recommended (see text).

Abdominal bracing[98]

Starting position: The patient lies supine with hips and knees well-flexed and palms on lower front thighs (Fig. 14.4)

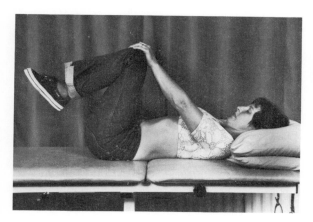

Fig. 14.4 Abdominal bracing (see text).

Exercise: While breathing freely, the action of pelvic tilting is resisted by the hands to initiate an isometric contraction of abdominal wall

Progression: With hands as before, but hips more flexed, the patient attempts to lift buttocks from plinth, against manual resistance as above.

Dorsal extensor muscles

Starting position (not illustrated): The patient lies prone with trunk on a flat surface such as a kitchen table, the edge of which is covered by a folded towel and approximates to the groin. The hips are flexed so that the toes may rest on the floor, with knees straight. By grasping the sides of the table, the trunk is stabilised; the legs are raised to the horizontal and held there, the isometric hold being maintained for increasing durations. (Fig. 14.5). As before, breathing should be free.

Progression: This is made by adding weight to the heels, e.g. a light cushion and then a heavier one; the method of performing the exercise does not change. It provides for powerful work by the erector spinae group, with the lumbar joints in what is virtually a neutral position.

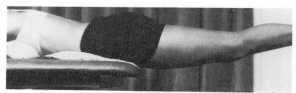

Fig. 14.5 Exercise for dorsal extensor muscles (see text).

(ii) Strengthening the segmental musculature in treatment of a hypermobile lumbar joint

The principle is that of stimulating small but important local muscle groups to work isometrically in maintaining the orientation in space of a single vertebra. This localised strengthening is of fundamental importance, because of clear evidence[94] that lumbar degenerative joint conditions are accompanied by changes in the relative populations of 'fast' and 'slow' fibres in the segmental musculature, e.g. multifidus.

Lateral technique

Starting position: The patient lies prone on the support; the therapist stands at the side and applies his thumbpads to that side of the spinous process of the upper vertebra of the segment concerned. The position is the same as for transverse vertebral pressure (Fig. 14.6).

Moderate but sustained pressure is applied to the bony point, the patient being instructed not to allow the vertebra to be 'displaced'. Initially, a considerable mass of paravertebral muscle is called into play to resist the displacing pressure, but with encouragement and practice the patient begins to localise the muscular effort to a surprising degree. Similarly, there is a need to consciously relax muscle groups which need not be called into play and to breathe in a quiet and relaxed way.

Isometric contractions are repeated to the opposite side, and progression is made by increasing the pressures being sustained, and the duration of the 'holds'. The exercise is repeated on the spinous process next below; where two hypermobile segments lie in one vertebral region, both components of each segment must be treated.

Sagittal technique

The patient sits across a plinth, with the buttocks at the rear edge. The therapist stands, crouches or kneels behind the patient, and applies both thumbpads to one spinous process. Moderate but sustained pressure is now applied in a postero-anterior direction, and the patient instructed to not allow the segment to be moved forwards. At first, this elicits a total response of all trunk musculature, but by encouragement to 'think and contract locally' the muscular effort does become much more localised. As before the patient should breathe freely and quietly, and learn to gently wriggle arms, hands, legs and feet to make the point about relaxation of all uninvolved muscle.

Progressions: are made as described above.

The L4–L5 and lumbosacral segments may also be treated with the patient in a prone position; the hips are flexed to 90° (Fig. 14.7) with the patient's

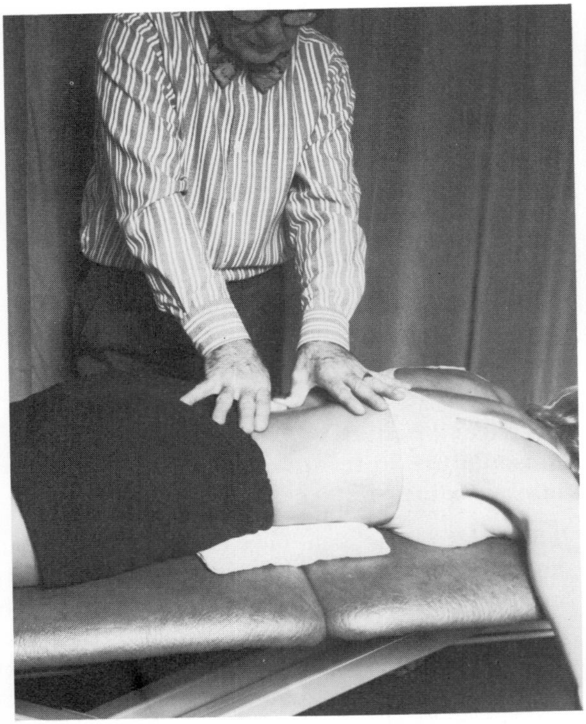

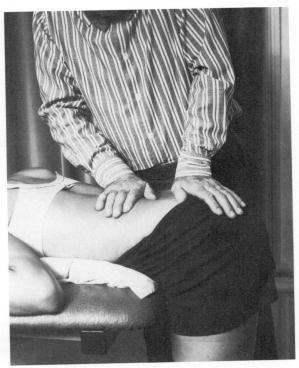

Fig. 14.6. Exercise for strengthening the segmental musculature related to a hypermobile lumbar joint. Lateral technique (see text).

Fig. 14.7 Segmental stabilisation exercise. Saggital technique (see text). It may be modified, of course, as a hold-relax technique to assist stretching of shortened soft tissues.

feet resting on the floor and the knees some three inches (7 cm) or more above it. The therapist stands at the side, level with the patient's pelvis, and places his cranial palm on the lumbar region immediately above the segments concerned. Moderate, but increasing and sustained pressure is applied to the patient's sacrum by the therapist's caudal hand. The patient must be discouraged from using hip and knee extensor muscles to resist the pressure; the legs should be wriggled about now and then to ensure they are relaxed and taking no part in the movement.

Home exercises: At one attendance, a relative can be taught to give the resistance; the postero-anterior pressures can be self-administered by the patient (Fig. 14.8) and many become highly adept at the exercise.

Other regions

Thoracic joint problems appear generally to need simple maintenance exercises for mobility (Figs. 14.9 (a) (b) (c)) than resisted exercises for stability, but where joint plan is arising from a hypermobile

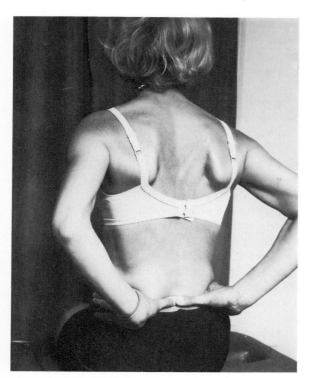

Fig. 14.8 Home segmental exercise, showing auto-resistance by the patient (see text).

segment, resisted exercises should form part of the treatment. They are less easy to administer than at the lumbar spine, but the principles are the same.

Paravertebral muscle of the *neck* may become weakened as a consequence of chronic degenerative joint changes. There are many methods of strengthening the musculature, varying from (i) somewhat heroic procedures involving the patient lying extended over a kitchen table with a looped towel suspending in space a brick, which is lifted up and down by neck extension, and (ii) proprioceptive facilitation techniques, to (iii) simple self-administered resistance by hand pressure. The latter method is quite efficient, quite effective and does not involve a search for building materials.

Strengthening exercises are by no means always indicated (but see p. 204); if localised manual mobilisation, traction and/or a cervical collar have produced relief of pain and freedom of movement, this will allow better muscle function, and thus simple postural-correction exercises and prophylactic advice are more appropriate than strengthening exercises for their own sake.

b. (i) Regional mobility exercises

These are well known to all therapists, and all that one needs to mention is the importance of ensuring that the type of exercise given does indeed affect the intended vertebral region. For example, the favourite group of prone-kneeling exercises, to mobilise the lower spine, have much more effect upon the thoracolumbar region than the lumbosacral segments.

Hydrotherapy provides the benefits of relaxing warmth, support and buoyancy, allowing easier voluntary effort and regional mobilisation of stiff spinal joints.

(ii) Segmental mobility exercises

These previously rather specialised techniques have, in the last few years, become more widely used, and a handy pocket-book text[22] describes some of them. For example, if the right hand is passed across the chest and around the left side of the neck, so that the palmar aspect of the right middle fingertip is placed against the *right* side of the C6 spinous process to stabilise it, active left neck rotation will mobilise the

C5–C6 segment. Again, if the patient sits in a high-backed chair, so that the spinous process of T3 bears precisely against the upper edge of the chair-back, extension of the head, neck and upper thorax, with a degree of 'chin-pulling-in', will exercise the small extension range of the T2–T3 segment much more than will a generalised thoracic extension movement.

A difficulty with segmental exercises is that many of the manual self-stabilisation techniques are not possible for the mature or elderly patient, by reason of shoulder joint restriction, for example. Sometimes, and in some patients, those who most need them are least able to do them. Ingeniously-devised segmental exercises, demonstrated by young models, often fall short of their face value when mature and chronically-stiff patients try to do them. Nevertheless, they are an important advance in the treatment of common vertebral problems.

c. Postural retraining and prophylactic exercises

Other factors given, individuals without vertebral joint problems are more likely to avoid them while they retain the natural resilience, extensibility and vascularity of their soft tissues, strong muscles which are well co-ordinated in isotonic or isometric contraction and reciprocal relaxation, and joints which are freely mobile.

While these are given to the young, the inheritance is often soon to be abused, by competitive trials of strength and endurance which begin the process of unequal muscular development, unequal tightness of connective tissue and certain restrictions of the 'global' mobility of joints.

Plain freedom from pain is not necessarily synonymous with the most efficient functioning of the physical machinery and in particular, the way in which we use our bodies is perhaps more a matter of enlightened physical education in human kinetics than pursuing the ideal of excelling in strength and endurance, and little else.

Low backache may coexist with excessive lordosis and a lax abdominal wall. Stabilisation of the lumbar spine in a less extended position, by isometric abdominal strengthening exercises while holding a corrected pelvic tilt, is effective in helping to relieve this type of backache, as it is in relieving low back and bilateral sciatic pain so often associated with

developmental and/or acquired spinal stenosis in mature people.

Spondylolisthesis at a lumbar segment need not cause symptoms, but when the condition does give rise to pain and surgical treatment is not immediately considered, inner range abdominal exercises combined with pelvic tilting will diminish the shearing stress and help to stabilise the faulty segment by reducing lordosis.

Conversely, a large number of patients, with recurrent low back pain after sitting, driving, bending and gardening etc. show a tendency to loss of lumbar lordosis, and lateral deviation to one or other side usually associated with the painful episode.

After correction of lateral deviation, if present, encouragement of lordotic postures is successful in preventing recurring back pain.[125]

(i) Cervical spine

Besides isometric exercises to help overcome symmetrical or asymmetrical tightness, or for other specific purposes, it is wise for healthy people to make two or three full-range excursions of the neck each day. Anterior cervical muscles frequently become elongated and weakened, and this is much easier to prevent than to reverse.

a. A mild traction effect, and prophylactic extension of the ligamentum nuchae, is produced when lying supine with the head on two pillows and the knees and hips bent; the head is smoothly raised and the chin depressed to the chest as closely as possible. After lowering smoothly to the pillow, the exercise is repeated 10–20 times.

b. A more positive exercise is that of sitting in a chair with the arms abducted and the palms, with fingers interlaced, resting on the forehead. While strictly maintaining a neutral neck position, the forehead is pressed against the hands to produce isometric contraction of the anterior neck muscles. The force of the contraction should be built up slowly and smoothly, and over one to three minutes daily.

Although generalised full-range movements (*vide supra*) are valuable for the neck as a whole, the occipitoatlantal joint may need localised home exercises, and while there exist localised exercise tehniques which involve somewhat exotic hand placings for fixation purposes, many patients are just not able to do them.[22]

c. While sitting with the hands lightly grasping the sides of the chair-seat, a simple lateral glide of the head and neck from side to side (like a Balinese dancer), exercises the craniovertebral junction more than the lower segments. If this is *then* followed by simple nodding exercises and full rotation from side to side in the same sitting position, the C0–C1 segment has been given an adequate 'home exercise' treatment in its important ranges. Five excursions in every direction are enough.

(ii) Cervico-thoracic region

Paradoxically, the key to relieving, as well as preventing, 'yoke' area pains which are clearly associated with thickened and tender upper thoracic vertebral joints, is that of attending to *shortened and tight pectoral muscles* as well as the joint problem. In general terms, manual segmental mobilisation

tehniques for hypomobility which are not complemented by exercises to maintain or improve mobility, are not enough; the cervicothoracic region is a prime example of this principle.

Simple exercises are:

a. Stand in a doorway with the arms abducted to 135° and the palms placed against the door jambs. Keep the elbows straight and push the chest (*not the abdomen*, which may painfully hyperextend the low back) through the doorway (Figs. 14.9 (a) (b) (c)).

This exercise is intended for tight pectoral structures, and is not suitable for a painful condition of the glenohumeral joint, unless there is no irritability and treatment has reached the stage of encouraging the last few degrees of elevation in 30° or so of abduction.

b. With the knees bent and feet resting on the support, place one palm behind the occiput and lie supine with the upper thorax over the edge of a stout table (a folded towel relieves painful pressure on the upper thoracic spinous processes). It will be found

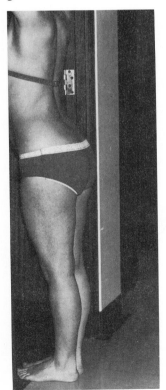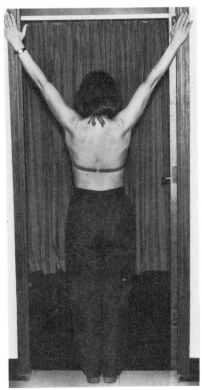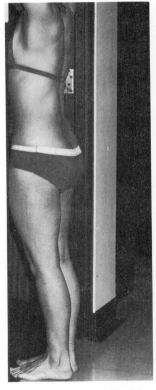

Fig. 14.9 A home exercise for stretching the pectoral muscles (centre). The chest is pressed forward, with the arms stabilised by the door jamb. Producing a lumbar lordosis by pushing the abdomen forward is incorrect (left); the normal posture of the spine should be maintained (right) and it is worthwhile spending a little time ensuring that the patient well understands the procedure.

that resting one ankle just above the opposite bent knee relieves a tendency to lumbar lordosis.[22] Allow the weight of the head, neck and arm to gently extend the upper thoracic region. The weight of the head should *not* be allowed to hyperextend the neck, by removing occipital support.

After a little practice, and reassurance, it should be possible to rest both hands on the abdomen, while the upper-most thorax, neck and head gravitate dorsally towards the floor, while minimal ventral cervical muscular effort prevents full neck extension (Fig. 14.10).

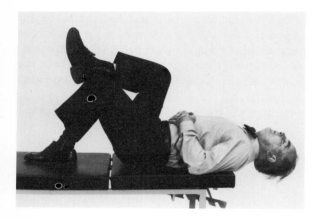

Fig. 14.10 A corrective postural exercise for chronically-contracted pectoral structures.

c. While sitting, reach the right arm round the left side, beneath the chin, to place the pad of the middle fingers on the *right* side of the C7 spinous process. Repetitively rotate the head and neck to the *left* side. By stabilising C7 (or C6 or T1) in this way, rotation mobility is exercised. Repeat to opposite side. Some patients are just not able to do this exercise.[22]

(iii) Thoracic spine

The position of relaxed leaning backwards in sitting, against the low back support of a standard office chair, is that in which the intravital disc pressures are lowest[1, 2] and office workers should take up this

position from time to time during the working day — many of them instinctively do.

a. A deep inspiration, while raising the arms to full elevation and leaning backwards in the chair, is also a method of reversing the effects of prolonged sitting in a hunched position. Relief from thoracic strain is also gained by lying supine on the floor, with the knees bent and the arms abducted to 135°.

The exercise for maintaining extensibility of the pectoral muscle group (Figs. 14.9 (a) (b) (c)) is also useful in this respect.

b. Extension mobility of the thorax, and the power of dorsal musculature, is maintained by the exercise of sitting in one's heels on the floor and bending forward to rest the forehead on the floor in front of the knees. The forearms are pronated so that the dorsum of the hands rest alongside the legs. Without altering the flexed posture of the lumbar spine, the thoracic spine is extended, the arms externally rotated and the scapulae approximated, as the head (maintained in a neutral relationship) and shoulders are raised to flatten the thoracic spine. The position is held for an increasing number of seconds as the patient becomes familiar with the purpose and technique of the exercise, which may be fairly strongly progressed by abducting the arms to 90°. Five to ten daily repetitions are enough (Fig. 14.11 (a) (b) (c)).

c. Side-flexion and rotation mobility, and mobility of the rib-cage, may be exercised by sitting on a stool or chair with the knees apart. While keeping the pelvis stabilised, one hand firmly reaches for the floor as the opposite arm is elevated to some 150° behind the plane of the trunk, and is looked at by turning head and trunk to that side. The exercise should be done smoothly and easily to full range without jerking. Repeat to opposite side, with 5 to 10 daily repetitions.

Nursing mothers are more prone to thoracic strain than may be recognised, and the exercises described are a useful preventive measure.

The benefits of swimming, badminton and squash are plain, yet patients often need reminding of what they know, i.e. the simple value of free activity. While Yoga exercises have a tendency to produce joint problems in the overenthusiastic, the cult is an excellent way of maintaining thoracic mobility, so long as the fervour to progress too rapidly in ability is kept in reasonable check by a good teacher.

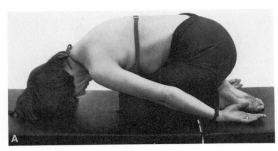

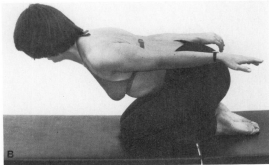

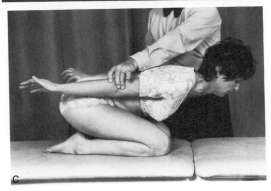

Fig. 14.11A, B, C An exercise for progressively strengthening the thoracic dorsal musculature and shoulder-girdle retractors (see text).

(iv) The low back

We have no therapy which can successfully and wholly compete with the infinite capacity of patient to reinjure themselves.

The unavoidable demands of life, e.g. suddenly reaching to protect a child at risk, having to change the wheel of a car, nursing a sick relative, a night in an unaccustomedly soft hotel bed, will occur sooner or later to induce a painful episode — prophylaxis can only reduce their frequency.

There is not necessarily a direct relationship

between the volume of literature on a particular subject and the orderly accumulation of facts about it; the prophylaxis of low back pain is one such example. The mountain of literature on the multifarious aspects of pathology of common spinal articular changes, particular disc changes, is massive enough to have become all things to all men — it is now so great that each can find in it what they might wish to find, while a great deal is yet unsolved.

The truth is that we do not know; this being so, we might get our best guidance from the thing we do know about, i.e. *the unique clinical presentation from patient to patient.*

The flexible application of principles which are clearly understood is probably better than highly detailed and 'military' instructions gloomily based on the dire need to keep the back straight at all times, or the back bent like a banana at all times.

Severe aggravation of the clinical feature of spinal stenosis, by lordotic postures, is well documented by Weinstein *et al.*[182] yet despite a considerable increase in awareness of the pathomechanics of spinal stenosis, patients with back pain and sciatica continue to be advised of the importance of maintaining, and even increasing, the 'natural' lumbar lordosis, sometimes without reference to that most dominant feature, *the particular nature and pattern of clinical features.*

Aside from habitual occupational stresses and/or single episodes of exciting trauma to which everybody is liable, low back pain appears generally more common in those with weak trunk musculature, somewhat tight hamstrings, a tendency to lordosis because of lax abdominal muscles, shortening of the psoas muscle and also the lumbosacral soft tissues. For these reasons preventive exercises should, in general terms, include those for:

Joint mobility, with an emphasis on flexion and extension
Abdominal and dorsal muscle strengthening
Stretching of the psoas muscle
Elongation of shortened hamstrings (to a degree normal for each individual)
Ability to correct forward pelvic tilt
Physical endurance (again to varying degrees suitable for the individual).

A simplified black-and-white division into two common types of low back pain presentation is perhaps justified in order to make the point, but it has its dangers, since the two simplified groups certainly represent less than 50 per cent of all patterns of low back pain presentation.

As an illustration we can describe a simplified 'A' group who stand with a pronounced lordosis and have a somewhat weak abdominal wall. Their pattern of recurrence is that of:

Pain across the low back, initially with some spreading to both buttocks

Aggravation of pain by standing, walking, and lying prone or supine and relief by sitting

All lumbar movements, other than flexion, provoke the pain

Flexion is painless, and free so far as tight lumbodorsal soft tissues will allow, with a localised low lumbar lordosis unchanged at the extreme of flexion

There are no neurological signs. Straight-leg-raising is fairly free, of equal range and not limited by pain.

Conversely, a simplified 'B' group, whose painful recurrences are more likely to be provoked by prolonged sitting and bending, tend to present with:

A degree of loss of lordosis

Sometimes with listing to one or other side

The amount of pain on sitting and the preference for standing depends upon the severity of loss of lordosis

Severe but temporary incapacity after driving for more than 30–45 minutes

Less provocation of pain on bending backwards (which, if possible, they nevertheless do cautiously) than on flexion

Pain on side-flexion is variable, but is usually greater on bending towards the side of pain

Reduced straight-leg-raising, sometimes bi-laterally and asymmetrically, but often on one side only

No neurological signs.

In Group 'A', the principles of exercise would be to stretch the psoas and also contracted lumbo-dorsal fascia, teach pelvic tilting, increase the power of abdominal muscles and lengthen short hamstrings (Figs. 14.12).

Stretching of the psoas muscle. When sitting and standing, *in vivo* manometry of the middle lumbar

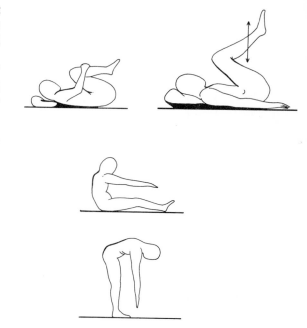

Fig. 14.12 Home exercises in the treatment of one type of back pain (see text). As pain diminishes and confidence improves, the exercise is changed to that of long-sitting and reaching for the toes, and then standing flexion.

discs reveals that they support heavier loads than can be attributed to gravitational compression, e.g. in a 70 kg man sitting upright, the L3 disc is carrying 140 kg, and when standing upright the load on L3 is 100 kg.[144]

Besides acting as a hip flexor, the vertebral portion of the psoas muscle also appears to take part in maintaining the upright posture, and by this activity adds a compressive effect upon the lumbar discs, in addition to that of gravitational force alone.

A simple 'maintenance' stretch of the left psoas muscle is achieved by lying supine on a firm surface and, grasping the right knee, pulling the knee onto the chest by full hip and knee flexion. The left lower limb is pressed onto the surface along its whole length. Repeat to opposite side (Fig. 14.13).

The exercise of pulling the knees onto the chest (Fig. 14.12) and its progressions will assist in maintaining flexion mobility, and in preventing tightness of the lumbodorsal fascia.

Backward pelvic tilting. These exercises need no description here.

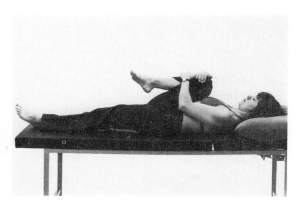

Fig. 14.13 Exercise to stretch left ilio-psoas muscle group (see text).

Abdominal muscle stengthening. Those exercises described in the treatment of a hypermobile lumbar segment (p. 200) are also suitable as preventive exercises.

Elongation of shortened hamstrings. The flexion exercises (*vide supra*) will assist this aim, but a more specific exercise is necessary. From standing with both feet parallel and a little apart, one heel is placed forward onto a support (stool, chair, seat, desk) as high as stability allows — the height will vary according to the individual. The hamstring muscles of the raised leg will be stretched as the standing-leg knee is bent, while both hands reach down the shin to the foot of the raised leg. Repeat to opposite side (Fig. 14.14).

In Group 'B' the principle of exercise is to restore full lumbar lordosis.[125]

Restoration of lordosis

For the patient whose painful episode is accompanied by some loss of the normal lumbar lordosis, a scheme of progressive extension will be suitable, following initial assessment.

From the prone kneeling position (Fig. 14.15 (A) (B)), with the hands placed forward of the shoulders, the hips and knees are gently extended by carrying the trunk slightly forward over the hands — the position is held for a few moments before the hips and knees are flexed again by backward movement of the trunk.

From a cautious beginning, by a dozen excursions every hour or so, the exercise is progressed by holding the forward position for longer and by increasing the amount of lumbar extension. The exercise is progressed to lumbar extension in standing.

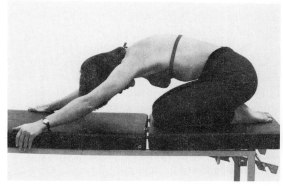

A

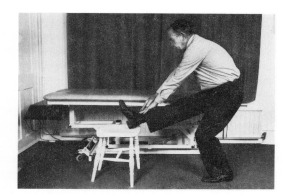

Fig. 14.14 Exercise to stretch tight hamstrings (see text).

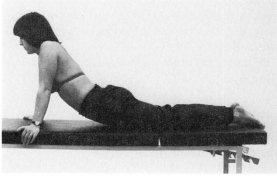

B

Fig. 14.15A and B Exercise for the restoration of lordosis of lumbar extension range (see text and also Fig. 11.46).

Extension mobility can be maintained by standing with the feet a little apart, supinating the forearms to place the palms on the lumbar region or iliac spines, and then leaning backwards as the pelvis is pushed forwards, so that the body's centre of gravity remains over the support area. Placing the palms higher or lower makes a slight but negligible difference to the effect (Fig. 11.46). (p. 149)

Lumbar extension posturing exercises are as valuable in prophylaxis, and 'de-fusing' of incipient low back pain episodes *in this group of patients* as they are in the treatment of established episodes, but should not be employed until lateral deviation or listing, associated with the onset of pain, has been corrected (p. 148).

N.B. Full and vigorous flexion or extension in standing, and full passive extension in prone lying, should be carefully approached until a passive physiological-movement test (PP–MT) has established that there is no segmental hypermobility reponsible for lumbar instability causing symptoms which may be aggravated by uninhibited and vigorous free movement.

Segmental hypermobility *per se* is no contra-indication to lumbar extension posturing drills, since much low backache in the presence of hypermobility is helped by these routines. Frank *segmental instability* which is manifestly responsible for symptoms is another matter — thus examination and accurate asssessment are vital.

Abdominal musculature, psoas tightness and shortened hamstrings may also require attention, as in Group A.

Physical endurance. The physically active person appears less likely to get backache. Recreation or work which involves 'global' mobility of joints is preferable to that which repetitively stresses one aspect of joints.

A more comprehensive scheme of exercises is given by Buswell.[22]

d. Exercise programmes to improve strength and endurance, and to restore confidence, do not require description here

e. Individual ergonomic instruction

The principles are well-understood by all physical therapists; the following suggestions refer to the low back.

With regard to lifting as such, after a simple exposition of the natural reaction of living tissues to physical insult, and the particular way in which this applies to the individual concerned, perhaps patients should receive no more written advice than can be contained on one side of a postcard.

For those with recurrent back pain, here indeed is the suggested postcard:

Analyse your work — relate your pain to what you do and how you do it
    No lifting if too heavy — get help
    No lifting without secure foothold
    No lifting by stooping with legs almost straight
    Stand close and grip well
    Always keep seat lower than head
    Hold low back in neutral position
    Lift without jerking
    Change foot position to turn with weight
    Don't stoop or reach to put it down

Where the hazards of specific industrial lifting and handling duties are well understood, and safety measures can be incorporated into preventive training, instructions can be highly specific, but for most individuals it is a matter of grasping and applying principles.

Prophylaxis is important, but it cannot prevent steady progression, to varying degrees, of the changes of degeneration. Degeneration as such is not disease, and the patients should never be given the notion that they have got a 'disease'.

The evidence is all around us — individuals who have survived a back-pain episode, got over it and pressed on regardless, albeit by sensibly avoiding the more gross type of physical insult, but by no means thinking carefully before they do anything at all.

It is gratifying to feel that out advice and detailed guidance may have been responsible for this happy state of affairs — but when we encounter cheerful, durable people who have got over a back episode and got on with their lives and no such advice or guidance has been given, there is food for thought. This is not to say that we should neglect our professional duties by ignoring potential hazard, but that while giving the patient instruction, we should instil confidence and not unwittingly undermine it. Thus the 'Lifting advice' postcard referred to above might have on its reverse side a further injunction:

Do the preventive exercise given
Avoid prolonged periods in one position (sitting, standing, driving, bending, decorating ceilings)
If you cannot, do the reverse for a bit, every so often
Your back is not falling to bits and will last as long as you do; get on with your life and don't become overconcerned about your back.

A more comprehensive text[70] discusses prophylaxis in depth.

2. AUTO TRACTION

Cervical auto-traction

The lack of sophisticated equipment need not preclude the use of rhythmic cervical traction. The patient sits beneath a double-pulley system attached overhead, and grasps either end of a spreader lying across the upper thighs. When the therapist has attached the harness and applied the maximum degree of tension required (best measured by a small spring balance in series), the cord is firmly secured to the spreader where it is held by the patient, thus maintaining the tension. By lifting the spreader gently from the thighs, the patient eases the tension applied, and by pressing the spreader down to the thighs again, reapplies the tension. The degree of cervical flexion, the poundage, and the 'hold' and 'rest' periods are variable according to the aim of treatment, and the muscle-work of repetitively pressing the spreader to the thighs does not increase the tension of the cervical musculature. An advantage is that the patient's thighs prevent application of a tension greater than that set by the therapist (Fig. 14.16).

Lumbar auto-traction

After reviewing some 20 existing, together with classical, methods of lumbar traction, Lind[116] suggested that many have one or more of the following shortcomings:
a. the design is complicated
b. medically correct treatment is difficult to accomplish because the patient is placed in a predetermined position on the traction table
c. the direction of the applied forces are usually fixed and the same for all patients
d. the magnitude of the force is only roughly chosen
e. the points on the body to which the tractive force

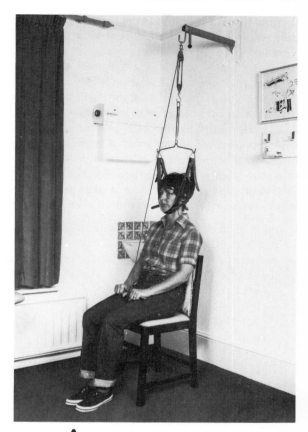

Fig. 14.16   Auto-traction for the upper cervical region (see text).

should be applied in order to have the intended effect on the relevant parts of the spine are not selected
f. some of these devices seem to rely on clairvoyant powers of the operator to avoid spinal and other injury due to excessive, if not wrongly applied, force
g. some are reminiscent of the rack of the torture chamber.

She formulated a precisely-detailed and multi-adaptable method of auto-traction, in which the supine, prone or side-lying patient, in a variety of subsidiary postures, is attached by a pelvic harness to one end of a multi-plane, split-section table, and applies the traction effect by pulling on a fixed bar with the arms, and at times pushing with the legs.

The system allows variations in applications of tension, and many modifications for individual requirements.

Auto-traction is based on the hypothesis that the cause of low back pain and/or sciatica is a mechanical 'conflict' between displaced tissue, of disc and adjacent nerves or other sensitive tissue, or incongruencies in displaced tissue. Refinement of diagnosis allows planning of the potentially most beneficial schedule of treatment for individual cases. Lind's electromyographic, radiographic and clinical study enabled the formulation of some 154 three-dimensional combinations of traction method, with selection highly individualised for each patient following comprehensive examination and assessment. Among the factors considered are:

— types of change in disc shape, without herniation, and with herniation
— presumed relationship of disc trespass to the nerve root, e.g.
  — medio-rhizal
  — latero-rhizal
  — sub-rhizal
— forward or backward postural tilt of pelvis
— roto-torsion or curvo-torsion (scoliosis) of the spine
— positional abnormalities of the sacrum relative to the ilia
— positional abnormalities of the ilia
— spondylolisthesis or retrolisthesis
— real and/or apparent leg length inequality.

For example, abnormal positions of the *sacrum* may be due to rotations about: (i) a transverse axis (forward or backward tilting) (ii) the sagittal axis (right- or left-forward rotation) and (iii) the vertical axis (clockwise or anti-clockwise rotation).

The positional abnormality is often due to a combination of all three rotations.

Similarly, radiographic projections of the *pelvis*, in the standing position, allow positional abnormalities of an ilium to be grouped as:
— ilium tilted forward
— ilium tilted backward
— 'pronation' of ilium
— 'supination' of ilium
since in a normal pelvis all transverse and vertical lines of reference are of equal length on the two sides and intersect at right angles. Real *differences in leg length* are determined by comparing the height of femoral heads on a plain erect radiograph of the pelvis, and apparent differences by noting the relationship of medial malleoli when lying with the legs extended.

Each of these factors, together with a full clinical examination, are taken into acount when selecting the initial trial-traction set-up, the force applied being decided by the patient himself. As with most other therapeutic methods, responses to initial treatment will guide subsequent applications.

Traction method

Taking: 'A' as the tilt, above (+) or below (–) the horizontal, of the head end of the traction table; 'b' as the same for the foot end; 'y' as the lateral tilt, to left or right, of the head end, a basic schedule of initial treatment positions is as follows:

Table 14.1 Schedule of treatment

Side of the lumbar spine on which compression is located		Prone Right a b Y			Prone Left a b Y			Supine Right a b Y			Supine Left a b Y		
Laterorhizal compression	Right	—	—	—	—	—	+	+	+	+	+	+	—
	Left	—	—	+	—	—	—	+	+	—	+	+	+
Mediorhizal compression	Right	—	—	+	—	—	—	+	+	—	+	+	+
	Left	—	—	—	—	—	+	+	+	+	+	+	—
Subrizal compression	Right	—	—	0	—	—	0	0	0	0	0	0	0
	Left	—	—	0	—	—	0	0	0	0	0	0	0

Reference should be made to Lind's full description of the method[116] or to Natchev's introductory handbook[148] and to Bighaug[12] for more detailed examples of application (Figs. 14.17, 14.18, 14.19, 14.20).

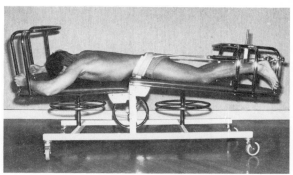

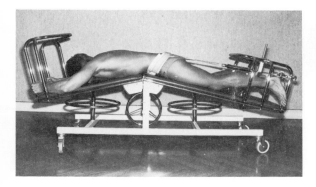

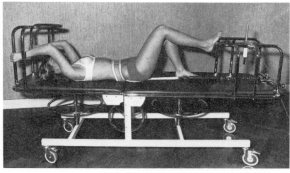

Fig. 14.19 In clockwise or right trunk rotation (note the laterally-tilted head end) the left side intervertebral foramina widen, tending to reduce nerve root compression.

Fig. 14.17 In lumbar flexion, there is a cranio-caudal increase of foraminal dimensions, and the possibility of reduced nerve root compression.

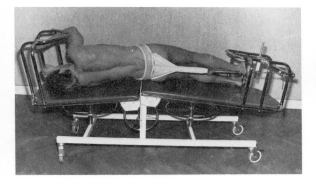

Fig. 14.20 Pushing with one or both raised legs, and thus actively contracting the hip extensors, reciprocally relaxes the iliopsoas muscles and thus induces lumbar spine flattening, which increases the vertical (or cranio-caudal) dimensions of the intervertebral foramina.

(Table 14.1 and Figure 14.17–14.20 are reproduced with permission from Natchev E. Pain Treatment and Auto-traction for Back Problems 1982 AB Spiraltryck, Stockholm.)

Fig. 14.18 In lateral flexion, there is widening of the intervertebral foramina on the convex side.

A relevant statistic is that the incidence of observations, by direct scrutiny at open operation, of nerve root/protrusion relationships is around 0.01 per cent.[70]

Some of the clinical workers (Malmström — see below — Evjenth and Hamberg[48]) with experience in the method have constructed modified tables, according to the same principle but incorporating additions and allowing different ways of achieving the same end (Figs. 14.21 (A) (B) (C), 14.22).

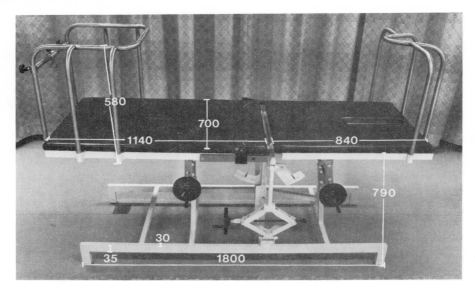

Fig. 14.21A A modified auto-traction table with push handles (folded down) for those patients unable to elevate arms sufficiently, or unable for other reasons to exert a pulling action with the arms (see Inset 14.21B).

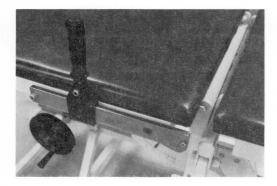

Fig. 14.21B Inset to Figure 14.21A

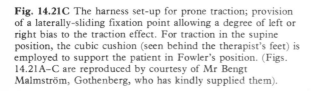

Fig. 14.21C The harness set-up for prone traction; provision of a laterally-sliding fixation point allowing a degree of left or right bias to the traction effect. For traction in the supine position, the cubic cushion (seen behind the therapist's feet) is employed to support the patient in Fowler's position. (Figs. 14.21A–C are reproduced by courtesy of Mr Bengt Malmström, Gothenberg, who has kindly supplied them).

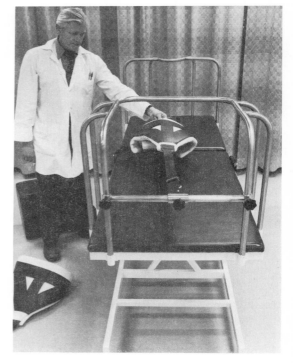

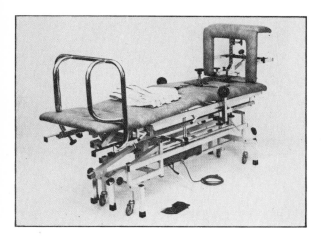

Fig. 14.22 This illustration of a multi-purpose treatment table, adaptable for auto-traction, is reproduced with permission from Evjenth O, Hamberg J 1980 Töjning av Muskler Vol II Tryckt hos Team Offset, Malmö. Courtesy of Masolet (UK).

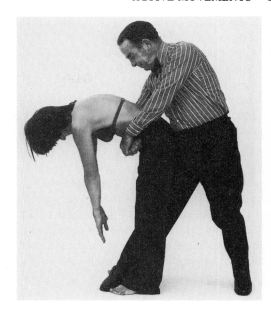

Fig. 14.23 Lumbar flexion resisted by placing a forearm across the patient's lower abdomen. Thus the usually gravity-assisted movement of flexion now requires a strong abdominal contraction, with consequent reciprocal relaxation of dorsal musculature.

3. ACTIVE EXERCISES TO STRETCH SHORTENED SOFT TISSUES

These are used to assist in stretching shortened soft tissues on one aspect of a vertebral joint, or vertebral district, and other body parts.

It will be evident that many of the exercises already illustrated in other contexts (Figs. 14.9–14.23) are also active stretching of soft tissues, so this aspect of both treatment and prophylaxis is a large one.

Passive stretching and post-isometric relaxation techniques should be accompanied by active movements to maintain the progress achieved. For example, contracture or shortening of the lumbar sacrospinalis muscle and associated connective tissue may be present and will require stretching; daily home exercises will complement manual stretching by the therapist.

Some forty years ago Mennell (1945)[135] described active exercises for stretching the ilio-tibial tract, and while this principle is not therefore new it has recently received some attention.[91] 'Many authors . . . over-emphasise morphological *joint* changes, whereas changes of function in the sense of so-called functional pathology of the motor system are still neglected.'[92] Some of the techniques are complementary to exercises with the therapist's participation (Fig. 14.23) and require purposeful active movement by the patient at home; others entail taking up a particular posture for short periods each day, so that the effect of gravity may counteract the postural tendencies accompanying joint pain (Fig. 14.10), yet others depend upon the posture itself rather than gravitational effects.

Janda[92] suggests that different therapeutic systems need not exclude each other, but that it is a question of emphasis—their application and combination depending upon a detailed, wide-ranging analysis and what we wish to achieve. He offers four principles of physiotherapy treatment of painful musculo-skeletal problems:

(i) Mobilisation of joints as necessary, mainly by passive soft-tissue techniques. Due to progress and improvement of these techniques, *the need for thrust manipulations has substantially decreased.*

(ii) Elongation of tight or shortened muscles by a combined technique, i.e. inhibitory or muscle-energy techniques which are believed to influence muscle fibres and muscle spindles, and by post-facilitation stretching during the short inhibition period, when it is believed that both muscle fibres and inert connective tissue elements are affected.

(iii) Strengthening of weakened muscles by neuro-physiological reflex methods, e.g. PNF.

(iv) Re-education of as good a movement-pattern as the patient is capable—this is difficult since it necessitates a well-motivated and co-ordinated patient and an extremely skilled therapist.

Janda also suggests that it is wrong to first try strengthening the weak muscle, since the shortened muscle is inhibiting its weak antagonist and treatment directed to strengthening is not rational until the 'tight' muscle has been released.

The purpose of this section is to illustrate exercises to assist in releasing tight musculature, with its connective tissue elements (Figs 14.24–14.29).

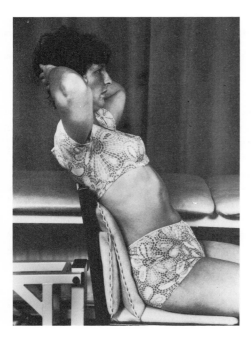

Fig. 14.24 Self-treatment of spasm or tightness of cranio-vertebral extensor muscles. With fingers on occiput and thumbs on zygoma, the patient maintains her head in normal orientation while the shoulders and torso are lowered backwards from the neutral position. Breathing out should accompany the backward movement of trunk, which should be held for a few seconds. Repeat the excursion 5–8 times.

N.B. It goes without saying that these home exercises for maintaining the extensibility of soft tissues are *contraindicated* until such time as joint pain, and reactiveness, have been relieved. They are a sequel, and not an accompaniment.

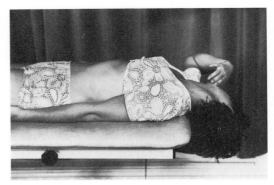

Fig. 14.25 Self-treatment of spasm or tightness of the left sterno-cleido-mastoid muscle. With the left hand a little under left buttock, the patient allows her head to fall into extension and right rotation, applying gentle pressure on her left mandible with fingers of the right hand. It is this hand which assists the head up after some 10 seconds of stretch. Repeat 3–5 times. The exercise is not suitable for patients with irritable upper cervical joints.

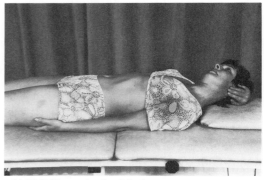

Fig. 14.26 Self-stretch of a tight levator scapulae muscle. With ipsilateral hand stabilised under the buttock, and head on a low pillow, the patient reaches round with opposite hand to apply the stretch on the postero-lateral occipital region. The position is maintained for some 10 seconds, and after relaxation is repeated 3—5 times.

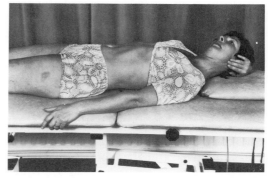

Fig. 14.27 To stretch the upper part of the left trapezius muscle, the position and procedure is virtually the same as in Fig. 14.26, except that the patient's ipsilateral hand now grasps the side of the plinth.

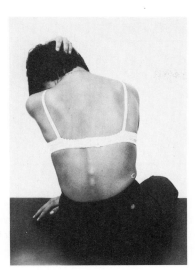

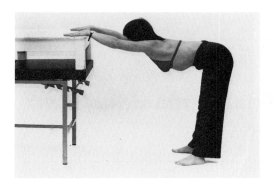

Fig. 14.29 An alternative home exercise for stretching the pectoral muscles. The patient stands with feet astride and, with the elbows kept extended, places the palms on a flat support at about chest height. By repetitively leaning backwards from the ankles, the chest is depressed to the floor, and the pectoral soft tissues repetitively stretched.

Fig. 14.28 The right thoracic sacrospinalis muscles group is stretched in a sitting position, with the trunk flexed, side-flexed left and rotated left. With right forearm lying across her thighs, the patient reaches left arm up and across her face to place her palm and fingers on the right occiput. The stretch is applied by gentle traction with the left arm.

15

What is manipulation?

The degenerative changes of spondylosis, osteo-phytic trespass, fibrosis, acquired stenosis, spinal root irritation, secondary contracture of soft tissue, segmental instability and segmental stiffness (for one reason or another) provide the major bulk of what we might term a family of 'abnormalities of movement', and since only 1 in 10 000 subjects progresses to the stage of myelography and major surgical procedures, i.e. 0.01 per cent,[70] conservative treatment is of the utmost importance.

A most superficial survey of the daily case-load of accident and emergency, orthopaedic, rheumatology, rehabilitation and sports injury clinics, and the multifarious needs of these patients with vertebral and peripheral joint pain in terms of passive and active movement techniques of one kind or another, suggests that to see manipulation proper as *only* the production of a click by facet-joint (or any other joint) gapping, is greatly to restrict its considerable and rightful place in physical medicine.

There is ample evidence that nociceptor activity giving rise to pain also generates extensive reflex effects; there is similar evidence that the simple passive movement of joints likewise generates reflex effects.

It is untrue that treatment by mobilisation and manipulation can be adequately discussed only on a mechanical cause-and-effect relationship; while we continue to regard musculoskeletal joint problems as simple mechanical ones, while we conceptualise only like mechanical engineers, our potential for better results will remain restricted.

Millions of asymptomatic individuals are walking about with mechanical joint problems.

We have every reason for progressing to the point where we begin to think like telecommunication engineers—since the most basic acquaintance with spinal joint neurophysiology and recent research findings indicate that the phenomenon of joint pain and its relief by mechanical techniques involve effects which transcend simple mechanical ones, e.g. widespread reflex changes in the degree of facilitation in spinal motor neurone pools, voluntary and smooth muscle tone, vasomotor and sudo-motor tone and alterations in pulse rate, cardiac output and blood pressure.

If we add to this the effects of treating chronic changes at the junctional vertebral regions, and that of modulating the chronic changes in texture and extensibility of the soft tissues, simple therapeutic concepts of 'putting back' things which are 'out', or hoping to routinely deal with joint pain by manoeuvres restricted to a single segment, begin to be seen as inadequate.

There are many alternatives to high-velocity thrust techniques.

Confident, gentle and skilful *handling* by whatever technique is a very powerful therapeutic weapon, and therapists who handle their patients with insight and understanding, and examine them attentively with care for detail, have already won half the battle; willy-nilly, they have already been psychologically cast by the patient in the role of 'the sympathetic handler who will make me better', and the confident and skilful therapist fulfils the role, satisfying a deep and unconscious psychological need. Only so far as this powerful psychological need is concerned, the actual clinical method of handling pales into insignificance; so much so that, even should the therapist not make the patient sign- and symptom-free, the burden of pain may be considerably relieved, and the patient calmed and reassured.

Although treatment of a single segment is often sufficient in the very early stages of dysfunction of that segment, where none existed before, the greater majority of joint problems present as a complex of chronic changes.

There is no magic in the manipulator's hand, there is no mystique of manipulation. But there is a central mystery, and *it lies in the variety of responses of the abnormal joint to the different things we do in the way of treatment by passive and active movement of one kind and another.*

Joints cannot read books, or understand theories about technique; what suits one joint problem will not suit another. We must learn to be humble in the face of this mystery, we must learn to listen to what the abnormal joint is trying to tell us — in short, we must learn to *assess.*

Questions of rationale

There is a disconcerting gap between observed mechanical effects of localised mobilisation techniques, extension postures, manipulation and/or traction on the one hand, and on the other precisely why our procedures relieve symptoms and restore function. In short, we simply do not know, and it is perhaps a disadvantage to students to suggest or imply that we do.

The best that can be said, about the precise means of therapeutic success, following any mobilisation, manipulation or other technique directed to a particular vertebral segment or district, is neatly and truly expressed by O'Brien[151], who suggested the phrase *'modifying the local environment.'*

This is as far as our certain knowledge goes.[70] For example, cervical, thoracic and lumbar rotation techniques are some of the oldest and most useful procedures known to therapists. Since Caxton (1422–1491)*, it has been difficult to find a 'manipulation' text which does not include them. Like spinal traction, the technique of regional lumbar rotation (Figs. 11.36, 15.1) is a prime example of manipulation being all things to all men; it is as old as the hills, and to the best of the author's knowledge there is no school of manipulation in the teaching of which it does not form part of the technique repertoire, in one guise or another. There are many slight variations of technique, of hand placing and method of contact with the patient; the effects are variously described as 'restoring the

*The innovator of printing in England

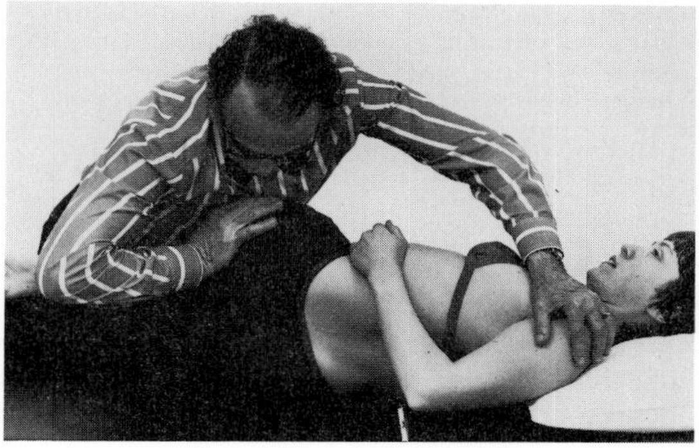

Fig. 15.1 Pose by model and therapist to illustrate a somewhat athletic thrust manipulation which is described as 'normalising the left sacro-iliac joint'. Despite the attempt at localisation by placement of the therapist's right hand on the patient's left ischial tuberosity, it is plain that a great many more structures are being influenced by the positioning technique. Notwithstanding osteopathic or chiropractic theories of facet and ligamentous 'locking' this is, in fact, a prime example of 'environmental manipulation' (see text).

normal configuration of the disc',[70, 186] 'shifting the nerve root off the disc', or 'correcting' unilateral sacroiliac joint asymmetry.[55, 76] Our difficulties arise because the techniques may indeed do just this, but the correlation between what has actually happened in the large family of soft tissue and joint structures influenced by the manipulation and what we may *believe,* or *hope,* has happened, is manifestly sketchy.

Any reasonably comprehensive review of the many modern texts on manipulation soon reveals that variations of technique, and the reasons for these, can sometimes be as plausible as the variety of explanations of effect.

Haldeman[76] has tabulated some hypotheses, from times past to the present, of the nature of therapeutic effects of manipulative therapy:

Theory	Author
1. Restore vertebrae to normal position	Galen (1958)
2. Straighten the spine	Pare (1958)
3. Relieve interference with blood flow	Still (1899)
4. Relieve nerve compression	Palmer (1910)
5. Relieve irritation of sympathetic chain	Kunert (1965)
6. Mobilise fixated vertebral units	Gillet (1968)
7. Shift a fragment of intervertebral disc	Cyriax (1975)
8. Mobilise posterior joints	Mennell (1960)
9. Remove interference with cerebrospinal fluid circulation	De Jarnette (1967)
10. Stretch contracted muscles, causing relaxation	Perl (1975)
11. Correct abnormal somatovisceral reflexes	Homewood (1963)

12. Remove irritable spinal lesions	Korr (1976)
13. Stretching or tearing of adhesions around the nerve root	Chrisman *et al.* (1964
14. Reduce distortion of the annulus	Farfan (1973)

Speculation and hypothesis, however well-informed and rationally-conceived, remain such, and teaching students how to perceive, and how to discriminate between fact and fancy, is much more important than 'teaching them how to manipulate'.

Benign joint problems are successfully treated in many ways, and there is no single universal system or philosophy of treatment. The mere presence of physiotherapists and manual therapists, osteopaths, orthopaedic physicians, chiropractors, naturopaths and bone-setters makes the point—besides the existence of various factions within these groups.

Thus it is wise to look at all aspects of work in this field because, in differing proportions, there is something valuable to learn from each.

As manual therapists get the experience to gainfully compare the rationale and treatment methods of others in the field, they will note how differing examination methods, and differing emphases on the relative importance of positive findings, accurately reflect differing views.[70]

Forms of extrapolation on the few available facts, and hypotheses, also vary considerably, a clear indication that our certain knowledge is all too limited.

There are particular ways of examining, allied to particular emphases in treatment and particular techniques. Examples of these are:

a. placing prime importance upon evidence of chronic muscle imbalance, or soft tissue dysfunction[91]

b. accurately noting the distribution and behaviour of pain, in relation to particular *physiological* movements and/or postures of the lumbar spine[125]

c. as above, including careful manual testing of accessory segmental movements, and noting their effects (if any) on the behaviour of symptoms[128]

d. a particular emphasis on *which* segmental movements, i.e. flexion, extension, rotation, of a vertebra may be restricted, and in what way[48, 168, 169]

e. observing the incidence of particular *patterns* of movement limitation in different joints, then formulating ideas and treatment rationale on this basis.[33] The *absence* of particular and common patterns also has import in this school of thought

f. special importance attaching to notions of possible 'malposition' or 'mal-alignment' of vertebrae, and the possible neurophysiological consequences. Hence X-rays are given more importance than just a means to exclude neoplastic and other diseases or gross mechanical defects.[73, 74, 76]

While these shorthand descriptions cannot be completely fair, they do give a salient principle of the different approaches mentioned. All philosophies of manipulative treatment incorporate all of the factors outlined above in varying degree, yet a recognisable emphasis on one or another of them will often easily identify the faction to which an individual clinician belongs.

The effort to understand others' rationale and procedure is well worth while, giving a more comprehensive grasp of the whole context of this work, besides improving one's own effectiveness, of course.

16

Recording treatment

Because of the prime importance of recording the nature and results of modern investigation procedures, which almost daily become more technical and comprehensive, the volume of accumulated medical information about one individual receiving hospital treatment is likely to be considerable.

There may be a tendency for the importance of this great amount of technical information to obscure its ultimate objective, and to diminish the importance of an equally valid necessity, i.e. an accurate and full notation of the therapeutic *results* of all this attention. This becomes a vital necessity when assessment of the effects of treatment procedures is made for the most part immediately after the procedures; the most effective use of mobilisation, manipulation and traction techniques depends upon precise observation of their immediate effects, and assessment of the meaning and importance of these effects.

Throughout treatment, the therapist must remain in full control of the proceedings and be awake to the significance of *changes* in the signs and symptoms as they occur, whether treatment occupies one or many sessions. Besides the prime consideration of the patient's welfare, there is the importance of learning by experience, and this is facilitated if retrospective analysis is made possible by the orderly habit of precise recording of each step in treatment, and of its effect.

Accurate recording is therefore an unavoidable necessity; all treatment procedures should be fully and precisely recorded, and a common system of expression and notation is desirable.

The currently available repertoire or vocabulary of techniques is something of a melting-pot, with several new and traditional systems mixed together. Thus there is a difficulty in that the number of manual and mechanical passive movement techniques runs into many hundreds at least; in the absence of an internationally agreed system of notation it is important that therapists use recording methods which are agreed, or at least readily understood, among those of their colleagues who may treat the same patient.

Notation methods arise naturally from what therapists do; where the variety of techniques is considerable, the notation system must be comprehensive and flexible.

Notes would come under several headings:

Examination
Mobilisation
Manipulation
Traction

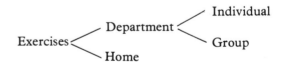

Adjunct treatments
Support.

EXAMINATION

See page 96.

MOBILISATION (grades I–IV)

Record at each attendance:

On left-hand side	On right-hand side
Techique used	*Patient's subjective*
Grade	*assessment of symptoms*
Vertebral level(s) treated	*(inverted commas)*
Number of times	*Therapist's objective*
Effects during application	*assessment of signs*

(if any)

and ending with *comments as a reminder for next attendance*

For example:

	'feels looser'
11 (C4) × 3	Ext. inc. by ¼ with less pain

If remains improved tomorrow, stop and check after 1/52. Wean from collar.

Thus, a complete but short account of treatment and immediate results is written at each attendance. Shorthand symbols for the techniques employed can save time, and are desirable so long as their meaning is agreed. (See Figs. 8.1–8.6.) Both persuasive correction of aberrant lumbar posture (p. 148), and manual stretching techniques for shortened soft tissues (p. 152) are recorded in the same way.

MANIPULATION (grade V)

There are many systems of annotating treatment procedures, yet they can be recorded exactly as above; where no symbol is used, or exists, it is wise to write a short description of the technique employed. Whatever recording method is used, it should include these factors:

— the segment treated
— the type of manipulation
— the direction
— whether a regional or localised effect was intended
— effects (unless it is planned that assessment be after a short period—this must be noted on the record).

Where a technique has been localised, the symbol 'localised V' (or 'loc V') should be used.

TRACTION (as an outpatient sessional procedure)

Recording should note:

— whether manual or mechanical
— apparatus employed
— position of the patient
— angle of pull or the suspension (attachment) point
— the segment(s) for which traction is given
— force of traction
— duration of traction
— whether sustained, intermittent or rhythmic; or manipulative (grade V)
— periodicity of pull and rest phases, if not sustained
— effects—if to be assessed immediately. If not, this must be noted.

The difficulty with traction is that there are innumerable ways of applying treatment, and therapists who employ many methods will need a fairly comprehensive recording system, which is flexible enough to meet most requirements.

To distinguish between continuous or sustained traction in bed, and traction treatment on an outpatient basis, the word 'sessional' is probably better than 'intermittent' alone, since the latter could apply to once daily outpatient treatment, or to two applications of sustained traction with a rest between, at a single outpatient attendance.

Manual traction can be specified by the letter 'M'; if this is omitted, the traction can be taken, by agreement of colleagues, to indicate mechanical traction.

If the gross position of the patient is indicated by arrows, e.g.

sitting or standing,   half-lying, and
(supine) lying or   (prone) lying,

'SRCT ⌐ (C2–C3)' would denote, 'Sessional rhythmic mechanical cervical traction in sitting for the C2–C3 segment', since it is unlikely that mechanical cervical traction as a sessional treatment would be applied with the patient standing.

'SMRLT ⌐ (L3)' would denote, 'Sessional manual rhythmic lumbar traction to L3', in either sitting or standing, which should be specified.

Where traction is employed as a grade V manipulative technique, the term 'grade V' is added after the segment to be treated.

For example, 'SMMT ↑ (T5) V sitt.' would denote,

'Sessional manual manipulative traction (T5) grade V in sitting.'

Similarly, 'SSCT ⟋ (C5–C6)' denotes, 'Sessional sustained cervical traction in half-lying for the C5–C6 segment.'

Whether the neck is slightly flexed to position the C2–C3 segment at the midpoint of its saggital movement, or further flexed in the half-lying position to do the same for the C5–C6 segment (see p. 161), depends upon careful palpation, and arrangement of the harness and suspension point during preparation for the treatment; therefore the precise positioning adopted is not capable of description unless the suspension point is a standard one, the harness is standard and the patient's position is standard, when degrees of flexion, or a neutral position, may then be recorded.

Nevertheless when cervical traction, for example, is applied in the lying or half-lying position, it is convenient to record details of the number and type of pillows used to support the neck, and these details will naturally follow symbols denoting the patient's position. When normal-sized pillows and small ones are used, the details can be expressed as follows:

'SSCT ⊢⟋ 1½ pillows'

'SRCT ⊢⟋ 2 pillows'

'SSCT ⊢→ 1 pillow'

'SSCT ⊢⟋ no pillow'.

Thus it is suggested that arrows are used to describe the *gross posture of the patient*, and not the *segmental posture of the joint* to be treated. By specification of the segment treated and the number of pillows used, another therapist subsequently treating the patient would know that the named segment must be so positioned in the sagittal plane that the traction is sustained with this joint in mid-position.

When giving *cervical* traction with standard apparatus providing standard suspension points and using a uniform position of the patient (i.e. degree of neck-flexion on the trunk), there is a method of writing a formula for arrangement of the head/neck angle. Using the Maitland[128] harness the number of strap-holes showing *beyond* the buckle can be expressed in the sequence, for example:

Mandibular — 3 holes showing
Occipital strap — 4 holes showing
Horizontal strap — 4 holes showing

Thus, the head/neck angle for a particular individual is written as '3/4/4'.

Slight flexion of the patient's hips and knees by the use of pillows for relaxation and comfort should also be recorded, and this may be noted by the symbol ⟋ 1 pillow or ⟋ 2 pillows; this is also of particular importance when treating the thoracic and lumbar segments.

1. Hence, provided the same apparatus is used each time, the recording of a sessional rhythmic cervical traction treatment in half-lying, for C4–C5, with a pull phase of 60 seconds and a rest phase of 30 seconds, could be as follows: 'SRCT ⊢⟋ 1 pillow (C4–C5) 3/4/4 8 kg 60/30 × 20 min ⟋ 2 pillows.'

2. Two sustained traction treatments at one session, with a rest between, can be written:

'SSCT ⊢⟋ 2 pillows (C7–T1) 2/4/4 20 kg × 20 min × 2 (rest 5 min) ⟋ 2 pillows.'

3. Autotraction (see p. 211) in the sitting position can be recorded as: 'SRCT auto ↑ sitt. (C1–C2) 2/3/3 5 kg 30/20 × 10 min.'

4. For sustained traction to a low thoracic segment in half-lying, on the Akron table (see p. 165), the recording could be: 'SSTT ⊢⟋ ½ pillow (T10–T11) 24 kg × 15 min ⟋ 1 pillow', indicating that a small flat pillow was used to support the head, and a normal-sized pillow supported the patient's knees in some flexion.

5. Rhythmic lumbar traction in the prone position, for example, would be written: 'SRLT ⊢→ (prone) (L4–L5) 20 kg 120/30 × 15 min.'

6. Sustained traction to L5–S1 in supine, with

some flexion, would be written: 'SSLT ├─────▶ (supine) (L5–S1) 30 kg × 15 min ──⁄── low stool.'

Auto-traction

(i) The cervical spine
This is referred to above.

(ii) Lumbar spine

When a purpose-built apparatus (Figs. 14.17–14.22 is being used, there are many factors to be recorded, since some 150 three-dimensional combinations of table angulations, strap attachments and patient's position are possible:

— disposition of table: the meanings of a, b, and y are given on page 212.
— position of patient: this is recorded as prone, supine or side-lying, together with particular limb positions
— attachment of harness: to obtain an emphasis of distraction on one or other aspect of an intervertebral joint, there must be many slight variations; these are recorded by taking an imaginary clock-face, in the plane of a horizontal section through the waist, as the reference. If the median point in the small of the back is 6 o'clock, then the anterior central abdominal point is 12 o'clock, the left side 9 o'clock and right 3 o'clock.

Because there are three phases to each traction 'pull', and the dispositions of both table and patient are altered for each phase, these must be recorded[148] e.g.

Protrusion of lumbo-sacral disc, medial to the right S1 nerve root

| | Right side lying | | | |
	Foot	Harness	Head	
Start	b – 4°	7 o'c	a – 8°	y = 0
Traction	b + 2°	7 o'c	a + 4°	y = 0
Pause	b + 1°	7 o'c	a + 2°	y = 0

Changes in symptoms are noted and recorded during traction, and changes in signs after it.

Post-isometric relaxation techniques

The use of combined postures, together with the three-dimensional active movements asked of the patient, make the need for fuller recording than with mobilisation techniques — until a universally agreed notation method is evolved.

To the form of recording for mobilisation (p. 99) there should be added the patient's position, the type of active movements employed and whether the 'direct' or 'indirect' method (p. 191) is used. The standard method of recording muscle strength, in peripheral and other nerve injuries, on a nil-to-normal scale of 0—5, can be useful here to record the *degree* of muscle activity asked of the patient. Plus or minus values of that scale, from 2 to 4– would be appropriate.

A suggested recording method might be:

First line	Segment treated	Posture	Preparation
	R L5/S1	Stride sitting	Flexion, left side flexion, left rotation

Second line	Times	Patient's movement	Muscle force (in brackets)	Type
	4	Extension, right-side flexion, right rotation	(3)	Indirect

and it could be recorded as:

				Result
L5/S1 Std. Sitt.		F–LSF–LR	⊥	changes in
4 × E–RSF–RR (3) Ind.				symptoms and/or
(+ effects during)				signs

Again:

				Result
L 1st Rib. Sup.Ly.		RSF–RR	⊥	changes in
5 × LSF–LR (2+) Ind.				symptoms and/or
				signs

In the first example, right-sided lumbar pain is restricting lumbar flexion, and in the second, the left first rib is elevated and muscle tightness is presumed to be the cause.

EXERCISES

The orderly nominating of each *type* or *aim* of exercise is a good habit, and it aids assessment. Headings are therefore:

Stability (Power) — Mobility — Stretch — Posture/ Balance/Control — Endurance — Handling.

A record should be kept of the nature of *group exercises,* whether for general strengthening of trunk and cervical musculature, physical endurance or training in lifting and handling techniques.

If we take the example of chronic lumbar pain in a young woman, due to a hypermobile L4–L5 segment, the manual mobilisation treatment (in this case solely for the relief of pain) would be recorded as previously suggested (p. 222). If static isometric contractions are chosen as home exercises for the *regional* improvement of muscle power, it is probable that the therapist has a tried and trusted handful of exercises with the required specific effect, but these should nevertheless be recorded; the aims, type, frequency and duration of exercises must be clear and reproducible for both therapist and patient.

For example, the prescription for an interim week of home exercises may be:

'*Stab:* —abdo. iso. ex. 10 sec hold × 8   ↗
12 × 4 daily

—neut. ext. iso. exs. 10 sec hold   ↗
12 × 4 × 8 daily'

and this indicates:

'*Stability:* abdominal isometric exercise with 8, progressing to 12, 10-second holds, 4 times a day neutral lumbar extension holds for the same periods' (see p. 201).

Progression of the exercise programme for the succeeding weeks should also be recorded. For any progressive scheme of exercises, patients should be encouraged, and shown how, to keep a simple graph of their progress, and to bring it with them on the next attendance.

There is no better reminder of the value of dogged persistence than a manifest indication of steadily increasing muscle power.

For improving the power and functional efficiency of *segmental* musculature, static isometric contractions, against resistance applied to vertebral apophyses, will need to be precisely recorded, and a simple method is to use the mobilisation symbols, differentiated by being enclosed in a circle, i.e.

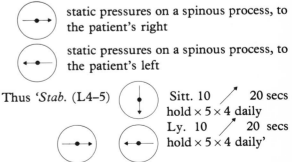

Thus '*Stab.* (L4–5)   Sitt. 10 ╱ 20 secs
hold × 5 × 4 daily
Ly. 10 ╱ 20 secs
hold × 5 × 4 daily'

would indicate, 'Segmental stability exercises for L4–L5, as isometric "holds" of 10, progressing to 20 seconds, against resistance applied centrally and transversely to the fourth and fifth lumbar spinous processes. Five holds at each of four sessions daily.'

The fact that the patient can self-administer the central posteroanterior static pressures, but may need an assistant to give the transverse pressures, does not invalidate the method of recording the programme of home exercises.

ADJUNCT TREATMENTS

Therapists will not need reminders of the necessity for careful recording of any adjunct procedure; with regard to insonation, Oakley (1978)[150] has provided an admirable example of precise recording of treatment.

Supports

The fact that a patient has been given an 'instant' lumbar support, which is to be worn for 5 to 10 days and no more, or is to be used only for gardening and long car trips, should be recorded, as should be a note of the effects, for future reference.

17

Indications

GENERAL INDICATIONS

In general terms, a joint problem is suitable for this treatment if the symptoms are aggravated by activity, some particular movements of the joint and certain postures, and relieved by rest and other ('antalgic') postures — these differ from patient to patient.

Sometimes patients have no immediately apparent articular signs (that is, pain on movement or limitation of gross movement), only an ache, and after passive mobility testing has localised the tight intervertebral segment(s) at a spinal level reasonably compatible with the distribution and nature of their symptoms, they will be found to respond well to passive movement techniques.

It must be remembered that some types of serious visceral and other pathology, for which these treatments are either contraindicated or pointless, have a tendency to simulate vertebrogenic problems and to refer pain to the neck and back; this pain is not as a rule aggravated by spinal movement but on occasion may be, e.g. in disease of thoracic viscera, some thoracic neoplasms and upper urinary tract lesions in women.

The indications for gentle, moderate or more vigorous treatment become more certain in an almost direct relationship to the number of factors which are accurately assessed. The more comprehensive the examination, the more likely is the appropriate treatment approach to become clarified, as the weight of emphasis one way or another gradually mounts up during the 'indications' examination. Therefore, it is of first importance to be thorough, but also to be quick and not to waste time; for this reason, it is good sense to become skilled in examination procedures as a vital first requirement.

The following INDICATIONS are given on the assumption that the patient has been through a diagnostic sorting procedure, that treatment by movement is appropriate and, so far as is possible, serious disease and significant mechanical defect have been exluded by X-rays.

The 'Rules of procedure' (p. 181) should be observed without exception.

1. PASSIVE MOVEMENT

(i) Massage

Detailed indications for massage, in its various forms, have been excellently described in many texts and general indications only are given.

Stroking and light effleurage is used as a preparatory regional treatment when excessive muscle spasm is present in an overanxious patient.

Stretching (B), kneading and petrissage are frequently necessary for the regional soft tissues overlying chronic joint problems; both longitudinal and transverse mobilisation of muscle are needed to soften them, improve their tissue-fluid exchange and local extensibility.

Inhibitory pressures are used for the relaxation or 'decontraction' of muscle spasm.

Vibrations are best applied mechanically.

Fine vibrations are used to reduce the chronic muscular ache resulting from a sustained tension, and are usefully applied to a muscle group *after* a stretching (A) technique.

Coarse vibration stimulates muscle groups which are antagonistic to those requiring stretching; also, some patients may need a vibratory treatment in preparation for instruction in self-applied isometric segmental exercise.

Transverse frictions may sometimes be necessary at the aponeurotic attachments on the nuchal lines of the occiput and at the medial border of the scapula. Their use for connective-tissue changes at the limb girdles, and more distally, has been well described.[32]

Circular frictions are occasionally indicated when acutely tender and discrete 'nodules' or fasciculi are accurately localised by the patient as a source of discomfort; these accessory treatments should never be used without primary elucidation and treatment of coexisting vertebral joint problems.

(ii) Maintenance movement —see page 123.

(iii) Localised mobilisation (Grades I–IV)

Indications for gentle treatment

In the history (elicit by observation and specific questions):

— much joint irritability
— most or all movements hurt severely
— particular postures hurt severely
— much limb pain
— not sleeping well
— cough/sneeze reproduce distal pain
— pain has been severe for some time
— postural spasm protecting the joint area

During testing (elicit by careful movement tests, noting degree of pain on movement, neurological test, careful palpation):

— pain sufficient to produce facial distortion
— spinal movement produces distal limb pain
— pain and/or paraesthesiae increase some seconds *after* the testing movement has been completed
— elicited spasm
— pain much increased after minimal examination
— pressure on bony points provokes distal pain/paraesthesiae
— the presence of neurological deficit, unless this is established to be of previous origin

Result of initial treatment:

— response to first moderate treatment is much increased pain.

Indications for more vigorous treatment, or increased grades (elicited as above)

History:

— moderate pain has been static for some time, and is generally unvarying in intensity
— no joint movement stirs it up much
— when stirred up, soon settles
— sleeping well
— little limb pain, or distal pain
— cough, sneeze or jar does not hurt
— no exacerbation in any particular posture
— no postural spasm

Testing:

— joint irritability obviously minimal, with no muscle guarding (elicited spasm) on movement
— spinal testing movements may be limited, but do not stir up pain especially
— limitation of movement is more by tissue-tension or by tissue-compression than by pain
— no neurological deficit, or deficit of previous origin only
— spinal pressure does not hurt much, or provoke paraesthesiae, distally or locally

Treatment:

The initial moderate treatment does not produce any aggravation of signs or symptoms.

Neurological signs. A neurological deficit, manifested by reflex changes, muscle weakness and sensory changes in the distribution of the involved root, need not of itself preclude the use of this treatment to the asociated joint(s) so long as: (a) no more than *one cervical root*, on that side, is involved in the upper limb; (b) no more than *one* of the *lumbar roots* is affected, on one side. If the neurological signs span two lumbar segments on one side this is still acceptable provided they are adjacent.

Restricted joint range, and pain at rest or on movement, can still be treated in the presence of the type of neurological deficit outlined above, provided the 'Rules of Procedure' (p. 181) are followed and so long as (a) and (b) are borne in mind.

The *degree of joint and root irritability*, rather than the presence of neurological signs in themselves, which may be old, is the main factor for assessment when planning treatment, and when irritability is marked, or signs are currently developing, the patient must be treated gently, and with caution, repectively.

N.B. Cervical and thoracic joint problems producing neurological symptoms and signs in one or both lower limbs are an ABSOLUTE *contraindication.*

Indications for more vigorous treatment (or building up to vigorous treatment) in patients with distal pain and signs of neurological deficit

In the history:

— when the state of affairs in the preceding week or fortnight has been static. If improving, there would be no need for vigorous treatment
— when their answer to, 'what makes the pain worse/better?' is that nothing does either, i.e. symptoms are generally unvarying in nature.

If the symptoms are easily exacerbated, one should be careful.

During examination:

— though movements may be restricted, and may reproduce pain distally, or proximally only, it is not *great* pain, even with overpressure. The harder it is to reproduce the pain, the more vigorous treatment can be
— straight-leg-raising is a useful test here. Even if SLR is restricted by 40° or more, and there is only a block with little pain, treatment can be more vigorous. A combination of limited SLR and limited flexion, with other factors pointing as outlined above is a good indication for vigorous treatment.

In treatment:

— if the initial gentle technique does not produce distal pain, or an increase of it, or a 'latent-period' exacerbation of pain *during* that session, then one can go ahead and build up to more vigorous treatment during the next attendance
— by the third session, one should be moving through the techniques fairly quickly, i.e. rotations, pressures, traction, etc. to find the most effective.

Temporomandibular joint

Manual treatment is indicated in:

— painful capsulitis due to bruxism, or traumatic stress
— hypomobility without derangement
— internal derangement
— joint pain, secondarily associated with benign upper cervical joint conditions
— asymmetry of closing and opening due to unilateral joint pain.

N.B. It is important not to waste time attempting to relieve pain which is clearly secondary to mal-occlusion problems. These are the province of orthodontists, to whom the patient should be referred. Manual treatment may be indicated for residual discomfort following orthodontic attention.

(iii) (b) Regional mobilisation (Grades I–IV)

Indications are:

— localised symptoms arising from degenerative changes and stiffening in several adjacent segments
— thickening, tightness and soft-tissue induration in several adjacent segments, not necessarily degenerative
— as a prelude to more specific treatment when the patient finds it difficult to relax (excluding marked irritability).

Massage techniques are often combined with the joint movement techniques; active mobilising and postural exercises are frequently required—some specific conditions are:

— ankylosing spondylitis in quiescent periods and preferably early in the course of the disease
— quite firm regional and specific manual mobilisation techniques assist the patient to offset stiffness and fixation by regular active exercises, among which respiratory exercises are important, as are movements for upper and lower limb girdles
— postural kyphosis of the thoracic spine, secondary to tightness of anterior structures
— lumbar region stiffness, as a sequel of arthrosis of the hip
— regional cervical stiffening in the subacute and

chronic stages of recovery from acceleration and deceleration trauma (whiplash). Localised conditions should be given specific treatment.

(iv) (a) Localised manipulation (Grade locV)

N.B. Grade V techniques should never be used in the presence of spasm which is protecting the segment being treated.

Indications

— as a progression from adequate mobilisations which have reached grade IV, where the latter have not achieved the fullest improvement in signs and symptoms considered possible
— in those joint problems where there are no articular signs, only an ache, and the tight vertebral segment has been localised by passive mobility testing. These cases should not be treated by manipulation if the limited movement at a segment is due to old pathology
— where pain is minimal and does not appear until near the end of the range
— localised symptoms of sudden onset (but see below). Localised manipulation must always be preceded by a passive test of functional mobility at each vertebral segment, to localise the level of movement restriction. As a working rule, apply the emphasis of the movement to the lower vertebra of the tight segment (e.g. at C7–T1, it is T1 which should be moved). Techniques are normally done to both sides.

When manipulative thrust techniques are employed for segmental stiffness, they should be done to both sides, although this does not apply to techniques with a bilateral effect. When they are used for asymmetrical restriction of movement, in cases where the opposite movement is free, the techniques are employed to free the restricted movement only.

If we take a further example, i.e. of restricted neck movement, in the absence of any factor precluding grade V techniques, the direction of the manipulative thrust depends, as always, on the direction and nature of restriction.

— If cervical left-side-flexion feels blocked on the left side, and right-side-flexion feels free and

unrestricted, i.e. movement which tends to *gap* the side of restriction is not affected, then a technique which encourages facet-*gliding* on the left side is indicated. Thus the technique employed would be ⤚⤙ taking care while positioning that left-side approximation is not too firmly applied, and applying the emphasis to the thrusting hand rather than the other. If both left- and right-side-flexion were limited, by a left block and a left pull respectively, the technique to use would be ⤚⤙ .

— If cervical left-side-flexion feels free and unencumbered, but right-side-flexion is restricted by tethering on the left side, the technique to use is ⤚⤙ , provided that adequate localised mobilisation had not been fully effective.

Precautions

Besides Contraindications, there are certain clinical factors which preclude the use of manipulation, and these are:

— hypermobility of the segment involved
— when joint irritability and painful movement are manifest
— the presence of spasm, protecting the joint being treated
— when segments *adjacent* to the main joint problems are either irritable, or hypermobile, and stresses applied by the positioning for manipulation would aggravate them
— inability of the patient to relax
— when the operator senses that the joint will not give — this is felt as a rubbery resistance to the final movement, and must in all circumstances be respected.

Since so much effective work is possible by the best use of *mobilisation and traction techniques which are under control of the patient,* perhaps grade V manipulative thrust techniques should be used in much the same way as rheumatologists use systemic steroid drugs — after extra deliberation and then with watchfulness and care.

As lengthening clinical experience is accompanied by more confidence in recognising indications for grade V manipulations, the therapist uses them more surely, safely and effectively, and with the minimum of vigour. This is no field for the sporting amateur, whose concept of what manipulators do appears to be that they spend all their clinical time producing dramatic clicks by exotic techniques.

(iv) (b) Regional manipulation (Grade V)

Although manipulative techniques *with a localised effect* may involve some movement of a whole vertebral region, this is not the same thing as routinely dealing with lumbar pain by 'environmental' manipulation of the lumbar spine, or routinely treating cervical pain by gross cervical spine manipulations, for example.

They are infrequently indicated; the author's practise is mainly to employ regional lumbar manipulation for those patients who have no detectable clinical signs of any importance, other than stiffness, but who have plainly lost confidence in the health and durability of their spines, and need to have its underlying functional soundness demonstrated to them. Even in these cases, vigour is unnecessary, although a purposeful flamboyance may impress the gullible.

(v) Correction of lateral deviation of lumbar spine

The procedure is successfully used for individuals with previously straight spines, in whom deviation of the trunk to one or other side is accompanied by low back and proximal limb pain, and also, when the aberrant posture can reasonably be associated with onset of the painful episode. Some loss of lumbar lordosis often accompanies the more immediately obvious lateral lumbar deviation.

The occasional patient may present with a laterally-deviated lumbar spine, a history of the postural deviation occurring after a painful flexion stress yet be in no pain at the time of examination.

(vi) Stretching (A)

This will be necessary for tightened soft tissue overlying, or associated with, chronic joint problems, e.g.

— the ligamentum nuchae and other posterior cervical structures

— the upper fibres of trapezius
— the scaleni
— the sternocleidomastoid
— pectoralis major and minor
— the concave side of lateral curves due to pelvic tilt in the frontal plane
— the psoas major, which is often unilaterally tight
— the lumbodorsal fascia and posterior lumbosacral structures
— the iliotibial tract.

Stretching (A) and regional mobilisation are frequently combined, since the indications are similar.

(vii) Manual traction

Other than those occasions when the patient may be unable to lie down, or the reassurance of manual contact is of some importance to the patient, indications are much the same as for regional mobilisation.

(viii) Mechanical harness traction

Rhythmic traction

Notes: (for all regions):

With more severe symptoms: relatively long periods of 'hold' and 'rest' should be employed (i.e. less movement)
As symptoms become less severe: shorter 'hold' and 'rest' periods are more effective (i.e. more movement)

Progressive traction techniques, in which a set maximum tension is applied gradually by small increments, and similarly released, find their best use in:

— the very gentle application of low, and later moderate, tension when treating root irritability by sustained traction
— accustoming a nervous patient, or one who has experienced indifferently applied treatment in the past, to traction
— the watchful application of traction to the patient with asthma, or other forms of respiratory distress.

Cervical traction

Traction can be used for any musculoskeletal conditions of the cervical spine, either alone or combined with manual techniques.

Sustained:

— where joint and/or root irritability is high
— recent or developing neurological signs, associated with irritability
— severe arm pain much reducing neck movements towards the painful side.

Rhythmic:

— acute joint derangements (but see irritability above)
— as a mobilising technique
— upper cervical problems not responding quickly to mobilisation (but see irritability above)
— much degenerative stiffness coexisting with evidence of gross changes
— the elderly osteoporotic and degenerative neck (probably more comfortably treated by gentle rhythmic traction than by contact techniques)
— established neurological signs *without* irritability.

Thoracic traction

In comparison with the cervical and lumbar regions the sphere of thoracic traction is restricted, while remaining a useful treatment method.

Sustained:

— where joint irritability is high

Rhythmic:

— widely distributed thoracic pain associated with advanced degenerative changes (but check irritability)
— thoracic joint problems producing symptoms not aggravated by active movement
— when manual mobilisation has not produced the fullest improvement considered possible
— as a mobilising technique.

Lumbar traction

Traction can be considered for most musculoskeletal conditions of the lumbar region, either alone or combined with manual techniques.

Sustained:

— any symptom, of gradual onset without trauma, which is localised to the lumbar spine or referred distally, and accompanied by pain rather than an ache
— low back and bilateral, symmetrical leg pain (change to rhythmic traction as symptoms settle)
— where joint and/or root irritability is high and root pain is severe

Rhythmic:

— where joint and/or root irritability is low
— localised pain from the lumbar spine, not limiting active movement
— a lumbar *ache*, often accompanying degenerative bony change, or postural deformities, or after old trauma
— localised lumbosacral pain, sharply aggravated by extension and side-flexion, but not flexion
— lumbar pain with a diurnal rhythm of slowly increasing throughout the day, after a pain-free early morning
— as a simple longitudinal mobilising technique
— where, in the absence of backache initially, the onset of pain is in the haunch or more distally, and is accompanied by dural tension signs (i.e. neck flexion and/or straight-leg-raising markedly limited by limb pain), traction in prone-lying may be more successful, in some, than in supine lying.

N.B. Repetitive, rhythmic traction techniques applied *manually*, other than oscillatory longitudinal movements, are more suitably categorised under Indications for regional mobilisation.

2. MANUALLY ASSISTED OR RESISTED ACTIVE MOVEMENTS

(i) Self-correction of lateral spinal deviation

When treating lateral deviation of the lumbar spine

(p. 188), teaching self-maintenance of the straightened lumbar posture is assisted by hand placings, and thus manual guidance in the early stages, to keep the pelvis stable and direct the lateral movement of the trunk. This method, of pro-prioceptive help for the patient to understand what is required, is not new, of course; it was used some thirty or more years ago in the postural re-education of neck and thorax deviation after thoracoplasty operations.

The method also assists in teaching the prophylactic exercise described on page 205.

(ii) Post-isometric relaxation techniques

These are best used when restriction of segmental and/or regional spinal movement is due to recent and easily-reversible muscle tightness. Thus the condition treated is a lesion of simple and temporary *tethering*, usually by a degree of recent and localised postural spasm (as opposed to elicited spasm, p. 107), and sometimes mild connective tissue shortening too. Muscle hyperactivity appears to be the essential abnormality. The techniques are less successful when restricted movement is presumed due to (a) an intra-articular or functional 'block' to movement (b) established soft-tissue shortening and (c) gross degenerative changes; and they are not suitable when joint irritability (undue reactiveness) is present.

3. ACTIVE MOVEMENTS

(i) Regional or localised active exercises

When the nature and the site of a vertebral movement-abnormality has been established, exercises are indicated as follows:

Segmental instability:
    regional, and segmental, strengthening exercises to assist in stabilising the hypermobile joint, e.g. isometric abdominal, back extensor and segmental exercises for lumbar instability.
Postural/mechanical insufficiency:
    postural retraining and strengthening exercises, to diminish the effects of gravitational stress upon a particular spinal segment, e.g. spondylolisthesis.
Segmental stiffness:

segmental mobility exercises, to maintain the range of movement at a particular segment following localised passive mobilisation.
Asymmetrical tissue-tightness:
    exercises to assist in maintaining the extensibility of contracted soft tissues on one aspect of a vertebral segment or vertebral region, e.g. unilateral tissue-tightness as a sequel to lateral pelvic tilt.
Symmetrical tissue-tightness:
    as above, where chronic bilateral contracture has occurred, e.g. (i) the lordosis syndrome, with chronic tightness of lumbosacral fascia and associated soft tissues, and (ii) tight pectoral structures.
Generalised or regional poor posture/balance/control:
    postural correction exercises.
Regional stiffness and muscular inco-ordination in the mature/elderly:
    training in light, rhythmic, co-ordinated regional movements to offset the tendency for facet-joint locking as a consequence of unco-ordinated or impulsive movement.
Recently acquired lateral deviation of the lumbar spine:
    self-administered corrective exercises to restore and maintain normal posture.
Backache due to generalised muscular insufficiency:
    progressive regional mobility and strengthening exercises to restore muscle power and physical endurance.
Spinal stenosis:
    postural retraining in backward pelvic tilt, and strengthening of abdominal muscles, for the standing and walking pain of spinal stenosis, when surgery for decompression is delayed or inadvisable.
Lumbosacral root adhesions:
    flexion exercises to assist in stretching an adhesed root, following the period of acute sciatic pain.
Pelvic joint asymmetry:
    postural positioning exercises to assist correction.

N.B. *Re-education of regional vertebral movement*

In a multijointed articulation like the vertebral

column, the restoration of better movement, after months and years of stiffness, may depend on something more than the simple mobilisation of joints. Frequently, patients seem to have a lost or diminshed proprioceptive sense of what the normally complex movement *feels* like, and in addition to segmental and regional manual or mechanical techniques they may need to have some simple re-education of movement. A little treatment time spent in this way often pays handsome dividends.

For example, the patient who bends the head back by just tilting the chin upwards with little lower cervical or cervicothoracic movement, may persist in doing this even when the stiff lower segments have been mobilised. Unjustifiably, the therapist may experience a sense of failure to realise aims of treatment, when in fact all that is now required is to restore the lost motor pattern, by exercises which emphasise neck rather than head movement.

(ii) Auto-traction

a. *Cervical spine.* Because the distraction is rhythmic, or at best intermittent, the indications are essentially as for rhythmic traction applied by a machine, with the patient sitting, half-lying or lying (Fig. 14.16).

b. *Lumbar spine.* In general terms, the indications are similar to those given for machine traction, with modifications according to the presumed nerve root/protrusion relationship.[148]

With the patient *prone:*

— protrusion lateral to the nerve root — one or both ends of the table are lowered and/or the head section rotated towards the side opposite the presumed herniated disc
— protrusion medial to the nerve root — one or both ends are lowered and/or the head section rotated towards the same side as the presumed herniated disc
— protrusion beneath the nerve root — one or both ends are lowered.

These angulations of the table are reversed when the patient is *supine.*

The method of auto-traction devised by Lind may also be modified for cervical and thoracic traction.[116]

In some cases, where the application of a thoracic harness may preclude orthodox lumbar traction, the auto-traction method would be suitable.

(iii) Active stretching of shortened soft tissues

Using carefully contrived positions, the patient is taught how to complement passive stretching techniques, by the therapist, with active exercises or actively-sustained postures as a home exercise regime.

Thus the indications are the same as for the passive stretching techniques (p. 149).

18

Contraindications

Because this heading refers usually to conditions or syndromes for which the treatment under consideration is unsuitable, more for reasons of the dangers involved than because of therapeutic pointlessness, the nature of the treatment should also be discussed.

When physical treatment can be modified to range from the most gentle to quite vigorous, the conditions which might be contraindications can be divided into two groups, i.e. (1) absolute contraindications; (2) those conditions requiring extra care in selection and application of treatment.

N.B. One overriding consideration is that any treatment which involves the production of movement or applied stress, either to body regions and tissues or in the form of increased pressures in vessels and vascular sinuses, is *contraindicated* in the absence of a thorough clinical and preferably a radiological examination to exclude organic disease.

1. PASSIVE MOVEMENT

(i) Massage and maintenance movements

Contraindications need no description here.

(ii) Mobilisation

A consideration of contraindications to mobilisation must include a review of the *purpose* of treatment.

For example, it is known that repetitive small-amplitude movements, applied rhythmically to joints, have an inhibitory effect on afferent impulse traffic from articular receptors subserving pain, and thus the purpose of treatment can be *to relieve pain*, e.g. the pain arising from a hypermobile segment, by the use of gentle mobilisation techniques. In this example there can be no intention to stretch tight tissues, break adhesions, restore displaced material or increase the range of movement.

Similarly, careful mobilisation guided by assessment can be of value for the pain associated with frank neurological signs in the territory of one root on one side. There can be no intention to try to reverse the serial tissue changes culminating in the neurological deficit, only to *relieve the symptoms of it,* and thereby minimise the degree of functional disablement.

Absolute contraindications to mobilisation are:
— malignancy involving the vertebral column
— cauda equina lesions producing disturbance of bladder and/or bowel function
— signs and symptoms of:
    spinal cord involvement
    involvement of more than one spinal nerve root on one side, or two adjacent roots in one lower limb only
— rheumatoid collagen necrosis of vertebral ligaments; the cervical spine is especially vulnerable
— active inflammatory and infective arthritis
— bone disease of the spine (if no more than a simple osteoporosis of ageing, see below).

The *rules of procedure* should be followed at all times:
— careful examination, including the mandatory questions
— economy of vigour in technique
— treatment guided by assessment and reassessment throughout
— discontinuing treatment which begins to produce deterioration in the signs and symptoms.

CARE is necessary in the following situations:

The presence of neurological signs. While following the rules of procedure, it is important to avoid treatment procedures which reduce the dimensions of intervertebral foramina on the side of the painful limb.

Rheumatoid arthritis. When prescribed, gentle mobilisation treatment can help the patient, provided:

— there is no acute inflammation
— the cervical spine is avoided and the dangers of ligamentous changes and the depletion of bone structure (especially the ribs) are borne in mind.

Osteoporosis. The condition may be due to one or more of several causes. A loss of approximately 40 per cent of bone salts must occur before osteoporosis becomes radiologically evident, and the ribs are especially vulnerable. Pressure techniques must be used with care.

Spondylolisthesis. This condition is often symptomless and unknown to the patient. If pain is arising from the affected segment, gentle mobilising can be helpful in reducing pain, but pressure techniques with a degree of energy are contra-indicated. The pain may be caused by soft-tissue changes of *adjacent* segments, and in these cases any techniques found to be effective in helping symptoms may be carefully used, while mindful of the possibly unstable segment.

Hypermobility has been discussed above.

Pregnancy. It is difficult to generalise, but the considerate and moderate use of pressure techniques is possible up to the sixth month and rotations of small amplitude up to the eighth month.

Dizziness which is produced or aggravated by neck rotation contraindicates the free use of rotation techniques in treatment, but does not preclude careful pressure techniques and traction.

Previous malignant disease in other than spinal tissues need not contraindicate mobilisation for spinal joint problems so long as the possibility of metastases can reasonably be excluded and treatment is prudent.

Polymyalgia rheumatica. So far as manual treatment is concerned, this should be regarded as an inflammatory arthritis of the axial and limb girdle joints; there is evidence to suggest that this is the case.[152] At times, prudent and considerate mobilisa-

tion may be indicated.[70]

(iii) Manipulation

Absolute contraindications (often because of co-existing disease) are:

— frank spinal deformity due to old pathology (e.g. scoliosis, or kyphosis due to adolescent osteochondrosis)
— most craniovertebral, and some lumbosacral, anomalies (e.g. lack of a stable lumbrosacral articulation)
— neoplastic disease of skeletal or soft tissue of the spine
— bone disease (e.g. osteomyelitis, tuberculosis, Paget's disease, osteoporosis, e.g. due to senility, prolonged steroid therapy, certain hormonal drugs, gastrectomy, or endocrine and other disorders)
— in the presence of calcification in thoracic intervertebral discs, it is probably wise to use manual techniques prudently, especially at the middle and lower thoracic segments
— inflammatory arthritis (e.g. rheumatoid arthritis, ankylosing spondylitis, septic arthritis)
— manipulative thrust techniques should not be used in the presence of gout
— physical involvement of the central nervous system (e.g. cord pressure *signs* in limbs, cauda equina lesions, neurological diseases such as transverse myelitis)
— an example is a positive Lhermitte's sign,[17] i.e. shooting paraesthesiae in the limb on sudden flexion of the neck. It is seen in disease of the cervical spinal cord, disseminated sclerosis and other demyelinating conditions
— cervical and thoracic joint conditions producing neurological *symptoms* in one or both lower limbs
— evidence of involvement of more than one spinal nerve root on one side, or more than two adjacent roots in one lower limb only
— advanced diabetes, when tissue vitality may be low
— vascular abnormalities (vertebral artery involvement, visceral arterial disease)
— congenital generalised hypermobility (Ehlers-Danlos syndrome)
— advanced degenerative changes

— severe root pain
— undiagnosed pain
— painful vertebral joint conditions, psychologically reinforced, where manual treatment or manipulation runs the risk of producing an obsessional neurosis of vertebral displacement
— warfarin sodium anticoagulant medication.

Further, there are certain clinical factors, confirmation of which is often elicited during examination by palpation, which *preclude manipulation* and these are:

— acquired hypermobility or instability at the segment involved
— when joint irritability and painful movement are manifest
— the presence of spasm which is protecting the segment being treated
— when segments *adjacent* to the main joint problem are either irritable, or hypermobile, and stresses applied by the positioning for manipulation would aggravate them
— inability of the patient to relax
— when the operator senses that the joint will not give — this is felt as a rubbery resistance to the final movement, and must in all circumstances be respected.

Pregnancy. A considerately performed manipulation to the cervical or upper thoracic spine may be indicated and necessary, but after the fourth month vigorous rotatory stress should not be applied to the thoracolumbar spine; manipulation should not be employed at *any* time if there is known possibility of miscarriage. Techniques of compression are probably best avoided in the later stages of pregnancy.

(iv) Correction of lateral deviation of the lumbar spine

The first attempt should be gentle, considerate and closely monitored; over-enthusiastic pressures at the initial attendance are unwise since the patient may faint. The technique is unsuitable if pain is increased, remains increased and/or migrates more distally during the corrective lateral shift, or has moved thus at the next attendance. It is less likely to succeed if the pain and the associated aberrant lumbar posture have been established for three or more months.

So-called 'root' pain, accompanying neurological symptoms and signs in a limb, is a contraindication, as are evidence of sphincter involvement and extreme pain with great apprehensiveness. The technique, with its accompanying lumbar extension posturing, is not suitable for the lordosis syndrome (where low back pain is a *consequence* of approximation of neural arch structures), lumbar spinal stenosis, spondylolisthesis causing pain and frank lumbar scoliosis due to causes other than a transient low back pain episode.

It should not be necessary to list those conditions already mentioned under 'Contraindications to manipulation', which also apply here, of course, nor mention that thoraco-lumbar junction lesions may also refer pain to the low back.

Scoliosis in youngsters can be due to osteoid osteoma, spondylolisthesis, severe disc prolapse, a trapezoidal L5 vertebral body, an uneven upper sacral surface. Also sacro-iliac 'shuffling' lesions in young women, when treatment should be directed to the pelvic joints rather than to the low back.

The lumbar extension posture must not be encouraged *until* the patient's spine is straight; attempts to increase lumbar lordosis in a laterally-deviated spine will provoke rather than ease the joint problem.

(v) Stretching (A)

Although stretching techniques may have a place in the overall management of mild idiopathic scoliosis, for example, this general disturbance of body architecture is not the same as localised soft tissue tightness on one aspect of a vertebral district, and thus the approach to stretching is not quite the same in these two clinical states.

Stretching is contraindicated for those muscle groups, with connective-tissue elements, which invariably tend to lengthening and weakening (see p. 150), and when postural spasm is protecting a painful and irritable vertebral segment. They are also contraindicated until the benign nature of the soft-tissue shortening has been established.

(vi) Traction

N.B. Care should be exercised in treating patients

who obtain dramatic relief from severe pain with the first application of traction.

Cervical traction

— those with marked irritability of the temporo-mandibular joint(s); uncomfortable pressure may be avoided by using a frontal/occipital harness in place of the more usual mandibular/occipital harness. The edentulous patient is often more comfortable with a gauze pad between dentures, or with a thicker pad replacing the denture
— marked ligamentous insufficiency, and segmental instability
— patients who are dizzy, nauseated and sick after the first careful attempt(s)
— patients who are unable to relax.

Conditions like neoplasms, active inflammatory arthritis, *rheumatoid erosions and instability*, etc. are not discussed, because the question of traction should not arise.

N.B. Without confirmation of rationale with the prescribing physician, spondylotic *cervical myelopathy* is a contraindication.

Breig[17] has described in clear detail the potential dangers of giving cervical traction, especially traction in flexion, in cases of cervical myelopathy.

When the free mobility of spinal cord and meninges is already restricted, or nervous tissue is distorted, by the space-occupying and/or tethering effects of degenerative or traumatic changes in the neck, a further increment of physical stress by traction may be critical.

Similarly, the arrangement of a pull, via the cervical harness, to affect the upper two-thirds of the thoracic spine (p. 163) should never be employed in the presence of frank cervical spondylotic change, cervical irritability or when neurological symptoms and signs, in one or both lower limbs, are considered due to the thoracic change; it is probably wise not to use traction, particularly in flexion, for thoracic joint problems when there is X-ray evidence of thoracic disc calcification at the level concerned.

Weinberger[181] makes the long overdue observation that heavy intermittent or rhythmic traction (or sustained traction) is contraindicated in the treatment of the 'whiplash' patient. It can well be traumatic, and a potent cause of the prolongation of symptoms — in short, unnecessary suffering.

Thoracic traction

Coexisting conditions may rule out:

— the patient's position, and
— the pressure of a snugly applied harness, with further pressure as tension is applied. Similarly, pregnancy may rule out harness pressure.

Effective traction may be difficult in:

— orthopnoea for any reason
— asthma and other forms of respiratory distress
— hiatus hernia
— recent thoracic and abdominal surgery
— old thoracoplasty.

Segmental hypermobility or instability generally contraindicate traction, unless the therapist is able to restrict longitudinal movement to less than the normal of this accessory range. This careful technique is occasionally used for the relief of pain, but is much better done manually.

Thoracic joint problems producing *neurological symptoms and signs in one or both lower limbs are an absolute contraindication.*

Lumbar traction

Because lumbar traction technique is very similar to that for the thoracic spine, the contraindications mentioned above for thoracic traction also apply here, of course.

Effective traction may be ruled out by coexisting conditions, e.g. pregnancy. Traction is used effectively for acute conditions of sudden onset in the cervical spine, applied in the line of painful deviation until a normal attitude is possible, but it is unwise to use traction for pain of sudden onset in the lumbar spine (acute lumbago) without a cautious and short initial trial to test the patient's reactions. The patient whose severe back pain is dramatically relieved with the first gentle pull should have the tension smoothly lessened without delay, otherwise a very severe pain reaction might occur. Also:

— recent onset of severe lumbar pain
— hypermobility or instability of lumbar segments
— undiagnosed pain

— persistent cough
— cardio-vascular conditions such as left ventricular failure or aortic aneurysm
— co-existing rib-joint lesion, which the thoracic band may provoke.

Generally, hypermobility or instability of a segment contraindicate traction, but it may be prescribed, together with abdominal strengthening exercises, for spondylolisthesis, for example, when it can be established that the olisthetic segment is responsible for the pain reported.

2. MANUALLY ASSISTED OR RESISTED ACTIVE MOVEMENTS

(i) Self-correction of lateral deviation of the spine

The contraindications are similar to those for passive correction (p. 237).

(ii) Post-isometric relaxation techniques

These are contraindicated, in the general sense, in all of those conditions already mentioned under 'Mobilisation' and 'Manipulation', of course (p. 235–236).

They are also unsuitable when irritability of the joint concerned is evident in the history and/or during physical tests, as undue reactiveness. While not absolutely contraindicated, they are less successful when tried for established soft tissue contracture, a presumed functional 'block' to movement and gross degenerative change.

3. ACTIVE MOVEMENTS

(i) Regional or localised active exercises

Again, exercises are generally contraindicated in those conditions mentioned under 'Mobilisation' and 'Manipulation', although it will be plain that an *appropriate* level of physical activity is better for the osteoporotic patient than is lying about, for example. Similarly, an active regime will better suit the patient with ankylosing spondylitis, and at times regional mobilisation can help.

While a general physical exercise regime has been shown to be of value in the long-term management of chronic rheumatoid arthritis[149] head and neck exercises are unwise for a particular group of these patients and even moderately vigorous trunk exercises are unsuitable for those with rheumatoid rib erosions.[70]

Hamstring-stretching exercises, and those for releasing an adhered lumbo-sacral nerve root, are indicated when the severity of 'root' pain has considerably diminished, but contraindicated until then, of course.

Thus contraindications are frequently a matter of timing and of degree, together with the clinical context in which exercises are being considered.

(ii) Auto-traction

Besides the contraindications already mentioned under 'Traction' (p. 237), there is no point in trying the techniques for those unable to co-operate, for whatever reason.

(iii) Active stretching of shortened soft tissue

Apart from the formal contraindications mentioned under 'Mobilisation' and 'Manipulation' (p. 235), severe pain, segmental or regional irritability and co-existing conditions which may be provoked by the applied stress are unsuitable for this treatment; it is also unsuitable for those patients who cannot learn to do them correctly, because over-enthusiasm may cause stress to innocent structures.

References

1. Andersson B J G, Ortengren R et al 1974 On myoelectric back muscle activity and lumbar disc pressure in sitting postures. Scand J Rehab Med 6: 104
2. Andersson B J G, Ortengren R et al 1975 The sitting posture: an electromyographic and discometric study. Orth Clin N Amer 6: 1
3. Arieff A J, Tigay E L, Kurtz J F, Larmon W A 1961 The Hoover sign. Arch Neurol 5: 109
4. Ariotti B 1981 Vertigo. In: Proceedings: The cervical spine and headache. Manipulative Therapists Assoc of Australia, Brisbane
5. Atkinson T A, Vossler S, Hart D L 1982 The evaluation of facial, head, neck and temperomandibular joint pain patients. J Orthop & Sports Phys Ther 3: 193
6. Barnett C H, Cobbold A F 1962 Lubrication within living joints. J Bone & Jt Surg 44B: 662
7. Barnett C H, Cobbold A F 1969 Muscle tension and joint mobility. Ann Rheum Dis 28: 652
8. Barnett C H 1971 The mobility of synovial joints. Rheum Phys Med 11: 20
9. Beresford-Jones R 1981 Migraine: the dental involvement. Country Publications, Carlisle
10. Bergquist-Ullman M, Larsson U 1977 Acute low back pain in industry. Acta Orthop Scand Suppl 170
11. Biemond A 1951 Thrombosis of the basilar artery and the vascularization of the brain stem. Brain 74: 300
12. Bihaug O 1975 Erfaring med autotraksjon. Fysioperateuten 42: 434
13. Bourdillon J 1982 Spinal manipulation, 3rd edn. Heinemann, London
14. Brain W R, Northfield D W C, Wilkinson M 1952 The neurological manifestations of cervical spondylosis. Brain 75: 187
15. Brain Lord 1957 The treatment of pain. SA Med J 31: 973
16. Brain Lord, Wilkinson M eds 1967 Cervical spondylosis. Heinemann, London
17. Breig A 1978 Adverse mechanical tension in the central nervous system. Almqvist & Wiksell, Stockholm
18. Brendler S J 1968 The human cervical myotomes: functional anatomy studied at operation. J Neurosurg 28: 105
19. Brodal A 1981 Neurological anatomy in relation to clinical medicine, 3rd edn. Oxford University Press, London
20. Brody I A, Wilkins R H 1969 The signs of Kernig and Brudzinski. Arch Neurol 21: 215
21. Buchan W 1982 John Buchan: a memoir. Buchan and Enright, London
22. Buswell J 1978 A manual of home exercises for the spinal column. NZ Manip Ther Assoc, Auckland
23. Cailliet R 1977 Rehabilitation management of the patient with low back pain. In: Buerger A A, Tobin J S (eds) Approaches to the validation of manipulation therapy. Thomas, Springfield, Illinois
24. Campbell D G, Parsons C M 1944 Referred head pain and its concomitants J Nerv Ment Dis 99: 544
25. Chusid J G 1973 Correlative neuroanatomy and functional neurology 15th edn. Lange Medical, Los Angeles
26. Clancy W G 1979 Shoulder problems in overhead-overuse sports: introduction. Amer J Sports Med 7: 138
27. Cohen H 1947 Visceral pain. Lancet 2: 933
28. Colachis S C, Strohm B R 1965 Cervical traction: relationship of traction time to varied tractive force with constant angle of pull. Arch Phys Med Rehab 46: 815
29. Colachis S C, Strohm B R 1965 A study of tractive forces and angle of pull on vertebral interspaces in the cervical spine. Arch Phys Med Rehab 46: 820
30. Colachis S C, Strohm B R 1966 Effect of duration of intermittent cervical traction on vertebral separation. Arch Phys Med Rehab 47: 353
31. Coutts M B 1934 Atlanto-epistropheal subluxations. Arch Surg 29: 297
32. Cyriax J 1980 Textbook of orthopaedic medicine Vol 11, 10th edn. Balliére Tindall, London
33. Cyriax J 1982 Textbook of orthopaedic medicine, Vol 1, 8th edn. Bailliére Tindall, London
34. Davis P R 1955 The thoraco-lumbar mortice joint. J Anat 89: 370
35. Deets D, Hands K L, Hopp S S 1977 Cervical traction: a comparison of sitting and supine positions. Phys Ther 57: 255
36. De Lacerda F G 1980 Effect of angle of traction pull on upper trapezius muscle activity. J Orth Sports Phys Ther 1: 4: 205
37. Denny-Brown D, Kirk E J, Yanagisawa N 1973 The tract of Lissauer in relation to sensory transmission in the dorsal horn of the spinal cord in the Macaque. J Comp Neurol 151: 175
38. Denslow J S 1944 Analysis of variability of spinal reflex threshold. J Neurophys 7: 207
39. De Séze S, Levernieux J 1951 Les tractions vertébrales: premiéres études experimentales et resultats therapeutiques d'aprés une experience de quatre années. Semaine des Hôpitaux des Paris 27: 2085

40. Doran F S A, Ratcliffe A H 1954 Physiological mechanisms of referred shoulder-tip pain. Brain 77: 427

41. Doran F S A 1967 The sites to which pain is referred from the commom bile-duct in man and its implication for the theory of referred pain. Brit J Surg 54: 7

42. Droz-Georget J H 1980 High-velocity thrust and pathophysiology of segmental dysfunction. In: Proceedings: Aspects of manipulative therapy. International Conference Lincoln Institute, Melbourne

43. Duncan D 1948 Alterations in the structure of nerves caused by restricting their growth with ligatures. J Neuropath & Ex Neurol 7: 261

44. Ebner M 1978 Connective tissue massage. Physio 64: 208

45. Editorial 1979 Stay young by good posture. New Scientist 82: 544

46. Elvey R L 1980 Brachial plexus tension tests and the pathoanatomical origin of arm pain. In: Proceedings: Aspects of manipulative therapy. International Conference Lincoln Institute, Melbourne

47. Epstein B S 1980 The Spine: a radiological text and atlas, 4th edn. Lea and Febiger, Philadelphia

48. Evjenth O, Hamberg J 1980 Töjning av Muskler. Vol. 1 Extremiteterna, Vol. 11 Ryggraden, Tryct hos Team Offset, Mälmo

49. Farfan H F 1973 Mechanical disorders of the low back. Lea and Febiger, Philadelphia

50. Fahrni W H 1966 Observations on straight-leg-raising with special reference to nerve root endings. Can J Surg 9: 44

51. Feinstein B et al 1954 Experiments on referred pain from deep somatic tissues. J Bone & Jt Surg 36A: 981

52. Feinstein B 1977 Referred pain from paravertebral structures. In: Buerger A A, Tobis J F (eds) Approaches to the validation of manipulative therapy. Thomas, Springfield, Illinois

53. Fordyce W E et al 1975 Operant conditioning in the treatment of chronic pain. Arch Phys Med Rehab 54: 399

54. Frankel V H 1965 Temporomandibular joint pain syndrome following deceleration injury to the cervical spine. Bull Hosp Joint Dis 26: 47

55. Fraser D M 1976 Post-partum backache: a preventable condition? Can Fam Phys 22: 1434

56. Friberg S, Hult L 1951 Comparative study of abrodil myelogram and operative findings. Acta Orthop Scand 20: 303

57. Frumker S C 1978 Head pain of dental occlusion origin: clinical screening tests. In: Proceedings: Second World Congress on Pain, Montreal

58. Fryette H H 1954 Principles of osteopathic technique. Academy of Applied Osteopathy, Carmel, California

59. Frykholm R 1971 The clinical picture. In: Hirsch C, Zotterman Y (eds) Cervical pain. Pergamon Press, Oxford

60. Gaymans F 1980 De bedeutung der atemptypen für die mobilisation der wirbelsäule. Man Med 18: 96

61. Gerschman J, Burrows G, Reade P 1979 Chronic oro-facial pain. In: Bonica J J (ed) Advances in Pain Research and Therapy 3: 317

62. Ghadially F N 1978 The fine structure of joints. In: Sokoloff L (ed) The joints and synovial fluid 1. Academic Press, London

63. Goldie I F, Reichman S 1977 The biomechanical influence of traction on the cervical spine. Scand J Rehab Med 9: 31

64. Goodridge J P 1981 Muscle energy technique: definition, explanation, methods of procedure. J Amer Osteop Assoc 81: 249

65. Goor C, Ongerboer de Visser B W 1976 Jaw and blink reflexes in trigeminal nerve lesions. Neurology 26: 1

66. Grant J C B 1958 Method of anatomy. Williams & Wilkins, Baltimore

67. Greenman P 1979 Manuelle therapie am brustkorb. Man Med 17: 17

68. Grieve G P 1976 The sacro-iliac joint. Physio 62: 384

69. Grieve G P 1978 Manipulation: a part of physiotherapy. Physio 64: 358

70. Grieve G P 1981 Common vertebral joint problems. Churchill Livingstone, Edinburgh

71. Grieve G P 1982 Lumbar instability. Physio 68: 2

72. Grieve G P 1983 The hip. Physio 69: 196

73. Gutmann von G 1970 X-ray diagnosis of spinal dysfunction. Man Med 8: 75

74. Gutmann von G 1971 Beitrag zur qualititaven analyse des röntgenbildes der halswirbelsäule im seitlichan strahlengang. Man Med 9: 197

75. Haldeman S 1978 The clinical basis for discussion of mechanics of manipulative therapy. In: Korr I (ed) The neurobiologic mechanisms in manipulative therapy. Plenum Press, London

76. Haldeman S 1980 Modern development in the principles and practice of chiropractic. Appleton-Century-Crofts, New York

77. Hanraets P R M 1959 The degenerative back and its differential diagnosis. Elsevier, Amsterdam

78. Harman J B 1948 The localisation of deep pain. British Medical Journal 1: 188

79. Harman J B 1951 Angina in the analgesic limb. British Medical Journal 2: 521

80. Hazlett J W 1975 Low back pain with femoral neuritis. Clin Orth & Rel Res 108: 9

81. Head H 1920 Studies in neurology. Oxford Medical Publications, London

82. Head H 1933 On disturbance of sensation with especial reference to the pain of visceral disease. Brain 16: 1

83. Heron L D, Pheasant H C 1980 Prone knee-flexion provocative testing for lumbar disc protrusion. Spine 5: 65

84. Hirsch D, Ingelmark B, Miller M 1963 The anatomical basis for low back pain. Acta Orthop Scand 33: 1

85. Hockaday J M, Whitty C W M 1967 Patterns of referred pain in the normal subject. Brain 90: 481

86. Hohl M 1974 Soft tissue injuries of the neck in automobile accidents: factors influencing prognosis. J Bone & Jt Surg 56A: 1675

87. Hood L B, Chrissman D 1968 Intermittent pelvic traction in the treatment of ruptured intervertebral disc. Phys Ther 48: 21

88. Hoppenfeld S 1979 Physical examination of the knee joint by complaint. Orth Clin N Amer 10: 3

89. Inman V T, Saunders J B 1944 Referred pain from skeletal structures. J Nerv & Ment Dis 90: 660

90. Janda V 1976 The muscular factor in the pathogenesis of back pain syndrome. Physiotherapy Symposium, Oslo

91. Janda V 1978 Muscles, central nervous motor regulation and back problems. In: Korr I (ed) The neurobiologic mechanisms in manipulative therapy. Plenum Press, London.

92. Janda V, Schmid H J A 1980 Muscles as a pathogenic factor in back pain. In: Proceedings: 4th Conference of International Federation of Orthopaedic Manipulative Therapists. Christchurch, New Zealand

93. Johnstone D R, Templeton M 1980 The feasibility of palpating the lateral pterygoid muscle. J Pros Dent 44: 318

94. Jowett R L, Fidler M W Histochemical changes in the multifidus in mechanical derangements of the spine. Orth Clin N Amer 6: 145

95. Judovich B D 1954 Lumbar traction therapy and dissipated force factors. Journal Lancet 74: 411

96. Keele C A, Neil E 1973 Samson Wright's applied physiology (12th ed). Oxford Medical Publications, London

97. Kendall P H 1955 A history of lumbar traction. Physio 41: 177

98. Kennedy B 1980 An Australian programme for management of back problems. Physio 66: 108

99. Kirk E J, Denny-Brown D 1970 Functional variations in dermatomes in the Macaque monkey following dorsal root lesions. J of Comp Neurol 139: 307

100. Kirkaldy-Willis W H, Hill J R 1979 A more precise diagnosis for low-back pain. Spine 4: 102

101. Knott M, Voss D E 1956 Proprioceptive neuromuscular facilitation. Hoeber-Harper, New York

102. Kostyuk P G 1968 Presynaptic and postsynaptic changes produced in spinal neuron by an afferent volley from visceral afferents. In: von Euler C, Skogland S, Söderberg U (eds) Structure and function of inhibitory neuronal mechanisms. Pergamon Press, Oxford

103. Korr I M 1978 Sustained sympathicotonia as a factor in disease. In: Korr I (ed) The neurobiologic mechanisms in manipulative therapy. Plenum Press, London

104. Kunert W 1965 Functional disorders of internal organs due to vertebral lesions. Ciba Symposium 13: 85

105. Lansche W E, Ford L T 1960 Correlation of the myelogram with clinical and operative findings in lumbar disc lesions. J Bone & Jt Surg 42A: 1483

106. Leading article 1973 Physiotherapy or psychotherapy. Lancet December 29: 1483

107. Leading article 1976 Trial by traction. British Medical Journal January 3: 1

108. Levau B 1977 Williams and Lissner's biomechanics of human motion 2nd edn. W.B. Saunders, Philadelphia

109. Lewis T, Kellgren J H 1939 Observation relating to referred pain, viscero-motor reflexes and other associated problems. Clin Sci 4: 47

110. Lewit K 1969 The course of impaired function in the spinal column. In: Proceedings: Faculty of Medicine and Hygiene Charles University, Prague

111. Lewit K 1976 Manuelle Medizin in Rahmen der Medizinschen Rehabilitation. Barth, Leipzig

112. Lewit K, Gaymans F 1980 Muskelfazilitations —und inhibitionstechniken in der Manuelle Medizin Teil 1: Mobilisation. Man Med 18: 102

113. Lewit K 1981 Muskelfazilitations —und inhibitionstechniken in der Manuelle Medizin. Teil 11: Postisometrische Muskelrelaxation. Man Med 19: 12

114. Lewit K 1981 Muskelfazilitations —und inhibitionstechniken in der Manuelle Medizin. Teil 111: Postisometrische Muskelrelaxation. Man Med 19: 40

115. Lidstrom A, Zachrisson M 1970 Physical therapy in low back pain and sciatica. Scand J Rehab Med 2: 37

116. Lind G A M 1974 Auto-traction: treatment of low back pain and sciatica: an electromyographic, radiographic and clinical study (thesis). University Med Diss, Linkopings

117. Lissiman M 1974 Clinical application of lumbar traction. In: Twomey L T (ed) Symposium: low back pain. Western Australia Institute of Technology, Perth

118. Lossing W W 1980 A natural treatment for lumbar disc syndrome. In: Proceedings: American Physical Therapy Association Congress, Phoenix, Arizona

119. MacConaill M A 1964 Joint movement. Physio 50: 359

120. Macnab I 1977 Backache. Williams & Wilkins, Baltimore

121. Macnab I 1978 Foreword. In: White A A, Panjabi M M. Clinical biomechanics of the spine. Lippincott, Philadelphia

122. McKee G K 1956 Traction-manipulation and plastic corsets in the treatment of disc lesions of the lumbar spine. Lancet 1: 473

123. MacKenzie J 1909 Symptoms and their interpretation. Shaw, London

124. McKenzie R A 1972 Manual correction of sciatic scoliosis. NZ Med J 76: 194

125. McKenzie R A 1981 The lumbar spine: mechanical diagnosis and therapy. Spinal Publications, Waikenae, New Zealand

126. Maigne R 1972 Douleurs d'origine vertébrale et traitements par manipulation, 2nd edn. Expansion Scientifique, Paris

127. Maitland G D 1972 Manipulation: individual responsibility. Physio South Africa 28: 2

128. Maitland G D 1977 Vertebral manipulation, 4th edn. Butterworth, London

129. Maitland G D 1977 Peripheral manipulation, 2nd edn. Butterworth, London

130. Maitland G D 1978 Movement of pain sensitive structures in the vertebral canal in a group of physiotherapy students. In: Proceedings: Manipulative Therapists Association of Australia Inaugural Congress, Sydney

131. Maitland G D 1981 Musculo-skeletal Examination and Recording Guide, 3rd edn. Lauderdale Press, Adelaide

132. Masturzo A 1955 Vertebral traction for treatment of sciatica. Rheum 11: 62

133. Mathews J A 1968 Dynamic discography: a study of lumbar traction. Ann Phys Med 9: 275

134. Mathews J A, Hickling J 1975 Lumbar traction: a double-blind controlled study for sciatica. Rheum & Rehab 14: 222

135. Mennell J B 1945 Physical treatment by movement, manipulation and massage, 5th edn. Churchill, London

136. Mennell J B 1952 The science and art of manipulation, Vol 2. Churchill, London

137. Mennell J McM 1960 Back pain. Little Brown, Boston

138. Mennell J McM 1972 Treatment of myofascial pain, secondary to facet-joint dysfunction, by cold. Man Med 10: 76

139. Miller J 1978 How do you feel? The Listener 100: 665

140. Mitchell F L, Moran P S, Pruzzo M A 1979 An evaluation and treatment manual of osteopathic muscle energy procedures. ICEOP Inc, Valley Park, Missouri

141. Moll J M H, Wright V 1971 Normal range of spinal mobility. Ann Rheum Dis 30: 381

142. Mooney V, Robertson J 1976 The facet syndrome. Clin Orth & Rel Res 115: 149

143. Mooney V, Cairns D 1978 Management in the patient with chronic low back pain. Orth Clin N Amer 9: 543

144. Nachemson A 1966 Electromyographic studies on the vertebral portion of the psoas muscle. Acta Orthop Scand 37: 177

145. Nachemson A, Elfström G 1970 Intravital dynamic pressure measurements in lumbar discs. Scand J Rehab Med Suppl No 1

146. Nachemson A 1980 A critical look at conservative treatment for low back pain. In: Jayson M I V (ed) The lumbar spine and back pain, 2nd edn. Sector, London

147. Nathan P A 1976 The gate-control theory of pain. Brain 99: 123

148. Natchev E 1982 Pain treatment and auto-traction for back problems. AB Spiraltryck, Stockholm

149. Nordemar R, Ekblom B, Zachrisson L, Lundqvist K 1981 Physical training in rheumatoid arthritis: a controlled long-term study 1. and 11. Scand J Rheum 10: 17 and 10: 25

150. Oakley E M 1978 Application of continuous beam ultrasound at therapeutic levels. Physio 64: 169

151. O'Brien J 1982 Biomechanics of the spine. Symposium: Manipulation Association of Chartered Physiotherapists, London

152. O'Duffy J D, Hunder G G, Wahner H W 1980 A follow-up study of polymyalgia rheumatica: evidence of chronic axial synovitis. J Rheumatol 7: 685

153. Ongerboer de Visser D W, Goor C 1976 Jaw reflexes and masseter electromyograms in mesencephalic and pontine lesions: an electrodiagnostic study. J Neurol Neurosurg Psych 39: 1

154. Oudenhoven R C 1978 Gravitational lumbar traction. Arch Phys Med Rehab 59: 510

155. Parsons K O 1945 Pain, its significance and assessment. Physio 30: 71

156. Parsons W B, Cumming J D A 1957 Mechanical traction in lumbar disc syndrome. J Can Med Assoc 77: 7

157. Phillips D G 1975 Upper limb involvement in cervical spondylosis. J Neurol Neurosurg Psychiat 38: 386

158. Piedallu P 1952 Problemés Sacro-iliaques. Homme Sain No. 2 (Biére ed) Bordeaux

159. Pomeranz B, Wall P D, Weber W V 1969 Cord cells responding to fine myelinated afferents from viscera, muscle and skin. J of Physiology 199: 511

160. Prowse K 1979 Medical chests — asthma, bronchitis and emphysema. Physio 65: 341

161. Radin E L, Paul I L, Lowry M 1970 A comparison of the dynamic force transmitting properties of subchondral bone and articular cartilage. J Bone & Jt Surg 52A: 444

162. Richardson J 1960 The practice of medicine. Churchill, London

163. Rocabado M 1977 Relationship of the temporomandibular joint in cervical dysfunction. In: Kent B (ed) Proceedings: 3rd Conference International Federation of Orthopaedic Manipulative Therapists, Hayward, California

164. Rolander S D 1966 Motion of the lumbar spine with special reference to the stabilising effect of posterior fusion. Acta Orthop Scand Suppl 90

165. Sandifer P H 1967 Neurology in orthopaedics. Butterworth, London

166. Saunders H D 1981 Unilateral lumbar traction. Phys Ther 61: 221

167. Schmorl G, Junghanns H 1971 The human spine in health and disease, 2nd USA edn. Grune & Stratton, New York and London

168. Stoddard A 1980 Manual of osteopathic technique, 3rd edn. Hutchinson, London

169. Stoddard A 1969 Manual of oesteopathic practice. Hutchinson, London

170. Sturrock R D et al 1973 Spondylometry in a normal population and in ankylosing spondylitis. Rheum & Rehab 12: 135

171. Sunderland S 1978 Nerves and nerve injuries, 2nd edn. Churchill Livingstone, London

172. Sydenham P H 1980 Measuring instruments: tools of knowledge and control. Peter Peregrinus, London

173. Taylor T K F, Weinir M 1969 Great-toe extensor reflexes in the diagnosis of lumbar disc disorder. British Medical Journal 2: 487

174. Trott P H, Goss A N 1978 Physiotherapy in diagnosis and treatment of the myofascial pain dysfunction syndrome. Int J Oral Surg 7: 360

175. Unsworth A, Dowson D, Wright V 1971 Cracking joints. Ann Rheum Dis 30: 348

176. Valtonen E J et al 1968 Comparative radiographic study of the effect of intermittent and continuous traction on elongation of the cervical spine. Ann Med Int Fenn 57: 143

177. Valtonen E J, Kiuru E 1970 Cervical traction as a therapeutic tool: a clinical analysis based on 212 patients. Scand J Rehab Med 2: 29

178. Van Adrichem J A M, Van der Korst G 1973 Assessment of the flexibility of the lumbar spine. Scand J Rheum 2: 87

179. Warwick R, Williams P (eds) 1980 Gray's anatomy, 36th edn. Longman, London

180. Weber H 1973 Traction therapy in sciatica due to disc prolapse. J Oslo City Hosp 23: 167

181. Weinberger L M 1976 Trauma or treatment? The role of intermittent traction in the treatment of cervical soft tissue injuries. J Trauma 16: 377

182. Weinstein P R, Ehni G, Wilson C B 1977 Lumbar spondylosis: diagnosis, management and surgical treatment. Year Book Medical Publications, London

183. Wigh R E 1980 The thoraco-lumbar and lumbosacral transitional junctions. Spine 5: 215

184. Wyke B 1979 Cervical articular contributions to posture and gait. Age and Ageing 8: 251

185. Yates D A H 1964 Unilateral lumbo-sacral root compression. Ann Phys Med 7: 169

186. Yates D A H, Mathews J A 1968 Reduction of lumbar disc prolapse by manipulation. British Medical Journal 3: 696

187. Young R F, Kruger L 1981 Axonal transport studies of the trigeminal nerve. J Neurosurg 54: 208

Further reading

This basic list of salient papers and books is arranged in sections to assist the student, and almost every reference quoted should be available in British medical libraries.

No review is intended, by inclusion or exclusion.

A more comprehensive list is given in *Common Vertebral Joint Problems* (1981) Churchill Livingstone, Edinburgh

Upper cervical spine

Sherk H H, Fielding J W 1978 The upper cervical spine. Orth Clin N Amer 9: 867–1127
von Torklus D, Gehle W 1972 The upper cervical spine. Butterworth, London

Cervical spine

Brain Lord, Wilkinson M 1967, Wilkinson M 1971 Cervical spondylosis, 2nd edn. Heinemann, London
Hirsch C, Zotterman Y (eds) 1971 Cervical pain. Pergamon Press, Oxford
Jeffreys H 1980 Disorders of the cervical spine Butterworth, London
Penning L 1968 Functional pathology of the cervical spine. Excerpta Medica Foundation, Nederland

Cervico-thoracic junction

Grieve G P 1981 Common vertebral joint problems. Churchill Livingstone, London
Nathan H, Feuerstein M 1970 Angulated course of spinal nerve roots. J Neurosurg 32: 349

Thoracic spine

Benson M K D, Byrnes D P 1975 The clinical syndromes and surgical treatment of thoracic intervertebral disc prolapse. J Bone & Jt Surg 57B: 471
Butler R W 1955 The nature and significance of vertebral osteochondritis. Proc Roy Soc Med 48: 895
Goldthwait J E 1940 The rib joints. New England J Med 223: 568
Grant A P, Keegan D A J 1968 Rib pain – a neglected diagnosis. Ulster Med J 37: 162
Nathan H 1959 The para-articular processes of the thoracic vertebrae. Anat Record 4: 605
Nathan H 1962 Osteophytes of the vertebral column. J Bone & Jt Surg 44A: 243
Nathan H et al 1964 The costovertebral joints: anatomico-clinical observations in arthritis. Arth & Rheum 7: 228

Nathan H 1968 Compression of the sympathetic trunk by osteophytes of the vertebral column in the abdomen: an anatomical study with pathological and clinical consideration. Surgery 63: 609
Schmorl G, Junghanns H 1971 The human spine in health and disease, 2nd American edn. Grune & Stratton, New York

Thoraco-lumbar junction

Davis P R 1955 The thoraco-lumbar mortice joint. J Anat 89: 370
Horner D B 1964 Lumbar back pain arising from stress fractures of the lower ribs. J Bone & Jt Surg 46A: 1553
Paige M J 1959 Manipulation in the management of the first lumbar root syndrome. Aust J Physio 5: 47

The lumbar spine

Emmett J L, Love J G 1971 Vesical dysfunction caused by protruded lumbar disc. J Urol 105: 86
Farfan H F 1973 Mechanical disorders of the low back. Lea & Febiger, Philadelphia
Fielding J W, Rothman R H 1977 The lumbar spine 11. Orth Clin N Amer 8: 3–223
Jayson M I V 1980 The Lumbar Spine and Back Pain, 2nd edn. Pitman Medical, Tunbridge Wells
McKenzie R A 1981 The lumbar spine: mechanical diagnosis and therapy. Spinal Publications, Waikenae, New Zealand
Macnab I 1977 Backache. Williams & Wilkins, Baltimore
Mooney V, Robertson J 1976 The facet syndrome. Clin Orth & Rel Res 115: 149
Newman P H 1968 The spine, the wood and the trees. Proc Roy Soc Med 61: 35

The pelvic joints

Grieve G P 1976 The sacro-iliac joint. Physio 63: 384
Harris N H 1974 Lesions of the symphysis pubis in women. British Medical Journal 4: 209
Harris N H, Murray R O 1974 Lesions of the symphysis in athletes. British Medical Journal 4: 211
Sandler S 1982 Innominate rotations: fact or fiction. Brit Osteop J 14: 101

Epidemiology

Billings R A, Mole K F 1977 Rheumatology in general practice. J Roy Coll Gen Prac 27: 721
Lawrence J S 1977 Rheumatism in populations. Heinemann, London

Wood P H N (ed) (1977) The challenge of arthritis and rheumatism: report of problems and progress in health care for rheumatic disorders. British League Against Rheumatism, London

Radiology

Epstein B S 1980 The spine: a radiological text and atlas, 4th edn. Lea & Febiger, Philadelphia
Murray R O, Jacobson H G 1977 The radiology of skeletal disorders, Vols 1–IV 2nd edn. Churchill Livingstone, Edinburgh

Biomechanics

Breig A 1978 Adverse mechanical tension in the central nervous system. Almqvist & Wiksell, Stockholm
Engineering aspects of the spine 1980 Conference proceedings: Engineering in Medicine. Institute of Mechanical Engineers, London
White A A, Panjabi M M 1978 Clinical biomechanics of the spine. Lippincott, Philadelphia

Arthrology

Warwick R, Williams P 1980 Arthrology section. Gray's anatomy, 36th edn. Longman, London

Osteoporosis

Frost H M 1981 (ed) The osteoporoses. Orth Clin N Amer 12: 473–737

Autonomic nervous system

Johnson R H, Spalding J M K 1974 Diseases of the autonomic nervous system. Blackwell Scientific, London
Shafar J 1966 The syndromes of the third neurone of the cervical sympathetic system. Amer J Med 40: 97

Vascular system

Dommisse G F 1974 The blood supply of the spinal cord. J Bone & Jt Surg 56B: 225
Dommisse G F 1980 The arteries, arterioles and capillaries of the spinal cord. Ann Roy Coll Surg Eng 62: 369
Herlihy W F 1947 Revision of the venous system: the role of the vertebral veins. Med J Aust 1: 661
Leading article 1967 Infarction of the spinal cord Lancet 11: 143
Williams D, Graeme Wilson T 1962 The diagnosis of the major and minor syndromes of basilar insufficiency. Brain 85: 741

Neurology

Bogduk N, Tynan W, Wilson A S 1981 The nerve supply to the human lumbar intervertebral discs J Anat 132: 39
Brodal A 1981 Neurological Anatomy in Relation to Clinical Medicine, 3rd edn. Oxford University Press: Oxford
Howe J F, Loeser J D, Calvin W H 1977 Mechanosensitivity of dorsal root ganglia and chronically injured axons: a physiological basis for the radicular pain of nerve root compression. Pain 3: 25
Korr I (ed) 1978 The neurobiological mechanisms in manipulative therapy. Plenum Press, London
Newton R A 1982 Joint receptor contributions to reflexive and kinaesthetic responses. Phys Ther 62: 22

Wyke B D 1981 The neurology of joints: a review of general principles. Clin in Rheum Dis 7: 223
Ysohizawa H, O'Brien J P, Smith W T, Trumper M 1980 The neuropathology of intervertebral discs removed for low back pain. J Path 132: 95

Pain

Bishop B 1980 Pain: its physiology and rationale for management (Parts I—III). Phys Ther 60: 13–91
Bogduk N, Lance J W 1981 Pain and pain syndromes, including headache. In: Appel S H (ed) Current neurology, Vol 3. Wiley, New York
Melzack R, Wall P 1982 The challenge of pain. Penguin, Harmondsworth
Watson J 1981 Pain mechanisms: a review Part I: Characteristics of peripheral receptors. Aust J Physio 27: 135
Watson J 1981 Pain mechanisms: a review Part II: Afferent pain pathways. Aust J Physio 27: 191
Watson J 1982 Pain mechanisms: a review Part III: Endogenous pain. Aust J Physio 28: 38
Wyke B D 1979 Neurological mechanisms in the experience of pain. Acup and Electro-Ther Res 4: 27

Examination

Grieve G P 1981 Common vertebral joint problems. Churchill Livingstone, Edinburgh
Hoppenfeld S 1976 Physical examination of the spine and extremities. Appleton-Century-Crofts, New York
McRae R 1983 Clinical orthopaedic examination, 2nd edn. Churchill Livingstone, Edinburgh
Maitland G D 1981 Musculo-skeletal examination and recording guide, 3rd edn. Lauderdale Press, Adelaide

Treatment

Bourdillon J 1982 Spinal manipulation, 3rd edn. Heinemann, London
Buerger A A, Tobis J S (eds) 1977 Approaches to the validation of spinal manipulative therapy. Thomas, Springfield, Illinois
Buswell J 1978 A manual of home exercises for the spinal column. NZ Manip Ther Assoc, Auckland
Cyriax J 1980 Textbook of orthopaedic medicine, Vol 11 10th edn. Balliere Tindall, London
Evjenth O, Hamberg J 1980 Töjning av Muskler Vol. 11 Ryggraden. Tryct hos Team Offset, Mälmo (English edition should be available during 1983)
Farrell J P, Twomey L T 1982 Acute low back pain: comparison of two conservative treatment approaches. Med J Aust 1: 160
Goodridge J P 1981 Muscle energy technique: definition, explanation, methods of procedure. J Amer Osteop Assoc 81: 249
Grieve G P 1976 The sacro-iliac joint. Physio 63: 384
Grieve G P 1981 Lumbar instability. Physic 68: 2
Grieve G P 1981 Common vertebral joint problems. Churchill Livingstone, Edinburgh
Grieve G P 1982 Neck traction. Physio 68: 260
Grieve G P 1983 The hip. Physio 69: 196
Idczak R M (ed) 1980 Aspects of manipulative therapy. Proceedings: International Conference Lincoln Institute, Melbourne
Janda V, Schmid H J A 1980 Muscles as a pathogenic factor in back pain. In: Proceedings: 4th Conference of Federation

of Orthopaedic Manipulative Therapists Christchurch. New Zealand

Maitland G D 1977 Vertebral manipulation, 4th edn. Butterworth, London

McKenzie R A 1981 The lumbar spine: mechanical diagnosis and therapy. Spinal Publications, Waikenae, New Zealand

Mennell J McM 1960 Back pain, Little Brown, Boston

Mennell J McM 1964 Joint pain. Little Brown, Boston

Mitchell F L, Moran P S, Pruzzo M A 1979 An evaluation and treatment manual of osteopathic muscle energy procedures. ICEOP Inc, Valley Park, Missouri

Stoddard A 1980 Manual of osteopathic technique, 3rd edn. Hutchinson, London

Trott P H, Goss A N 1978 Physiotherapy in diagnosis and treatment of the myofascial pain dysfunction syndrome. Int J Oral Surg 7: 360